# The Fetal Matrix: Evolution, Development and Disease

New discoveries reveal how crucial interactions that determine our destiny occur before birth, when our genes interact with their environment as the embryo and fetus develop. These processes – in the matrix of the womb – are evolutionary echoes of mechanisms that allowed our hunter–gatherer ancestors to survive. These exciting insights into predictive adaptive responses suggest new ways of protecting the health of the fetus, infant and adult. If inappropriate they can trigger obesity, diabetes and heart disease, formerly thought to result solely from adult lifestyle. The new concepts in this book are crucial to understanding the daunting public health burden in societies undergoing rapid transition from poverty to affluence. They add an important new dimension to evolutionary theory. Synthesising developmental biology, evolutionary history, medical science, public health and social policy, this is a ground-breaking and fascinating account by two of the world's leading pioneers in this important emerging field.

Professor **Peter D. Gluckman** is Professor of Paediatric and Perinatal Biology, Director of the Liggins Institute (for Medical Research) and Director of the National Research Centre for Growth and Development, at the University of Auckland.

Professor **Mark A. Hanson** is Director of the Developmental Origins of Health and Disease Research Division at the University of Southampton Medical School, and British Heart Foundation Professor of Cardiovascular Science.

# The Fetal Matrix: Evolution, Development and Disease

Peter Gluckman

University of Auckland, New Zealand

Mark Hanson

University of Southampton, UK

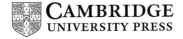

CAMBRIDGE
UNIVERSITY PRESS

PUBLISHED BY THE PRESS SYNDICATE OF THE UNIVERSITY OF CAMBRIDGE
The Pitt Building, Trumpington Street, Cambridge, United Kingdom

CAMBRIDGE UNIVERSITY PRESS
The Edinburgh Building, Cambridge CB2 2RU, UK
40 West 20th Street, New York, NY 10011–4211, USA
477 Williamstown Road, Port Melbourne, VIC 3207, Australia
Ruiz de Alarcón 13, 28014 Madrid, Spain
Dock House, The Waterfront, Cape Town 8001, South Africa

http://www.cambridge.org

First published 2005

Printed in the United Kingdom at the University Press, Cambridge

*Typefaces* Minion 10.5/14 pt. and Formata      *System* LATEX $2_\varepsilon$   [TB]

*A catalogue record for this book is available from the British Library*

*Library of Congress Cataloguing in Publication data*
Gluckman, Peter D.
The fetal matrix: evolution, development, and disease / Peter Gluckman and Mark Hanson.
   p.   cm.
Includes bibliographical references and index.
ISBN 0 521 83457 0 – ISBN 0 521 54235 9 (paperback)
1. Development biology.   2. Embryology, Human.   3. Human evolution.   4. Medicine, Preventive.
5. Medical genetics.   I. Hanson, Mark.   II. Title.
OH491.G584    2004
612.6′4 – dc22    2004045815

ISBN 0 521 83457 0 hardback
ISBN 0 521 54235 9 paperback

Time present and time past
Are both perhaps present in time future
And time future contained in time past.

T. S. Eliot, 'Burnt Norton'

**māt'rix**, n. (pl. *–ices*) womb; place in which thing is developed; formative part of animal organ; mass of rock etc. enclosing gems etc.; (biol.) substance between cells; mould in which type etc. is cast or shaped. [L, f. *mater* mother]

*Oxford English Dictionary*

# Contents

# Preface

This is a book about a rapidly developing idea that has very important implications both for evolutionary biology and for medicine and public health. It offers clues to a better understanding of the origins of many diseases and their prevention and also provides additional insights into important biological processes relevant to evolutionary and life-history theory.

Ideas in science do not often develop in a manner that Fleet Street would have us believe. Science is not normally about 'breakthroughs' and brilliant scientific insights springing from nowhere. It is a most unusual event for scientific understanding to arise in the 'Eureka!' mode, where a single scientist has a flash of inspiration, jumps out of his bath and runs down the street screaming with excitement. Imagine the streets of Boston or Oxford if science was really like that!

Most science is in fact rather boring, in that each advance in understanding is made by the painstaking and careful work of scientific teams operating in collaboration and competition (often simultaneously!) with each other. Their observations gradually provide greater insights into a particular field. Therefore scientific progress must be measured by a series of small steps – some experimental and some conceptual. It is most unfortunate that the media-driven perception of science on one hand, and the competitive nature of restricted research funding on the other, force scientists to hype and to present scientific progress as isolated 'Eureka moments'.

Despite this caveat, increases in scientific understanding of a field are not linear but episodic. When there is significant progress it often comes because new technologies have been applied. One such technology has been the use of DNA-related techniques to study gene expression and regulation. In turn this has led to the human genome project that produced the surprising result that we have only about 35 000 genes – not enough to explain the myriad proteins and functions within the body. In turn this led to greater attention to post-genomic regulation and that, in turn, to how environmental factors influence genomic function. Whereas evolutionary theory had originally been developed in the absence of knowledge and understanding of modern genetics, the robustness of the Darwinian model has been confirmed and extended by this growing knowledge.

Other key technological advances have included a variety of new methods that allow us to study body function non-invasively in increasingly precise ways and even, as we shall see, before birth. They range from all sorts of clever imaging methods, including some – such as CAT scans – that just look at the shape of an organ, to methods such as magnetic resonance spectroscopy that allow molecular functions to be studied in the living animal or human.

In parallel, there have been massive advances in our ability to study the earliest processes of conception, implantation and early embryonic development. A particular focus of this book is on understanding of early life, of the embryo, fetus and newborn. Because of these new reproductive technologies, there has been an explosive increase in our knowledge of this period of life in recent years.

The dominant approach to modern science is the Baconian model of hypothesis-creation and testing. This can emphasise a rather narrow approach to obtaining new information. In it, specific hypotheses are generated that can either be confirmed or refuted experimentally. The experiments are designed to test the idea, and the model is modified in light of the results. So science progresses in a day-to-day manner. Hence, most ideas in science just seem to evolve – no single person is the real inventor – rather multiple groups of researchers converge on a problem, offering thoughts and insights and experimental data, and the theory gradually develops.

But ideas in science are not just about getting new data. New theories or models come from thinking about both old and new data in different ways. New thinking is often more important than new data. While research-funding bodies focus on supporting the generation of new data, often in a very reductionist manner,[1] it is the broader integrated synthesis of new ideas from data across several fields that frequently does most to advance our understanding of biology. Perhaps not surprisingly, when this approach is taken, there can be a shift in thinking of such magnitude that a field of science changes significantly and rapidly. The ideas of natural selection and their role in evolution developed by Darwin and Wallace are a dramatic example of such a revolutionary synthesis. They involved observations in geology, biogeography, palaeontology and taxonomy, and they irreversibly changed how we think about biological processes. Often, as in that case, the data on which the new idea is constructed come from very disparate fields, and the new idea arises from the fortuitous recognition of relevance across domains that do not normally overlap. Charles Darwin's work was not done in isolation – evolutionary thought

---

[1] A reductionist approach in science is based on the idea that an understanding of how a system works will be gained by breaking it down into its component parts, and then studying them separately. The opposite approach is to take an integrative approach.

had been progressing since the work of his own grandfather, Erasmus. What Darwin (and Wallace) did was firstly to demonstrate that evolution was a fact; secondly that one species could evolve into another; and thirdly to provide mechanistic bases (natural and sexual selection) for these related processes.

This book is about a significant shift in biological thinking. It builds on the work and ideas of both ourselves and others. About 15 years ago, it was first suggested that some adult diseases had their origins partly in fetal life. A raft of experimental work and epidemiological and clinical observation has followed that has led us to a reasonable understanding of the biological processes underpinning this link. But as we have considered comparative perspectives and as developmental biology and evolutionary thinking have converged, we have given greater thought to the broader biological significance of these observations.

When we started to write this book three years ago, our intention was to focus on a description of the data suggesting a role for early development in the origins of disease, and its implications for disease prevention and treatment. However, as we worked together discussing the available data and extending our understanding into broader fields, we recognised an increasing gap between evolutionary thought and human medicine, with neither field sufficiently informing the other. Most evolutionary biology books, especially those with a developmental focus, largely keep away from the human, and from human disease theory. Conversely human biology has become dominated by genomic thinking, and the new paradigms of gene–environment interactions – well accepted in comparative biology – have been little considered. Our research forced us to bridge this gap. As we did so, we recognised that a more general framework is possible for thinking about aspects of early development and its consequences for health, disease and biological theory. We have called this new framework the concept of *predictive adaptive responses.*[2] So now this book has two major intersecting themes – one about general biological processes of responses to the environment during development and one about the developmental origins of disease.

The book derives from three related considerations – *how* do species survive short-term environmental changes, *when* do species make critical adaptive choices and *what* are the implications for human biology. As we shall explain, new insights into the first two questions, coming from diverse sources such as molecular genetics, experimental physiology, clinical medicine and epidemiology, led us to formulate the concept of predictive adaptive responses. The fundamental idea is that early in life, primarily in the embryonic, fetal and perhaps the postnatal period, mammals make irreversible choices in their developmental trajectories – not primarily to deal

---

[2] What is in a name? While we hesitate to put a catchy name to what indeed is a complex idea with a number of antecedents (see chapter 3), the practicalities of communication require a short and specific name to describe the phenomenon addressed. The rationale for this choice is given in chapter 3.

with the immediacy of their environment at the time when they are making the choice – but rather because they are *predicting* the environment into which they will be born or grow up, and in order to maximise their chance of reproductive success as an adult. Such a model explains how species can survive transient environmental change and it is therefore of broad evolutionary significance. But as we shall see, when put into the human context it also explains the origins of many common diseases including heart disease and Type 2 (or adult onset) diabetes mellitus. In turn, this radically changes our concepts of how and when to intervene in populations to reduce the burden of disease. We will argue for a far greater focus on maternal and fetal health.

This book draws on understandings of different areas of science including evolutionary biology, developmental biology, life-history theory, fetal development and clinical medicine. It describes the recent exciting discoveries that led us to posit this idea. But this is not a book only about theoretical biology, it is also about the practical applications of this idea to prevention of disease and to understanding the ecology of disease across the planet. It has significant implications for those involved in public health policy.

Three major themes are covered: developmental biology and fetal and perinatal physiology; clinical epidemiology; and evolutionary biology. In chapters 1 and 2 we provide a description of how the early phases of life progress in humans and other mammals, of what can influence or affect embryonic and fetal development, and what might be the life-long consequences of the effects of those influences. In chapters 4, 5 and 6 we give a description of how events in early fetal life can impact on later life and, in particular, lead to a greater risk of diseases such as heart disease and diabetes. The implications of this for both the developed and developing worlds are discussed in chapters 9 and 10. The exciting experimental, clinical and epidemiological science underlying the above observations led us to reflect on the significance of why we have evolved mechanisms that operate in early life but that can have adverse consequences in later life. The idea is introduced in chapter 3 and expanded upon in chapters 7 and 8.

One important conclusion is simple: in fetal life strategies are chosen based on a fetal prediction of the postnatal environment in which the individual will eventually live and reproduce. If the fetus makes the right prediction all will be well; if it does not then problems will ensue. Understanding how this happens and why evolution has preserved such a mechanism is an important part of this book. The consequences for our species are particularly dramatic because perhaps for the first time in our evolutionary history, humans now inhabit an environment in which we have not evolved to live.

Accordingly, we hope the book will appeal to a diverse set of readers – both lay people and scientists, those interested in disease and disease prevention, in pregnancy and, specifically, in a healthy start to life,[3] or in broader evolutionary biology. Inevitably, when a book is written for a range of readers, for some the technical detail in one area will be too much and for others, insufficient. We have tried to write the book so that it can be read in its entirety, or as individual chapters. We have also tried to give a brief explanation of technical terms, but also to structure the book so that more technical sections can be skipped. We hope that the totality of the book is stimulating and thought-provoking to the reader.

This book and our ideas build on the enormous contributions of scientists throughout the world, many of whom are our friends and colleagues, and we are grateful for the many interactions we have had with them. Our own experimental work is based on the contributions of numerous colleagues, fellows and students and we each are privileged to work with truly intellectually exciting and scientifically rigorous groups. All have helped build towards the ideas we have synthesised in this book. We acknowledge, in particular, the following. In Auckland: Frank Bloomfield, Bernhard Breier, Wayne Cutfield, Jane Harding, Mark Harris, Paul Hofman, Mark Oliver and Mark Vickers. In Southampton: Fred Anthony, Caroline Bertram, Lee Brawley, Felino Cagampang, Iain Cameron, Cyrus Cooper, Caroline Fall, Keith Godfrey, Lucy Green, Hazel Inskip, Shigeru Itoh, Alan Jackson, Catherine Law, Rohan Lewis, Christopher Martyn, Jim Newman, Hidenori Nishina, Clive Osmond, Takashi Ozaki, David Phillips, Kirsten Poore, Malcolm Richardson and Tim Wheeler.

Around the globe we thank Sir Patrick Bateson (Cambridge, UK), Dennis Bier (Houston), Carlos Blanco (Maastricht), John Challis (Toronto), Johan Eriksson (Helsinki), Terrence Forrester (Jamaica), Dino Giussani (Cambridge, UK), Nick Hales (Cambridge, UK), Guttorm Haugen (Oslo), Torvid Kiserud (Bergen), Anibal Llanos (Santiago, Chile), Sally MacIntyre (Glasgow), Steve Matthews (Toronto), Michael Meaney (Montreal), Julie Owens (Adelaide), Lucilla Poston (London), Jeffrey Robinson (Adelaide), Kent Thornburg (Portland, Oregon), Jaakko Tuomilehto (Helsinki), Marelyn Wintour (Melbourne) and Ranjan Yajnik (Pune). We particularly wish to thank Professor David Barker for his contribution in making the original epidemiological observations, for stimulating the biological insights from which much of our thinking and research has arisen and for his ongoing personal support of our research.

Hamish Spencer (Dunedin) and John Newnham (Perth) kindly read portions of the book and provided feedback from evolutionary and clinical perspectives, respectively. We thank Andrea Graves and Cathy Pinal for assisting with the research and Andrea and Donna Chisholm for also providing some literary input. Bron Parnall, Deborah Peach and Karen Goldstone patiently typed various sections of the

---

[3] See D. J. P. Barker, *The Best Start in Life* (London: Century, 2003).

manuscript. Peter Silver from Cambridge University Press and our agent, Mandy Little, have been most supportive at various stages throughout the project, and Frances Peck at Cambridge University Press made painstaking corrections to the typescript.

We are privileged to work at two Universities, Auckland and Southampton, that have allowed us to build significant research enterprises focused on the questions detailed in this book. It is pleasing to see our personal interaction as authors reflected in growing joint research enterprise between our institutions in this field.

Writing a book when the two authors are at opposite points on the globe has meant strong commitments from our families. We chose to write together, and all parts of the book (actually every paragraph) is the product of our joint effort. To our wives, Judy and Clare, and our children, Katie, Josh, Antonia and Jack, we are most grateful for forbearance with our many absences and long nights on the phone (by definition it was always night for one of us!).

PDG
MAH
Auckland, Southampton and places in between
August 2003

# Shaping our destiny: genes, environment and their interactions

This book is about a set of biological responses we have termed *predictive adaptive responses*, and their implications for understanding evolutionary processes, health and disease. These concepts flow from our more recent insights into one of the oldest debates in biological science.

Since the time of Hippocrates, there has been discussion about which characteristics are primarily genetic in origin, and thus immutable, and those characteristics that are plastic in nature, and thus can be influenced by the environment. The impact of modern molecular, genomic and developmental biology on our capacity to understand and address the issues that arise from this big question has been enormous – it is that explosion of biological understanding in the last 30 years that underpins this book. But as we have eradicated many causes of premature death, at least in the developed world, we have become much more conscious of the ongoing impact of environmental influences. In the enthusiasm for modern genetics, this has been much less studied. Yet it is critical we understand that it is the *interaction* between our environment and our genes that determines our destiny. It is now naïve to think about genes (nature) and environment (nurture) in a dichotomous way. We now comprehend that the manner in which the environment affects gene expression on one hand, and how genetic variation affects the response to the environment on the other, is the basis of biological destiny.[1]

However there is a newly emerging dimension to our understanding – namely that the interactions between genes and environment very early in life have a predictive role in defining how any subsequent interactions will be resolved. It is the nature of those predictive interactions early in life and their consequences that is the real focus of this book.

---

[1] This is well illustrated in the title of the book by Matt Ridley, *Nature via Nurture* (New York, NY: HarperCollins Publishers Inc., 2003).

In the early chapters of the book we examine how genes and environment interact to control our development.[2] We look at the relative roles of genes and environment, and we start to ask the questions of when and why these interactions occur, and what are the consequences – not just the immediate consequences at the time of the interaction, but consequences for the entire life history of the individual. It is the answers to these questions that led us to the formulation of the concept of predictive adaptive responses. But first let us use some comparative biological and human examples in order to illustrate what we really mean by gene–environment interactions.

## Lessons from the Antipodes

Australia was colonised relatively late in British colonial history. A penal colony was established at Botany Bay in 1788, but soon afterwards organised colonisation of this vast continent by working class British people wishing to improve their lot was encouraged. Rather than moulding to their new environment, the settlers tried to reproduce their familiar environment within the new colony. Many plants, birds and animals were brought to the new land. One food source these settlers could not do without was rabbits! After several failed introductions, 24 wild rabbits from the English countryside arrived in Australia aboard ship in 1859 and were successfully released.[3] The rabbit population increased far more rapidly than did the human population, as they had few natural predators and little competition for food. They spread across the continent to occupy a wide variety of environmental conditions, from lush farmland to semi-desert, and at sea level and in the mountains. As is well known, they rapidly became pests of such proportions that shooting or trapping them was inadequate, and Australia had to resort to creating hundreds of miles of fencing, and then to biological warfare (by introducing myxomatosis and, when that failed, the rabbit *calicivirus*) in an attempt to control the rabbit pest. What had seemed like a good idea initially became a nightmare, and the success of the Australian rabbits is an often-quoted example of the perils of interfering in a natural environment. No one had realised the tremendous ability of the rabbits to adapt to their new environment and to multiply accordingly. The Australian farmers expected the rabbit population to be no more extensive, and no more of a nuisance, than on a nineteenth-century English farm. But this unfortunate and unintended experiment with nature provides us with an insight into biological adaptability.

---

[2] Those readers with a working knowledge of genetics, developmental biology and evolutionary theory may prefer to skip chapters 1 and 2.

[3] It is thought that the rabbits were introduced as food for foxes, which were also introduced by the settlers. The problems of the British passion for fox-hunting are still debated today!

It turns out that, despite the originally homogeneous stock of rabbits brought to Australia, they are now very diverse in appearance. Throughout the country they vary in size and shape, body-fat content, coat colour and even in enzyme biochemistry. Research on body shape has revealed some intriguing differences. Rabbits born in the hotter and more arid parts of the country have less body fat than those living in the cooler regions. This is a very helpful adaptation because the insulating properties of fat are reduced in the hot climate, and increased in the cooler climate. Apart from body insulation, rabbits regulate body temperature by active means, and an important mechanism utilises the extensive blood supply to their ears, because when they are hot they can increase this blood flow in order to lose more heat, and, when cold, the flow can be reduced. Interestingly, it turns out that rabbits living in the arid parts of Australia have longer ears than those from the cooler climes.

How could such consistent changes in ear length and body fatness have arisen? Clearly they are appropriate adaptations to the environment. Presumably ear length is influenced by multiple genes, and in each generation different profiles of gene expression[4] will lead to some variation in ear length. If there were no survival advantage related to ear length then there would be no difference in ear length between rabbits from different geographical regions. However, in the hotter climates the animals with variation favouring longer ears survived better and thus were more effective reproducers; gradually ear length evolved to be longer in the hotter regions. This is a classic example of how genes and environment have interacted over time to produce two breeds of rabbit with different characteristics that confer a relative advantage or disadvantage in a particular environment. This is evolution in action within a species, producing population or group diversity. Animal breeders do this all the time – although in this case the environmental selection is not passive (that advantage comes to the animals because they can survive in the environment more easily) but is active and driven by the breeder.[5]

For many years after Darwin first proposed that the dual processes of natural and sexual selection drove the change in structure of organisms and ultimately led to new species formation, there was much doubt that selection could explain adaptation, because it was generally believed that these changes would be too imperceptible between generations. Then in the 1970s biologists returned to the Galapagos Islands, the source of many of Darwin's insights, and observed how the finch's beak changed

---

[4] Gene expression is a technical term referring to when a gene is active because it is being actively transcribed by the cellular systems to initiate formation of RNA, which in turn initiates specific protein synthesis. Genes are activated and turned off in a complex regulatory framework within a cell – they need not be fully on or off. Thus genes can be highly active with high rates of expression or conversely have low rates of expression.

[5] The success of selective breeding is related to the genetic determinants of the traits of interest. The fewer genes, the easier the selection. If a characteristic is not genetically determined it cannot be selected for. That is why racehorse breeding is such an uncertain business!

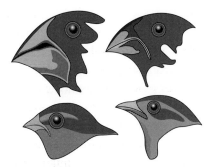

Fig. 1.1       Within a species, variations in phenotype can confer a survival advantage in a given environment, or in the face of an environmental change. The beaks of one species of finch in the
Galapagos Islands are a good example. They were instrumental in the development of the
theory of natural selection by Darwin. Redrawn from F. J. Sulloway. *Journal of The History
of Biology* **15** (1985), 1–53.

in a *single* generation in response to drought. Much to their surprise they found that
a single episode of drought was sufficient to cause a 5 per cent change in beak size –
because the deepest beaks were best for attacking the tough seeds that survived the
drought. But because more males than females survived the drought, the females
became choosy about their mates, and the successful males were those that had the
largest and the deepest beaks. They therefore had more progeny. So sexual selection
added to natural selection: the next generation also had 5 per cent deeper beaks
than their immediate ancestors. But after it rained it was the young finches with the
smaller beaks that were more likely to survive, because juveniles were more able to
eat soft seeds. The influence of selection became diluted and lost after the rains (see
Figure 1.1).

So there are tensions in selection processes. Environmentally-induced shifts
in appearance (phenotype) only stabilise when the environment is permanently
shifted in one direction or another. As we shall see, much of this book concerns
the reality that individuals do not develop in a stable or uni-directionally changing
environment – but more about that after we define what we mean by 'environment'.

### Evidence of gene–environmental interactions in development: a brief comparative anthology

Yellow dung fly are spread worldwide. Females lay their eggs within cattle dung on
which the hatched larvae feed. The most important environmental influence for the
dung fly is therefore the amount of cattle dung available! Where there is a limited
supply of dung, there will be competition for laying sites between dung flies within
one species and between species. To deal with this, the developing insects accelerate

their maturation and mature at a smaller body size – in other words they 'trade off' growth to reproduce. When dung is readily available, they grow larger and take longer to mature. The entire life cycle of growth, development and reproduction of the dung fly has been changed by the temporary environment of the larvae.

Similar environmentally-induced developmental changes are found in various locusts and grasshoppers. Many locust species respond to overcrowding and shortage of food by migrating. But to migrate they have to change their body form and their metabolism. Their wing shape and size must be different to fly long distances and they need to use fat as a high-energy fuel to migrate over long distances. They also need to be able to eat a wider range of plants. But these changes, while determined in the larval stage, only have their importance once the locust is fully developed. So this poses an interesting and fundamental question – are decisions made in early life that relate to the ability to survive in later life? There is an obvious advantage to the locust in an overcrowded situation in being able to fly away to a new source of food. It is thought that the larvae detect chemical signals (pheromones), which induce such morphogenic changes and a variety of other morphogenic changes to create body form and function appropriate to migration, rather than the alternate sedentary form. They also use a change in body colour to signal the change to other locusts, and indeed to predators (see Figure 1.2).

These two examples, both involving insects, show that environmental influences acting early in life can create changes which persist throughout life and have their primary advantage in later life by ensuring the capacity to reproduce. These are examples in evolutionary terms of true adaptations, where an adaptation is defined as a response that can be demonstrated to promote reproductive fitness.

Similarly in some species of reptile and fish, environmental influences can have a profound and permanent effect on the appearance of the animal – namely whether it will be a male or female. Unlike in mammals and birds (where anatomical gender is determined by the different chromosomal arrangements in males and females), in species such as the Mississippi alligator or the green back giant turtle it is the temperature of the incubated egg that determines gender. If the egg clutch is buried in sand in a position that keeps it warmer, the embryonic turtles will be female. If the nests are in a situation leading to cooler eggs, the hatchlings will be male. In alligators it is the other way around! We do not know whether the site of the nest is actively chosen by the mother so as to ensure male or female offspring but the possibility is intriguing.

Can similar phenomena occur in mammals? It has been found that coat thickness in the offspring of the meadow vole depends on the season of their birth: if they are born in the spring their coats are thinner than if they are born in the autumn. Thus their fur coats are appropriate for the climatic conditions that are likely to occur in the months following birth. It is not the temperature at birth that determines coat

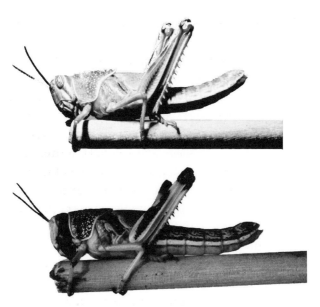

Fig. 1.2    Locusts develop with strikingly different body colours when their population density changes. The so-called 'solitary form' (top) is much lighter than the 'gregarious form' (below), which occurs in juveniles when the population density increases. This precedes swarming and migration, but it also indicates to predators such as lizards that the locust population has reached a point where they may be eating plants containing compounds toxic to the predators. (Photograph courtesy of Professor S. Simpson.)

thickness, because it is roughly the same in spring and autumn. Experiments show that it is hormonal signals from the mother responding to altered day length that determine the offspring's coat thickness while it is still a fetus. The biology of the fetal vole is responding to information from its mother about changing day length and *predicting* the appropriate coat thickness to have in the coming months after leaving the nest. This cannot be solely genetically determined – otherwise all voles born to the same parents would have the same coat length. Information is being processed so that the genes that determine coat thickness change their degree of expression *in expectation of a future environment*, the nature of which is *predicted by some aspect of the current environment*.

Intriguingly, Charles Darwin also touched upon this point in *The Origin of Species by Means of Natural Section*, first published in 1859. In a section on the Laws of Variation, he noted that 'it is well-known to furriers that animals of the same species have thicker and better fur the further north they live; but who can tell how much of this difference may be due to the warmest-clad individuals having been favoured and preserved during many generations, and how much to the action of the severe climate?'. One wonders what he had in mind when he then refers to 'the definitive action of the conditions of life' and contrasts them with the process of natural selection – was he pre-empting our current discussion?

There is evidence that such environmental interactions also exist in humans. Japan extends over many degrees of latitude. This creates a climatic range from the cold northern islands such as Hokkaido to the sub-tropical southern islands such as Okinawa. When the Japanese army invaded the tropics in 1941 they discovered that heat stroke was more common amongst those soldiers who had been born in the northern islands than in those born in the south. Heat stroke occurred more often because these soldiers could not effectively use one of their key means to reduce body heat – that is sweating – and they simply sweated less than those who adapted well. This led to the discovery that the number of active sweat glands is set soon after birth and does not change through life. But the ability to determine the number of active sweat glands is a once-and-for-all choice in development – once determined it is irreversible and one has to cope with that number of active glands throughout life. It was the number of functional sweat glands that differed between the different groups of soldiers. Those who were born in a cool climate had less active sweat glands and those born in a warm environment had a greater number of active glands. This example also illustrates how a *critical window* in development occurring early in life can have life-long consequences. The number of sweat glands that are set to become active is determined by an adaptation to the local environment at birth, and the choice made at that stage, as a result of a transient gene–environmental interaction determining sweat gland activation, has life-long consequences.

Clearly the number of active sweat glands is not genetically determined. Indeed, examination of the total number of sweat glands in the skin shows that all Japanese have similar numbers – the difference is that some become activated and some do not. This is determined by the degree of innervation of the sweat glands by the sympathetic nervous system. It is the actual environment at a critical period in early development that sets the number of active sweat glands. If this were a genetically determined phenomenon, then over a relatively small number of generations individuals would have the number of active sweat glands determined by their ancestors. But it is obvious that this is a highly adaptive response, making it possible to adjust the number of active sweat glands to a new thermal environment within a generation. Perhaps this high degree of adaptability to differing environments explains why in human prehistory human migrations over long distances could occur rapidly with such success. For example, the Americas appear to have been settled from Alaska to Tierra Del Fuego within a period of perhaps only 1000 years from the initial crossing from Eastern Siberia to Alaska over the Beringa land-bridge. The active sweat gland adaptation is helpful both to the neonate, who also needs to thermoregulate and be able to lose heat, and to the adult – that is, it has both immediate and long-term advantage. But of course the long-term advantage is only there provided the environment does not change.

The story of the Japanese soldiers demonstrates well how a past adaptation that made sense in one environment can influence one's ability to survive in a new environment. Such examples may seem extreme but, as we will see later in the book, they may be of contemporary relevance to the changing patterns of disease in many countries where nutrition is rapidly shifting from a poor to a relatively rich plane. We must conclude that the genetic make-up of the individual animal or human is not the only factor that determines either its appearance or its capacity to respond to a given environment. And, as we have already seen, there is a strong developmental component to how these interactions are determined.

So the balance between genetic determinants and environmental influences, the so-called gene–environment interaction, is at the heart of both how an individual thrives or does not thrive in any given situation. The deep beak of the finch was advantageous for the adult and disadvantageous for the infant. It was advantageous in a dry environment and disadvantageous in a wet environment. This is an important concept – just because selection has induced an adaptation does not mean that this adaptation will always be advantageous. Perhaps the most obvious example is one first used by the famous geneticist Richard Dawkins in his book *The Extended Phenotype* (see further reading, p. 218). The moth and many other nocturnal insects have evolved with an adaptation to fly towards light – this allows it to escape from a cave. While this makes sense when seeking food, flying into fire or an electric light is a terminal fate for many moths – clearly not, at that final self-immolating moment, an advantageous adaptation! These considerations are found at every level in the biological realm, both plant and animal, and the human cannot be considered differently.

We must now turn our attention to two important definitions: phenotype and genotype.

## Phenotype

*Phenotype* is the term used to describe the actual appearance and function of an individual organism. Most commonly the term is used to describe physical characteristics (for example, tall or short, fat or lean etc.). We will frequently refer to the physical phenotype at birth that encompasses the various measures that can describe size at birth – weight, length, head circumference etc. However, the term *phenotype* is actually more general than just a reference to physical measurements – it extends to include the entire status of the animal or human in physical, functional and biochemical terms. Thus a schizophrenic individual and a person suffering from depression might be considered to have different personality phenotypes. Similarly a person with high blood-sugar levels due to diabetes and a person with normal blood-sugar levels have different biochemical or metabolic phenotypes. We will use the term *phenotype* in its most generic sense – that is, to describe the sum total of the biochemical, functional and physical characteristics of the animal or human at the point of observation. An obvious question that will appear recurrently throughout this book is 'What determines phenotype?' It is obviously not only the genetic make-up of the individual. Imagine two cloned female calves.[6] They will develop as absolutely identical twins – they have the same *genotype* – that is, they are identical in so far as the genetic information they carry. But imagine that, after birth, one calf is raised on good pasture and is kept well 'drenched' to reduce gut parasite load, and the other is raised on very poor pasture and gets a large intestinal parasite burden. The first calf will grow into a large fat healthy cow with good reproductive performance and a high capacity to make milk – to the farmer's delight. However the second calf will be a 'runt' – it will grow poorly – its mature body size will be smaller, it will have less muscle mass and poorer condition and is likely to be a poor producer of milk and indeed calves. Its destiny is more likely to be sold for pet food early in its life. Thus while these two calves have the same genotypes, they certainly do not have the same adult physical phenotypes, and their destinies will be very different. Furthermore the major determinant of their different destinies was their nutritional and health environment after birth – but more about that later.

Identical twins are essentially the human natural equivalent of the cloning experiment we have just described. At the two- or four-cell stage the fertilised embryo splits and two embryos arise, which then develop into two fetuses – each with the same genotype. Yet identical twins are not identical in every respect. Even if two twins look the same to the less familiar, their mother can always tell them apart, because they have different personalities or slightly different mannerisms or one will be a bit heavier or a bit taller – indeed at birth identical (or *monozygous*) twins seldom have the same birth weights, and they sometimes differ by several hundred grams. These differences in phenotype are usually magnified during life, so that more and more we find it easy to tell them apart. Similarly, their biological destinies will tend to diverge. While if one twin develops adult-onset diabetes mellitus, the other is more likely to do so, this is by no means inevitable. The same is true for heart disease, cancer and so on.

---

[6] Cloning is an imprecise word because it has several meanings. However the cloning we describe here is the scientifically classical way in which embryos are divided to produce genetically identical offspring. It is based on in vitro fertilisation, then when the embryo has reached the two-cell stage, the two cells are dissected apart under a powerful microscope, without harming either, and they are then transplanted back into the donor mother, when each then fully develops into a calf.

So while there is understandably much interest in the role of genes in determining our fate (and the fate of the cow) it is obvious that genes cannot provide an understanding of everything in life – this is a major message in this book.

## Genotype

Genes are a relatively new concept. Darwin guessed that there must be discrete heritable elements and this was established by Mendel in 1865. The term gene was coined by a Danish geneticist, Wilhelm Johannsen, in 1909. It was only in the 1950s that the discovery of the double helix by Watson and Crick explained how genes could replicate, and this introduced the idea of the genetic code embedded within DNA. As is well known, Mendel was a monk who became fascinated by the ways in which characteristics in a species could be passed from one generation to the next. He had started life as a science teacher and his mathematical perspectives allowed him to identify some simple rules from some very complex biology. He was fortunate to become a monk in a monastery where the Abbott was also a committed scientist with interests in selective breeding of apples and sheep! Because Mendel's work was essentially lost for many years, we are left with many gaps in our knowledge of his life. One anecdote suggests that he had to modify his experimental model rather early in his studies, as he first started to examine the characteristics of a rat colony which he bred in the cellars of the monastery at Brno. The monastery apparently did not feel it appropriate for a monk to be engaged in an activity which involved so much sex, and so Mendel changed to the study of peas in the monastery garden. Presumably the Abbott was not aware that sexual reproduction also occurs in plants! For posterity, it was very fortunate that Mendel made the switch of species, for it would have been very hard in the rat to demonstrate inheritance of characteristics in the way that he was able to do in the pea. His studies of green versus yellow characteristics, or smooth versus wrinkled skins are examples of characteristics inherited by single genes that exist in only two forms (or alleles), dominant or recessive.[7]

---

[7] The concept of dominant or recessive genes comes from Mendel. Assume a gene can exist in one of two forms (alleles) – let us say Y or y, which have their origin in the sequence details of the DNA. As each gene is carried in two copies (one inherited from each parent) there are 4 possible arrangements: YY, yy, yY and Yy depending on the gene inherited from the mother or father – both being Ys in the first case, both ys in the second, and one of each in the last two cases. Let us assume Y makes peas yellow because it causes the peas to express a gene that makes the pigment yellow, but y is an inactive gene that makes no colour. If Y is a dominant gene then the presence of one Y gene will make the pea yellow. So peas with the genetic make up YY or yY or Yy will all be yellow and the yy will be green. If, however, the Y gene is recessive and therefore needs two copies to be fully active and visible, then the YY peas are yellow and the yy peas are green, and the Yy and yY peas are not very yellow, or are green. Note that whether the peas were yellow or green would determine their phenotype; and yellow phenotypes could have a range of genotypes (YY, Yy or yY if Y is dominant, or only YY if Y is recessive).

Genes encode the genetic information that determines whether the individual will grow to become a rabbit or a human. The total repertoire of genetic information in an individual's genes is called the *genotype*. These two species have the majority of their genomic DNA in common, as do all mammals. The genome houses a bank of information that describes evolutionary history, so that closely related species have an even higher proportion in common – it is over 97 per cent identical between humans and chimpanzees. But even distantly related species such as humans and fruit flies have at least 50 per cent of their genes in common. We even have considerable genetic material in common with the lowly flatworm. These similarities have helped the progress of genetic research enormously as fruit flies and flatworms are easy to breed and to manipulate genetically.

If follows that even very small changes in the DNA may produce drastic phenotypic effects on the individual. This is well established for the structural changes that may occur in very short segments of DNA and that are termed mutations: in the fruit fly these can give rise to animals with no wings, or even to those with double the normal number of wings. The point is that wingless or double-winged fruit flies are still fruit flies (because they can interbreed with other fruit flies) in terms of their genotype, even though their phenotypes vary considerably, just as was true for the long- and short-eared rabbits. And, just as for the rabbits, these phenotypic differences determine survival. Clearly, having non-functional wings is not great for the survivability of fruit flies escaping from a predator.

Genes are comprised of sequences of DNA[8] that carry the information necessary to tell cells how to make chains of amino acids, which form proteins. There are two copies of each gene in every cell except the gametes (sperm and ova). Each copy is known as an *allele*. For most genes both alleles are active – if they are identical in nucleotide sequence (i.e. homozygous) then only one gene product is formed. If there is a polymorphism or a mutation in one allele but not in the other

---

[8] DNA, or deoxyribonucleic acid, itself is a chain of nucleotides that are simple molecules combining a sugar with an amino acid. There are only four nucleotides: adenosine, guanine, thymidine and cytosine or A, G, T and C. Normally, DNA exists as two chains that spiral around each other in a beautiful manner termed the 'double helix'. The information in one chain is always sufficient to inform the sequence of the second chain in the helix because if there is a C on one chain it must pair with a G on the other; if there is a T it must pair with an A. This sequence-matching is critical to the processes of DNA replication, which must occur each time any cell divides. The basis of the genetic code is that groups of three nucleotides form the genetic alphabet. The complex machinery of the cell deciphers this code, which contains essentially a set of instructions of how to build proteins from constituent amino acids. Each triplet of DNA codes for a specific amino acid. The code also informs where a gene starts and where a gene stops. It codes for the structure of the protein that the particular gene represents and instructs the synthesis of the protein through the cellular machinery involving RNA (ribonucleic acid, a very similar chemical structure to DNA). Proteins are simply chains of amino acids, and all genetic information acts by coding for protein production. Body function is ultimately determined by the pattern of proteins that different types of cells make. Some proteins are structural such as the actin and myosin proteins in muscle, some are hormones such as insulin, others are enzymes that regulate the chemical pathways of the body, affecting the making and breaking down of fats, sugars and proteins, and some are control factors which in turn control the function of DNA and RNA themselves.

(i.e. heterozygous) both gene products may be formed or the abnormal may inhibit the production of the normal. Between genes are large portions of DNA that do not actively code for proteins. Some parts of this are the site where molecules called transcription factors bind with DNA to signal to a gene whether it should be activated or not. Within genes there are also portions of active (exonic) and inactive (intronic) transcribable DNA that offer further complexity in regulation and allow one gene to code for more than one protein. DNA is packaged in chromosomes. In multi-cellular organisms there are two copies of each chromosome, except the sex chromosomes, in each mature cell, and one copy in the gametes. In species that use chromosomes for sexual determination (birds and mammals), in one gender (females in mammals, males in birds) the two sex chromosomes are identical, and in the other gender there are two different sex chromosomes (X and Y chromosomes in mammals) in each non-gamete cell.

There are only about 35 000 genes in the human genome – but 35 000 protein switches are not in themselves enough to regulate the complex range of body functions that need to be regulated, particularly if they are just on/off switches. The complexity is created in a number of ways. Firstly, while there may be only 35 000 genes, there are various mechanisms to switch on or off part of the alphabet within a gene (generally called splicing variants) so as to produce more than one peptide from a gene. Secondly, transcription factors not only turn a gene on or off, but can regulate the degree to which it is turned on (i.e. expressed) or turned off.[9] Thirdly, after the protein is made, the intracellular machinery may lead to enzymatic processing, breaking it up into smaller bits or leading to addition or subtraction of phosphate groups (which is a way in which molecules transfer energy) or by addition of sugar moieties to the protein. These latter processes are called *post-translational* (i.e. occurring after the translation of the genetic code) modifications and lead to a very large number of possible proteins. It is this complex orchestra of processes – translational and post-translational – that leads to the complexity of biological processes in the human body.

## Variations in genotype

There is much variation in the individual genome (i.e. genotype) and it is this variation that is the genetic basis of our differences in function and appearance. For

---

[9] For example, while every cell has the gene for making insulin, it is only in the cells of the pancreatic islet that transcription factors act to turn the gene for insulin on. These transcription factors in turn are regulated by other transcription factors and by information coming from other cells near by or far away. In the case of the insulin-making cells of the pancreas, the transcription factors telling the cell to synthesise insulin were turned on at a critical point in development and from that point on the cells were activated to make insulin; non-islet cells were inactivated from making insulin. But throughout life other transcription factors, activated by high-or low-sugar levels and by hormones, continue to modulate the rate of insulin production and secretion by the islet cells.

example, the genotype of a Bantu and of an Icelander are different in the genetically determined expression of genes that determine the amount of melanin present in skin. Both genomes can make melanin – otherwise the Icelander could never get a tan when he or she went on holiday to Tenerife – but under normal conditions the amount of melanin in the skin cells is very different and this is genetically determined. Another example is the genes coding for cell-surface proteins on blood cells, which are detected in blood typing. Siblings may be similar in many respects but have different blood groups, depending on the parental blood groups. These differences are due to differences in the genetic code in the genes responsible for the blood group antigens of the two individuals.

The most common cause of genetic differences is a change in a single nucleotide in a gene. In some cases this sequence change causes overt disease. For example, in the case of phenylketonuria (PKU), a single change in the nucleotide sequence of one particular gene causes a change in the amino acid sequence of an enzyme that normally metabolises phenylalanine. As a result, toxic levels of phenylalanine build up in the infant's body when he or she eats protein foods, and these toxic levels cause brain damage.[10] In many cases of individual genotypes for which single nucleotide changes have been found, there is little or no obvious functional significance of the change.[11] The different consequences of a single nucleotide change occur because a change in nucleotide may or may not lead to a change in the amino acid encoded: there is considerable redundancy in the genetic code,[12] and the amino acid change may not change the function of the protein.

When the genetic change leads to an obvious change in function or appearance we term it a mutation. When the change is very subtle it is called a polymorphism.[13] Most polymorphisms are of no fundamental consequence. The large number of polymorphisms provide the basis of DNA-fingerprinting used by the police. However, while polymorphisms do not necessarily cause disease they can influence the amount of a protein secreted, or the action of a protein. For example, milk production in dairy cows is stimulated by growth hormone, and the different milk

---

[10] This is a very risky but treatable situation and it is why all newborn babies are screened for PKU by the heel-prick Guthrie test.

[11] Such single point changes in sequence are often called SNPs (single nucleotide polymorphisms and pronounced as "snips").

[12] For example, both GGU and GGC code for the amino acid glycine so there is absolutely no difference in the functional outcome of a code reading GGU or GGC. On the other hand UGC codes for cysteine and UGG codes for tryptophan, so the protein readout for the one change (C to G) in the nucleotide can lead to a change in the amino acid sequence of the protein.

[13] Mutations and polymorphisms are essentially overlapping terms. By custom, when the genetic change leads to overt disease it is called a mutation, when it merely leads to a non-obvious biochemical change, it is called a polymorphism. As we get better at genetic diagnosis we are finding that the definitions are not that easy to keep separate. Mutations also involve a broader range of genetic defects including deletions of pieces of DNA and DNA changes that lead to premature stopping of transcription etc. Both polymorphisms and mutations can involve alterations in single-base pairs or in the length of repeating pieces of DNA.

production in two breeds of dairy cow is caused by a polymorphism in the growth-hormone receptor. This polymorphism is thus very valuable.

## The element of chance

Sperm and eggs (ova) only have one copy of each autosome and one sex chromosome. At fertilisation the egg and sperm fuse to create a one-cell embryo containing – in humans – 46 chromosomes, which then has the capacity to develop fully into a mature human being. It is the mixing of genetic material at fertilisation, a process termed *recombination*, that is central to the process of maintaining mammalian diversity and thus is crucial to evolution.[14] It provides one chance element in the evolutionary process, somewhat like shuffling the cards. The other is genetic drift.[15] This inter-generationally driven variation in genetic mix is the basis of variation on which evolutionary selective processes operate.

Chromosomes line up in matched pairs during cell division in the cells that will form the egg or sperm. This lining up has the prime purpose of ensuring that the right number and the complete portfolio of chromosomes end up in each cell. Obviously one copy of each chromosome and one X chromosome must end up in each egg. The same happens in each sperm, except that there can be either an X or a Y chromosome present. Thus the correct and complete repertoire of 46 chromosomes forms the fertilised egg. If the individual has three copies of one chromosome, profound developmental abnormalities can occur – for example, many cases of Down's syndrome are due to the fertilised egg having three copies of chromosome 21. Most abnormalities of chromosome number are fatal to the development of the embryo – the exceptions generally involve the sex chromosomes but abnormality of number always has phenotypic effects.[16] But this lining up has a second purpose: it allows genetic recombination by one-to-one swapping of genes between the two chromosomes of different parental origin, without losing the

---

[14] Not all species reproduce in every generation in this sexual way in which genes from mother and father are mixed. For example, bacteria can reproduce by splitting in half – so that each daughter bacterium is identical to its parent; as well as by sexual reproduction. The processes of reproduction across species and, in particular, in microbes and other single-cell organisms is fascinating but beyond this book.

[15] Genetic drift is a concept largely outside the focus of this book. It is the process by which, in populations over time, the mean frequency of various alleles may shift by random chance. The rate of genetic drift depends on the population size (greatest when it is smallest), generation length (greatest when it is short) and litter size (greatest when small). Genetic drift arises because, particularly in small populations with low reproduction per generation, not all alleles pass by chance in equal proportion from one generation to the next. Thus over time some rarer alleles may get lost or in some cases, if carried by a dominant male for example, magnified.

[16] For example, a person with 45 chromosomes with only one X chromosome has Turner's Syndrome – the person is an infertile female with inactive ovaries and a number of skeletal and tissue abnormalities.

integrity of the full repertoire of genes.[17] Thus the variation in gene sequence can change from generation to generation.

This is the power of recombination – it ensures ongoing variation in the phenotype of each generation of the organism, but still complete functionality and integrity of the species. It is this variation created by polymorphism that is the infrastructure on which Darwinian selection occurs within a species. As we are learning, if the genotype varies between individuals then the nature of the gene–environment interaction can also vary across individuals for any given environmental stimulus.

## From genotype to phenotype

We have already introduced the concept that genetic determinants alone do not generate the phenotype – there are important environmental influences. Throughout this book we will use the term 'environment' in a somewhat broader sense than its most obvious and traditional usage. The environment of an organism is the sum total of all factors that can affect the organism – we can call this the macro-environment. For example the amount and type of food available is an environmental factor, a high likelihood of predators in the neighbourhood creates a risk/stress environment etc. For a given cell, the micro-environment is determined by the concentrations of sugar and oxygen and other nutrients in the blood stream and the tissue space surrounding the cell. The cellular environment is further determined by the cells lying next to it – for example, a liver cell lying immediately next to a blood vessel has a different environment from a liver cell surrounded by other liver cells. The fetal environment, as we shall see in chapter 4, is largely determined by the function of the placenta, and in turn by the mother's physiological function, which is in turn determined in part by her macro-environment.

This book is about *how* and *when* the environment acts on the genome to lead to specific phenotypes, and how these processes generate health or disease. A major thesis of the book is that the most important of these interactions operate at the

---

[17] Imagine two teams of rugby players wearing different uniforms but each in numbers from 1 to 15 according to their playing position. Each team is to swap two players with the other team and the swap occurs with the person lined up opposite. If the two number 9s and two number 15s changed, there still would be two complete teams each with one half back (number 9) and one fullback (number 15). Each could go off and play a good game of rugby. But if the teams did not line up properly at the start, then the number 15 in one team might have swapped with the number 9 in the other team, so that after swapping neither team would be fully functional. Recombination is this process of swapping when lined up correctly. Imagine the same exercise of aligned recombination going on after every game in a league. By the end of the season every team would still be an intact rugby team of 15 players covering every position but the membership of the teams would be very different. By chance, some teams may be very strong and some very weak but most would be of rather similar capability.

earliest stages of life and that we have grossly underestimated the importance of these interactions.

## Disease and genes

Few diseases are purely genetic. In those that are, the chromosome is abnormal or an important gene is critically disrupted in a major way. Down's syndrome (trisomy 21) is an abnormality of chromosome 21: this can happen in two ways but in each case the critical feature is that there are three copies instead of two of some genes that are located on chromosome 21. One of these ways – carrying three copies of the chromosome 21 (usually two from mother and one from father) is greatly increased in mothers over 35, and this knowledge is important in reducing the risk of having a baby with Down's syndrome. Other diseases are due to an abnormality of a single gene – for example, cystic fibrosis. This is a fatal disease in which the lungs and pancreas are particularly affected by very thick secretions of mucus. It occurs if both copies of the gene for a protein-channel within the cell wall that moves chloride between the outside and inside of the cell are abnormal. If one copy of the gene is normal, then so is the subject; if both copies are abnormal owing to a mutation (not necessarily the same mutation), then the disease is manifest. This is an example of an autosomal recessive genetic disease – i.e. the autosomes (chromosomes that are not the sex chromosomes) are involved; it is termed recessive because both genes (i.e. one from each parent) must be affected for disease to be present. Some diseases are dominant, in which case even if one allele is normal, it cannot block the devastating effect of the partner's abnormal gene. An example of this is Huntington's disease, which either affected parent has a 50 per cent chance of passing on to his or her progeny because disease arises if one copy of the paired alleles is abnormal at the relevant gene locus. Huntington's disease is caused by a mutation in a section of a gene that codes for a protein in the brain, and this changes the number of repeats of the sequence that codes for glutamine. This leads to an abnormal form of the protein, particularly in part of the brain known as the basal ganglia and in the cerebral cortex. It stimulates brain-cell degeneration in adult life and leads to a tragic and irreversible decline into dementia, movement disorder and death.[18] Each of these examples – trisomy 21, Huntington's disease and cystic fibrosis – is a disease where destiny is cast from the point of conception and nothing that happens later will change it.

---

[18] Huntington's disease illustrates other points relevant to this book. Because the disease does not manifest until after reproductive age, there is no selection (other than conscious cultural/social selection) against the defective gene. While both parents can pass on the Huntington's mutation, with a 50 per cent probability, children who inherit the gene from their father are more likely to get the disease earlier than if they inherit the gene from their mother. This demonstrates a degree of imprinting of the Huntington allele (for explanation see chapter 2). The Huntington-disease gene is found on chromosome 4 and the mutation is due to an insert of extra repeats of the nucleotide sequence CAG (which codes for glutamine) into a normal brain protein, making it abnormal.

## Environment, genes and disease

However, most disease is not simply genetic, even if it has a genetic component. Most often, genetic make-up creates an altered risk or propensity for a disease, but it requires environmental factors to come into play for the disease to be exhibited. Even so-called purely genetic diseases can have an environmental component. For example, the most common genetic abnormality in the world is glucose-6-phosphate-dehydrogenase (or G6PD) deficiency. It is estimated that G6PD deficiency afflicts some 400 million people, particularly those of African, Mediterranean or Asian ancestry, but it does occur in about 1 in 1000 Northern Europeans. The disease is caused by an abnormality on the X chromosome in the gene coding for the enzyme G6PD. If you are female then both copies must be abnormal to produce the disease. If you are male then you only have one X chromosome and so you cannot be protected from the disease by having a normal copy on the other chromosome, unlike in the female. This pattern of disease is called 'recessive sex linked', and other examples are haemophilia and red–green colour blindness. The enzyme G6PD is present in all cells but is particularly important in blood cells where it is essential for making glutathione; this is one of the molecules we endogenously use as an antioxidant.[19] Depending on the precise mutation, the vast majority of people with G6PD deficiency have no symptoms unless certain environmental factors occur. If the individual with the mutation eats fava beans or is given a particular anti-malarial drug called primaquine, then the red blood cells break down and there is a severe attack of haemolytic anaemia[20] with multiple and sometimes fatal consequences.

The point we are making is that G6PD deficiency is a genetic disease in which nothing usually happens unless there is an environmental trigger – the disease phenotype is precipitated by a specific interaction between the environment (e.g. fava beans) and the genotype (the faulty G6PD gene). This is a dramatic example of what is likely to be the most common way in which genetic factors predispose to disease – they change the way in which environmental factors impact on the function of the body.

Genes have been related to many common diseases such as diabetes and heart disease. Usually there are multiple genes involved and the genes are not in themselves causal. They create a risk situation in which a particular set of genetically determined changes in body function, together with environmental factors, creates disease. For example, many genes are known to alter the sensitivity of the body to insulin – but except in one or two very rare mutations, single-gene defects or changes do

---

[19] Antioxidants scavenge the small amounts of highly negatively charged oxygen produced as a by-product of normal metabolism. This charged oxygen is highly toxic, and if it accumulates leads to too much oxygenation of fats and proteins and to cell death.

[20] In haemolytic anaemia the red blood cells, which carry oxygen through the body, rupture.

not actually cause 'Type 2' diabetes.[21] Instead, polymorphisms or mutations in the many components of the cell machinery affect the sensitivity of a cell to insulin. Generally the disease phenotype will not be exhibited, irrespective of genotype, without an environmental factor acting. For example, a high-fat and carbohydrate diet, obesity (which by stretching fat cells makes them more insulin resistant) and a lack of exercise induce the appearance of diabetes. The genotype merely changes the sensitivity to the environmental interaction. As we shall see in chapter 4, the diabetes story is highly relevant as it is now clear that predictive adaptive responses play an important role in determining the sensitivity of this interaction.

Phenotypes clearly affect the disease risks for an individual organism: the rabbit with short ears is at greater risk of overheating in a warm environment; short people appear to be at greater risk of heart disease; people with truncal obesity are at greater risk of diabetes. But phenotype can also confer benefits: tall people are more likely to get better jobs; lions with longer manes are more likely to be sexually dominant and attractive to the lioness; the bower bird with the most impressive dance and the most impressive collection of objects is more likely to attract a mate; the peacock with the longest tail is more likely to attract a mate; and being thin, not smoking and being physically fit reduces the risk of heart disease and diabetes.

Some diseases are obviously environmentally determined and depend on a single environmental effect, but even in these there are variations – for example, thyroid cancer was markedly increased in people close to Chernobyl because severe irradiation causes cancerous changes in thyroid cells. But not every individual exposed to the same level of radiation got cancer – some other factors, perhaps environmental, perhaps genetic, changed the sensitivity of the individuals to the same environmental stress. Similarly, food poisoning is almost purely environmental but there may be individual variations in the degree of susceptibility to the infection or in response to the toxins. Conversely, some diseases are predominantly genetic – for example, thalassaemia or cystic fibrosis – but the disease course in such illnesses is influenced by the individual's external and internal environment.

So not every one who is obese gets diabetes, not everyone who is short gets heart disease, not everyone who smokes gets lung cancer, just as only those with a

---

[21] Type 2 diabetes mellitus is caused by insulin resistance. Type 1 diabetes is caused by insulin deficiency. Insulin is a hormone secreted by the pancreas into the circulation. It acts to reduce blood glucose by actions on fat cells, liver cells and muscle cells – which, under insulin stimulation, turn glucose into fat and incorporate it into muscle and liver, where the glucose is stored as glycogen. Insulin acts on cells by binding to receptors. Receptors for hormones are proteins either on the cell surface (in the case of insulin and other protein hormones) or inside the cells (in the case of steroid hormones) – they are equivalent to a lock and key where the hormone is the key and the receptor is the lock. Just as the lock only works with the key in it, the receptor is only activated by the hormone binding to it. This starts a train of intracellular events that ends in altered gene transcription. Insulin resistance can be relative or absolute but is the phenomenon whereby for a given amount of insulin, less activity in terms of metabolic or other actions is seen. Insulin resistance can be caused by faults anywhere along the pathway of insulin action.

particular genetic make-up will have an adverse reaction to eating fava beans. Yet, some thin and fit non-smokers have heart attacks. What is going on? How can we explain this complexity? While much of this variation has been rightly explained by genetic polymorphisms, it is now clear that earlier environmental influences can have an echo throughout life. This is the dominant theme of our book.

## How the environment influences phenotype

We have seen that the genotype is determined when the conceptus is formed, and both genotype and phenotype determine the propensity to disease. It thus follows that gene–environment interactions that determine phenotype must be critical elements in determining the destiny of an individual. Indeed that is the basis of evolutionary processes.[22]

The Darwinian framework, which has stood the test of time, involved several key ideas. First, species are adapted to the environments in which they live. Because of genetic variation (although Darwin did not know about genes, he had the key idea), some species would be more suited for one environment and others less. Those that were more suited would survive and be able to reproduce (natural selection). Gradual changes would make the species more likely to survive comfortably in a specific ecological niche and the appearance of the species would thus gradually change.

The famous example of natural selection was the finches of the Galapagos Islands. They led Darwin to recognise that some beak shapes were better suited to certain food sources in the different environmental niches across the islands. Darwin recognised that if there were genetic variation in the determinants of beak shape, then over time those better-nourished birds having the right beak shape would be more likely to survive. We could predict that their genes would come to dominate in the gene pool. Over time all the birds would end up with the optimal beak shape.

Technically, natural selection can be defined as an altered frequency of a particular genetic allele in a given population. At the point at which the diversity in the gene

---

[22] Evolution was an idea that developed quite quickly. It was not just one person's idea – several thinkers and scientists including Darwin's grandfather, Erasmus, had started to grapple with the ideas of geological time, changing environments, the fossil record, and the stability of species. These had created real challenges to the then dominant, purely theological model of creation. In the 1830s and 1840s Darwin gradually formulated his ideas of the processes that drive evolution. They were based in part on the climate of thinking and the impact of Malthus, in part from observations made on the relationship between fossils in a region and the current species found in the same region, and in part through his studies on geographical isolates such as the species found in the Galapagos. These ideas, while known to the cogniscenti, remained largely unknown to the public for nearly 20 years. Then Alfred Wallace, Darwin's contemporary and friend, in writing to him in 1858 showed that he had essentially developed a similar set of ideas. Darwin was spurred to publication – a behaviour not unfamiliar to modern scientists! Both of these thinkers, by marrying experimental observation with some brilliant insights, expounded a complete theory in what was the most critical and compelling paradigm shift that has ever occurred in biological thought.

pool was such that the paternal and maternal chromosomes from newly evolved variants could not align properly to allow cell division and gamete formation with the other variants, then a new species would have emerged.[23]

Darwin recognised that there was another form of selection, which we now call sexual selection. As selection is essentially all about preferential passage of one's genes, then genetically determined characteristics that make that more likely to happen will be selected. Thus the male lion's mane evolved because a long mane was meant to show the female that a particular male was stronger and thus his progeny were more likely to survive. One theory is that the mane is heavy and, like a thick scarf in a warm climate, having a long mane was presumably meant to illustrate to the female that the male was sufficiently strong to put up with such impediments. Indeed there are good scientific data that male lions with long manes are more likely to survive and have fewer injuries. But more importantly, for whatever reason, females were more willing to mate with male lions who had genes that somehow code for longer manes, and thus over time all male lions came to have longer manes. The same argument has been used to suggest why peacocks have developed long heavy useless tails, which presumably make flying more energy sapping. It is interesting to speculate which attributes in male and female humans might have originated in a similar way!

So evolution can be defined as the process by which genetic characteristics that have been selected as being advantageous are amplified by mating advantage, created either by greater survivability or by sexual attraction. But the environmental factors are both physical (e.g. food supply) and social (e.g. attractiveness to the other gender). Selection is, at one level, an example of the genotype–environment interaction leading over generations to an altered phenotype. At another level it can be seen as the process by which a species manages to adapt to an environmental change. Presumably the finch with the curved beak evolved because its ancestors flew to a new environment with a food supply which had changed from one that was easy to eat with a straight beak to one easier to eat with a curved beak; or maybe the birds did not move but the food supply changed because of some environmental change. Either way, gene pool survival in the face of an environmental change is made possible by the process of evolution.

Much of the latter part of this book will be concerned with the speed, direction and permanency of environmental change. The time-base of the response also varies greatly. For example, when we get overheated we sweat. This is a normal physiological response to an acute environmental change and is an example of homeostasis, the minute-by-minute changes in body function we make to the myriad of environmental influences to which we are exposed. At the other extreme are

---

[23] Species definition remains a complex and controversial topic, but it is not one for this book.

the adaptations brought about by Darwinian processes, which lead essentially to permanent changes in phenotype and which enhance reproductive fitness. These are the true adaptations[24] – for example, the altered beak shapes of finches. Intermediate between these are changes that are induced during development by environmental influences. But all these responses have an immediacy in that the response is obviously and immediately advantageously linked to the concurrent environmental selection.[25] Alternatively it is possible that the environmental response has no immediate advantage but has its advantage at some later time. The changed coat thickness of the meadow vole had no advantage to the fetus but clearly only has advantage later in life – as we will see this is *the* central characteristic of a predictive adaptive response.

Environmental change can obviously be permanent or transient, acute or chronic, and the implications of these differences will become obvious. If the change is very rapid and large and there is no phenotypic variation, then species extinction is likely if homeostatic mechanisms cannot cope. But if the environmental change is gradual, or if the possibility of survival of the less fit is realistic, then the environmental impact on the species may be very different. Darwinian selection is based on the inherent presence of variation, and on the presumption of some advantage of one phenotype over another; in addition, there must be a genetic heritable element to the origin of the phenotype that confers advantage.

But short-term catastrophic environmental changes do happen. Asteroid impacts created the equivalent of nuclear winters overnight and are thought to have led to the extinction of the dinosaurs. But not all species died out in those catastrophic periods – for example, proto-mammals survived. Similarly many species are faced with changes in food supply as a result of drought or flood or other transient environmental change. For a species to survive this kind of transient and remote environmental change it cannot rely on evolution, because evolution acts over many generations to produce a significant phenotypic change. As we shall see, predictive adaptive responses are a non-genomic mechanism that can be used. Through them, a mother can inform her fetus of a future adverse environment; the fetus makes a phenotypic change that is adaptive for the predicted environment and thus survives to reproduce.

---

[24] Adaptation is a word that causes some problems and confusion. In common parlance adaptation is a response to the environment that has immediate advantage. However, part of this book is about evolution, and in evolutionary biology adaptation has a particular meaning – the advantage must be demonstrated in terms of an improvement in reproductive performance (i.e. fitness). By and large we have avoided the common use of the word and tried to stick to the evolutionary definition. Certainly this is the case in any section concerned with evolutionary biology. But to make things easier for the reader, occasionally, as here, we have used it in its more commonly understood sense. Hopefully there will be no confusion to either lay or technical readers!

[25] Homeostasis is another form of immediate response to the environment, but acting over a very short time base.

A key concept that has recently emerged is that a single genotype can give rise to a range of phenotypes, depending on the environmental influences that have operated previously (during development) or are operating currently. The technical term for the range of phenotypes that can be induced by a genotype is the *developmental reaction norm* – or *norm of reaction* – a concept we shall return to in chapter 7. This does not mean that the full range of phenotypes can be induced in any particular situation but it does emphasise the role of development and environment in the induction of phenotypic variation.

## Timing the interaction

It is often cheaper to knock down an old building and then to build a new one, than to perform modifications to the old building to convert or modernise it. In just the same way, the most cost-effective period (in terms of energy use) in the life cycle for modifying phenotype is during early development: it is more efficient for nature to grow a rabbit with long ears than to modify an adult rabbit with short ears to enable it to survive in a hot environment. Because in any environment energy resources such as food are usually limited, a species will opt for the low-cost solution to a problem. This in itself will give it an evolutionary advantage over other species competing for the same food.

Hippocrates was the first to make a key point about developmental biology; namely that events occurring early in life have great consequences because they can be amplified later in life. Prune a seedling's main stem and it will be manifestly deformed as an adult tree; prune an adult tree and the impact is cosmetic. So is it with gene–environmental interactions. In general, insults occurring early in gestation will have greater effects than those occurring later in gestation or after birth. For example, infection with rubella in early pregnancy is likely to lead to severe malformations, but the effects of maternal rubella infection in late pregnancy may be limited to impaired fetal growth; and after birth the disease is, in most cases, benign.

Exposure to certain drugs as an embryo will lead to permanent developmental changes; exposure to the same drug as an adult will only have effects while it is being administered. For example, stilboestrol is a synthetic form of oestrogen that was tried in the 1960s as a treatment for recurrent miscarriage. It can be safely used as a replacement oestrogen in non-pregnant adult women but if a female fetus is exposed to it, that fetus will have a high risk of developing a rare form of vaginal cancer in adolescent or adult life. In some way fetal exposure to stilboestrol affects the developing vaginal mucosa (lining) and makes it more likely to develop a cancerous growth many years later.

As we will see in the next chapter, the capacity of an environmental stimulus to interact with the genome may be limited by the stage of development of the organism. There may be a particular window of development in which the stimulus can have impact – we call this a *critical window*. The critical window for stilboestrol to affect the vaginal mucosa is clearly the first half of fetal life.

We propose that there are two kinds of adaptive response that the embryo or fetus can make to environmental change. The first is well recognised, in that it is obvious that the developing organism has a set of homeostatic and adaptive responses that are used to respond appropriately to environmental changes and allow it to survive the immediate environmental challenge. These are discussed in chapter 2. The second kind of response is suggested by the example of the meadow vole and its coat thickness. Could it be that the developing organism makes responses to its environment, not for immediate survival advantage or need but in anticipation of its future? Such responses may or may not be manifest immediately as phenotypic change but are manifest subsequently. We propose that the fetus uses current environmental information to predict aspects of its future environment and thus resets its developmental trajectories to optimise its future performance (in Darwinian terms, particularly reproductive performance) in adult life. This would be a very clever strategy for species survival in a rapidly changing environment, and we will present many examples to show that this is in fact the case. But what if those adaptations are irreversible – that is, once made they cannot be undone even if the environment is no longer as predicted or if the prediction is wrongly made? This is what happened to the Japanese soldiers from the North when they suffered heat stroke in the tropics. As we shall see, even though most predictive adaptive responses are relatively subtle, those that are irreversible – when put into the context of a changed environment – can be very important causes of disease. Such adaptive responses must be distinguished from the potential for environmental stimuli to disrupt normal development (see chapter 2).

## Predictive adaptive responses

Understanding the processes of how the environment interacts with the developing genome is a critical challenge for modern biological and medical science. *Predictive adaptive responses,*[26] which we will abbreviate to PARs, is the term we have

---

[26] There is a difficulty in knowing what to call the biological processes underpinning PARs. One word to describe this linkage between an early environmental stimulus and later manifestations of changes in physiology is 'programming'. Such a term has the risk of implying a particular mechanism and also that the response is encoded within the command, which it probably is not. It has its obvious derivation from the concept of software programming, but therein lies the problem. Programming implies a physical

created to describe the second type of environmental response referred to above. PARs are the processes by which the environmental interactions in early development lead to changes in the physiological and physical phenotype of the developing egg/embryo/fetus/infant, not primarily for immediate survival advantage but in expectation of future advantage in a particular predicted adult environment. The theoretical basis for this idea will be developed in chapter 7 where we will demonstrate its importance in understanding biological determinism.

Why do we contend that PARs are such important processes? While they evolved as a mechanism for short-term adaptation of a species to environmental change, the reason for our focus on this phenomenon, and indeed a reason for writing this book, is because understanding the processes of PARs leads to a greater understanding of the biology of health and disease.

Many diseases have their origin, at least partly, in the prediction going wrong. That is, the irreversible plastic changes made as a result of an early gene–environmental interaction may turn out not to be appropriate later in life. This occurs when the egg/embryo/fetus 'perceives' its future environment to be in a certain range but it is born into a different environmental range. For example, the fetus might make a phenotypic adaptive response in the expectation of a future poor nutritional environment and yet it is born into an environment of nutritional excess. Indeed we propose that such a paradigm is a major cause of many lifestyle diseases including heart disease and adult-onset diabetes. *How* the developing organism makes these adaptive changes; why they evolved, why the fetus gets it wrong; *why* this can lead to disease; and *what* we need to do about it are central themes of this book. Because PARs occur only during early development we must start our enquiry with a consideration of the earliest stages of development – from egg to newborn.

separation between the hardware (perhaps in biological terms the protein structure of an organ) and the software (maybe hormonal) that controls it. Such a separation does not exist in biological reality – the processes of plasticity change both the structure and function of the organs (via changing their gene expression) and in doing so change their control systems. The other problem with 'programming' is it implies that once the programme is running, it will execute its function and has very little flexibility. It resembles the ballistic model of a ball that has been thrown. You can take all the time you need to plan the trajectory of the ball, but once it leaves your hand you have lost control of it. It may be blown off course by wind. Biological processes do not work like that, whether predictive or not. They can only ever operate in the context of the challenge that they are attempting to meet. How they will operate – for example how nervous discharge will increase, blood hormone levels change etc. – depends entirely on the environmental challenge. They are all about the ongoing interaction between the ball and the wind, as if the ball could continue to be steered to its target like a laser-guided missile. Nevertheless there is a lack of suitable alternatives. We could invent a new word based on the abbreviation PAR (which we will use) and create a verb 'parring' or 'to par'. We will resist this temptation and the risk of being confused with a golfing manual, and stick to programming, despite its limitations!

# 2

# Mother and fetus

In the previous chapter we saw how the interaction between genes and environment might determine whether or not the individual survives under varying conditions. The leaner body shape and the longer ears of one group of rabbits aided survival in the arid regions of Australia. We introduced the concept that different phenotypes can arise from the same genotype. Towards the end of chapter 1 we started to introduce two additional concepts about such interactions – the first is that gene–environment interactions are more likely to have a major impact on phenotype if they occur early in life; the second is that an irreversible change in phenotype acting early in life can have consequences if the environment later changes. Before expanding on these concepts we need to describe the basic processes of development.

## The timetable of development

The word 'development' means different things to different people, including scientists. To the embryologist, it implies the processes of laying down the key components of the body – the genesis of the limbs, the primitive brain and the internal organs such as the heart and gut. The genetic code for these processes, and the ways in which it can be modified by environment, are actively researched areas. To the child psychologist, however, development suggests the stages of behavioural, physical and mental attainment that human infants and children go through, namely learning to walk, to utter their first words etc. These apparently distinct uses of the word 'development' are not really contradictory, because development is a continuous process that starts with the inherited genotype and proceeds until the mature phenotype has been formed. But within the continuum of development, it is important to consider the timing of specific processes such as when locomotion develops, and we can see that different species have evolved to handle this in different ways. They must all achieve the objectives of developing tissues, organs and control systems, and of fine-tuning this development in relation to the environment in which the individual lives. It has generally been considered that such environmental influences are more prominent after birth than before because the postnatal mammal has much more information about its environment than the fetus.

We could argue, therefore, that prenatal processes would primarily be genetically determined with less influence from the environment, and that the fine-tuning of control systems would be better restricted to the postnatal period, when the environment can be accurately assessed. But clearly this is not the case. That species can vary so greatly in their level of maturity at birth implies a continuum of gene–environmental influences extending from conception to maturity. For example, newborn kittens, rabbits and mice are blind and relatively vulnerable at birth, unable to crawl far from the protective nest into which they were born. Newborn lambs, in contrast, run around within minutes of being born, have good vision and hearing and can follow the ewe around. We can speculate that these differences owe a good deal to the habitat and lifestyle of the species. The 'precocial' species such as the lamb must give birth to offspring which can recognise their mother and keep up with her as she grazes. The ewe will have to keep an eye on them, and will not be able to do this for more than two or three lambs, the maximum viable number for non-artificially bred sheep. 'Altricial' species such as rodents must leave their offspring in the nest while the adults forage for food, often nocturnally. It would not do for the pups to go wandering off on their own, and we cannot really imagine a cat hunting effectively with four or five newborn kittens in tow. In the marsupial, another approach has been adopted as the neonate is extraordinarily immature compared to other mammals – it is essentially still an embryo. Mother carries the joey in her pouch for many months.

Thus among mammals there is a spectrum of developmental maturity at birth according to the life-history strategy evolution has chosen as appropriate for that species. This is fascinating, from both an evolutionary and comparative perspective, and in terms of understanding developmental physiology. For example, we believe that the neural processes that underlie the development of vision are reasonably similar in kittens, humans and sheep, albeit occurring at very different times in relation to birth. We might imagine that environmental experience will only allow us to 'learn' to see after we are born, and there is some truth in this. But clearly the lamb has learnt to see in the relatively dark and restricted world of the uterus: it has its eyes open at birth and can show advanced three-dimensional visual perception. Much of this development must therefore be innate. Human neonates clearly have the capacity for visual recognition soon after birth, whereas kittens are blind. Our point is that genetic processes, environmental interactions, ecological niches, and the necessities of survival are inextricably intertwined in determining the strategy for a given species.

It is worth thinking a little at this stage about how such processes of determining the specific developmental timetable might have operated in human evolution – a topic we shall return to in chapter 8. The human developmental timetable was set in central Africa where *Homo sapiens* evolved.[1] The adult human skull has to be large in order to house the large forebrain that characterises our species. But because of the upright posture developed for walking upright, the pelvic birth canal must be relatively narrow. Therefore, in contrast to most other primates, the human fetus is born at a state of relative immaturity of brain growth and thus body function. A human baby is highly dependent on its mother for a long time after birth – for example, it has no independent ability to move about until long after birth, in contrast to all other primates. Furthermore, full communicative skills with other human beings are not developed until well into childhood, in contrast to other primate species. Obviously this relates to the complexity of speech and language used by humans. Similarly, the complexity of our neural function means that the knowledge necessary for maximal capability in our social and physical environment takes many years to learn. Thus sexual maturation must be delayed while the necessary skills are acquired. The social structure of human societies has evolved in parallel to sustain this long postnatal period of development. The human is relatively unique among primates in that life span exceeds, at least for females, the span of reproductive competence. This may relate to the importance of adult memory and knowledge to the survival of the hunter–gatherer through environmental crises. Similarly in elephants, it is the knowledge of the matriarchal grandmother that provides the herd with memory of geographical features such as waterholes.

## The pre-implantation embryo

The processes of how development proceeds from a single fertilised egg into a fully formed fetus to independent life as a newborn, and then its growth and maturation to adulthood, must be the most fascinating story in all biology. All the required information must reside in the 35 000 genes present in the single fertilised egg (zygote). Yet that single cell must divide and re-divide; the cells must transform from undifferentiated stem cells into specific cell types; they must move and re-divide or die so as to form organs; they must then start to function in the appropriate way at the appropriate time; and the organism must make major changes in its function as it develops through each of these stages. As we have already suggested, the developing

---

[1] The first hominids appeared about 5 million years ago. *Homo sapiens* evolved about 150 000 to 250 000 years ago but did not disperse out of Africa until about 65 000 years ago. Early hominids such as *Homo erectus* had spread through Asia and Europe a million years earlier but eventually died out.

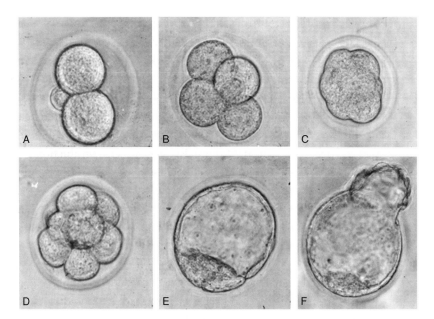

Fig. 2.1     Early embryo development. The first division of the fertilised egg gives rise to two cells (A) which divide to four cells (B) and divide again (C) to eight cells (D), and so on. At the 32-cell stage (E) the cells of the inner cell mass which will form the embryo are at the bottom, with the blastocoele cavity above. Both are surrounded by trophoectoderm cells, from which the placenta will form. The embryo then 'hatches' from the blastocyst (F) to continue development. (Photographs courtesy of Professor T. P. Fleming.)

embryo, fetus, infant or child is clearly not immune to its environment – indeed its biological destiny is affected greatly by early gene–environmental interactions.

Immediately after fertilisation the single-celled conceptus starts to undergo cell division. Initially all the cells are pluripotent, all with the same characteristics, and the embryo is only a ball of cells. But soon the embryo develops a polarity – this establishes which aspect is top (or dorsal), which is bottom (or ventral), which is front (or rostral), which is back (or caudal), and which is left and which is right. A cavity forms in the conceptus, which is now called a blastocyst. The embryo develops on one wall of the cavity – other components of the blastocyst form the placenta and other supporting tissues. Placental formation requires this component of the blastocyst to grow out and come into contact with the maternal uterine wall and, in species such as humans, indeed to invade it – a process termed trophoblastic invasion.[2]

<hr />

[2] The placenta is a particularly variable organ in structure between different mammals – placentae can be classified in several categories according to their structure and how many layers of membranes and tissues separate the maternal and fetal circulation. But all placentae subserve the same functions – transferring nutrients to the fetus, extracting waste from the fetus, secreting hormones to alter maternal physiology to

The developing conceptus has by this stage travelled down the Fallopian tubes into the uterus. The uterine wall has been prepared by the influence of the hormone progesterone produced by the corpus luteum (that part of the ovarian follicle left behind when the egg is released). The blastocyst implants into the uterine lining – this implantation allows some hormonal signals to be sent to the ovary to tell it to continue to make progesterone – if the ovary does not because there was no implantation, then progesterone production fails, the uterine lining will degenerate and menstruation will occur. Eventually progesterone production by the corpus luteum in humans is replaced by that from the placenta and it is this production of progesterone and some other hormones that prevents further ovulation while the woman is already pregnant.[3] It is also the basis of progesterone-based contraceptive pills and injections, whereby progesterone sends a false signal to the ovary as if pregnancy existed.

How do embryonic cells become specialised into all the diverse cell types that form a body and, when they have, why do some cell types stop multiplying? If we knew this for a specific tissue, say the liver, we might be able to devise ways of arresting the unwanted, excessive cell division that forms the basis of liver cancer. And an understanding of cell specialisation from the pluripotent stem cells could provide a way of treating the loss of neurons in the brain that accompanies Alzheimer's disease, because maybe we could inject stem cells into parts of the brain that have deteriorated. This of course might mean using such stem cells from the patient, but the problem is not insuperable as it is now known that all tissues (including the brain) retain some of these stem cells throughout life, even if under normal circumstances some tissues (especially the brain) do not use them for natural repair. Even more exciting is the possibility that we could grow from a patient's stem cells[4] a replacement organ such as a kidney for transplantation purposes, avoiding all the complications of transplant rejection. After all, the embryo can grow two kidneys, so why can't we do the same in the laboratory?

We do not want to go much deeper into studying these issues, fascinating though they are, because they are beyond the scope of our topic. But there is one crucial issue that we must focus on, and that is the way in which gene expression is controlled

support the pregnancy and yet creating an immune barrier between mother and her genetically different fetus.

[3] In some species such as the goat, the corpus luteum continues to be the major source of progesterone throughout pregnancy, and luteolysis is part of the process of parturition in such species.

[4] Stem cells are cells that theoretically can differentiate into any of the cell types of the body, because they remain in a 'primitive' state. All cells of the very early embryo are stem cells, until they become committed to trophectoderm (placenta) or inner cell mass (the embryo and then fetus). Once 'committed' to a line of development, e.g. to muscle or fat, cells cannot de-differentiate and be transformed into another cell type. Some tissues must retain stem cells throughout life, as they continually produce new cells, e.g. the blood cells formed in the bone marrow or the sperm formed in the testes. It was traditionally thought that tissues in which cell division is not seen in postnatal life, e.g. the heart or the brain, do not contain stem cells. However, this idea has been shown to be wrong. Much effort is now devoted to finding ways of growing new brain or heart cells in adults. The therapeutic consequences will be enormous.

in these early embryonic cells, because this provides one of the earliest, and most dramatic, examples of the gene–environment interactions that are central to this book. At its simplest, we can put it this way: all the cells of the early embryo at the morula/blastocyst stage (when it is just a ball of cells) will have the same genotype, yet already these cells are showing signs that they will develop differently – e.g., the inner cell mass and trophectoderm cells. So clearly some processes are acting to make cells express various parts of their genomic DNA differently even at this stage.

## Embryonic development

Once implantation has occurred, embryonic development progresses through a complex sequence of layering and folding, followed by organ differentiation and limb formation, until by mid-gestation the fetus has an appearance comparable to the adult human. This initial phase is generally termed embryogenesis and is considered largely complete in humans by about 14 weeks. The stages of development after 14 weeks are generally considered as the fetal stages. This is a somewhat artificial divide as, for all organs, development of structure and function continues until well after birth. However, the gross anatomical structures such as the heart, the liver, the gastrointestinal tract etc. are largely developed in the embryonic stage.

The processes involved in how the pluripotent single-cell embryo develops into a complex organism constitute the science of developmental biology. We have learned how the genetic code primes the primitive cells to start making chemical signals that either tell a cell what it should do or tell a neighbouring cell how to relate to it. Genes are turned on and off in a complex but orchestrated manner. The cells show division, migration and differentiation. Differentiation is the process by which a cell becomes specialised – a fat cell acquires the machinery for making and storing fat, a pancreatic islet cell develops the machinery for making, storing and secreting insulin, and so on. Once a cell has differentiated, it cannot de-differentiate (except under some cancerous conditions): if a cell line has differentiated into primitive blood cells, its progeny will all be forms of blood cell. Some cells, once fully differentiated, lose the capacity to proliferate – this is the case for neurons – any new neurons formed in the adult brain are derived from resident stem cells, cells that remained dormant from embryonic life in an undifferentiated state. Other differentiated cells such as skin cells can proliferate throughout life.

Another key process in development is cell death. In the course of the process of progressing from a simple ball of cells into a very complex structure, cells may have a temporary role in signalling or in providing structural support, but then must be removed. The processes of doing so are termed apoptosis[5] or programmed cell death. It is initiated by intracellular or transcellular signals not different in essence from other components of developmental signalling. For example the hand forms with webs between the fingers but then apoptosis occurs to destroy the webbing so that separate fingers remain.

In the brain far more brain cells are made than are finally present at birth and the others die by apoptosis. Some of the neurons that become apoptotic are those that fail to make connections to other neurons and thus have no functional capacity. It appears that if the neuron does not receive trophic support in the form of a growth factor from a target neuron, it will enter the apoptotic cascade. Other neurons only have a temporary role in regulating the migration to the cortex of neurons from the main proliferative zone deep in the brain and then die. Apoptosis is not only an important process in normal development but also it is a major pathological mechanism induced in disease processes. For example, in Parkinson's disease some cells in a critical part of the brain called the substantia nigra undergo apoptosis inappropriately and degenerate.

The regulation of these different processes of development is exceedingly complex and involves a host of signalling molecules. Many of these are transcription factors that alter the gene expression pattern of a cell, either inducing or suppressing transcription. These factors are in turn induced by the environment of the cell – where the cell sits in relation to other cells, what chemical signals it receives from those cells, its nutritional and metabolic milieu, etc. This carefully synchronised and complex score has evolved so that the cell's performance is usually nearly perfect. It is quite astonishing!

Given that our interest lies in how the environment can impact on the developing organism, to what extent can the embryo detect and respond to its environment? There is increasing evidence that, from the fertilised egg stage, such gene–environment interactions do indeed occur. Prior to implantation the environment of the pre-embryo is that of the Fallopian tube and intrauterine space. Concentrations of glucose and hormones can be sensed by the developing blastocyst. For example, one of the earliest groups of receptors to develop on the surface of the embryo at a four-cell stage are receptors that respond to growth factor concentrations in the lumen of the Fallopian tube which, in turn, are determined by maternal secretions from the lining of the tube. The developing embryo will change the relative assignment of cells to the inner cell and outer cell mass according to whether

---

[5] The word apoptosis is derived from the Greek words *apo* (meaning off) and *ptosis* (meaning falling). It is now recognised that cells contain within them ways of 'committing suicide' rapidly if required to do so. One mechanism, for example, involves activation of an enzyme called caspase-3, which in turn leads to DNA degeneration. Programmed cell death is at least as important in development as cell division, because most organs have a redundancy of cells in them during development.

it perceives problems in glucose supply. The consequences for this on longer-term function can be very striking: as will be seen later in the book there is evidence in the rat that poor maternal nutrition at this stage produces offspring with higher blood pressure!

The pre-embryo and very early embryo also change the expression of a variety of genes and thus subsequent development in response to low oxygen levels. Low levels of oxygen are a very powerful stimulus for the growth of the trophoblast cells, which are actively invading the lining of the womb to create the placenta at this time. Once this invasion has occurred, blood starts to flow through the maternal side of the placenta and it becomes not only a provider of nutrients to the fetus but a powerful transducer and determinant of the fetal environment. The relatively sudden increase in the oxygen levels in the fetus at this time forces it to make enzymes that protect it from oxidative damage; failure to do so will produce detrimental effects not only on the fetus but also on the placenta, and this may play a part in the development of the disease pre-eclampsia. The crucial point is that for about the first few weeks of human pregnancy the developing embryo is nourished by diffusion of nutrients from the mother's reproductive tract and its secretions, not by the placenta. We know very little about this nutrition in early life, and considerably more research is needed into how this unique environment affects early development.

## The placenta

Once formed, the placenta is the key transducer of information from mother to fetus and vice versa. The presence of a placenta is one of the defining characteristics of mammals. Most species of birds have an egg that is incubated in a nest – it is the egg that provides the nutrients to the embryo from the yolk sac although vascular outgrowth, somewhat like an umbilical cord and placental bed, develops. Oxygen diffuses through the eggshell to that outgrowth. Some non-mammalian species do give 'live birth' but in most of these cases the egg is merely incubated within a specialised organ in the mother and there is no nutritional connection between the mother and the egg. The exception are some lizards and skinks in which a placenta forms by which nutrients pass from mother to the fetus. This reptilian placenta must have evolved separately from the mammalian placenta. Despite its critical importance to mammalian survival, the placenta is a surprisingly poorly understood organ. Fascinatingly, there are also enormous variations in the shape and structure of the placenta across species.

The placenta forms from one part of the blastocyst. In the human the placental or trophoblastic tissue proliferates and invades through the lining of the uterus into the mother's blood vessels supplying the uterine wall. By 12 to 14 weeks the placenta is fully functional and mature. It is important to note that maternal and fetal blood are never in direct contact. Nutrients from the mother, such as oxygen and glucose, must leave the maternal blood vessels, enter placental tissue, and then pass through this tissue into the fetal blood stream. Conversely waste products such as carbon dioxide must leave the fetus in a reverse manner. There can be many problems associated with this transfer process and we shall be referring to these throughout the book.

It is clear that placental function can influence fetal growth. It is also important to realise that placental size is set by mid-gestation, many weeks before the maximum period of fetal growth. The growth of the placenta will therefore determine the supply of nutrients to meet fetal demand. From a teleological point of view, it could therefore be advantageous to grow a large placenta if the aim is to grow a large fetus. Later in this chapter we will discuss how competition between maternal and paternal genomes can set the trajectory of fetal growth. This is done through a process called genomic imprinting and similar processes also regulate some aspects of placental growth.

While gross placental size is established by mid-gestation, placental function continues to develop across pregnancy. So there is scope for the fetus to signal to its placenta if its need for nutrients is not being met, and this may cause changes in placental gene expression for amino acid and glucose transporter proteins, alter the amount of blood supply etc. The more we learn about this time of life, the more dynamic and interactive it turns out to be. The dialogue between the fetus and its placenta, effectively unknown to the mother, is very vigorous.

The placenta is not only about nutrient transfer; it is also an important source of hormones that influence both maternal and fetal function. From about the seventh week onwards the human placenta will make the hormone *chorionic gonadotropin*, which enters the fetus and stimulates the developing testis of the male to make testosterone – this in turn is a critical step in the development of the external genitalia of the male. If the male fetus cannot respond to chorionic gonadotropin because of a genetic defect in the function of the receptors for this hormone, then the penis and scrotum cannot develop and, even though the sex chromosomes identify the fetus as a male, it will not have a complete male phenotype. The infant will have female external genitalia with a small blind-ending vagina, but with testes rather than ovaries in the groin, and no uterus or cervix.

## The fetal environment

It is traditional to use *embryo* to refer to the developing organism prior to completion of gross organ formation and *fetus*[6] for the later stages of intrauterine life. Most

---

[6] One of the strangest debates is over the spelling of the word fetus. We get particularly annoyed when journal editors insist that foetus is the correct spelling – it is not! Even the spell checker on this computer insists on 'foetus'. The word fetus comes directly from the latin *fetus*, meaning 'offspring'. F*oetus* is thus

of our information about fetal physiology comes from studies in sheep. Scientists choose to study sheep because they have large fetuses and it is possible to identify periods in fetal life roughly approximating to those of human development. Like humans, sheep generally only have one or two fetuses. Techniques have been developed over the past 40 years for direct measurement of fetal functions in the sheep by operating on the uterus, inserting catheters and measuring instruments into the fetus, allowing mother and fetus to recover from surgery, and through these means observing the fetus in its normal environment. Obviously, where possible, scientists have sought to confirm their conclusions with appropriate human studies but these must, by their very nature, be limited. Ultrasound techniques allow imaging of the fetus, and assessment of fetal movements and fetal blood flow. Occasionally, for diagnostic reasons, human fetal blood can be sampled directly from the human fetus in utero. Having said that, the resolution now possible on ultrasound allows us to 'see' fetal expressions and to confirm that much of what we have learnt from the study of the sheep is directly applicable to the human fetus.

During the latter half of pregnancy the fetus has several tasks. It must continue to grow and mature its various organ systems, it must prepare for the challenge of birth, it must ensure that critical systems (such as breathing) are ready to work

etymologically incorrect even though the Oxford dictionary allows it as an alternative spelling. Many years ago this was best put in a poem by the obstetrician Geoffrey Chamberlain.

'SIR, –
The unborn child is not to blame
For bastard spelling of his name
The Romans knew their Latin best.
To Virgil, Ovid, and the rest
He was a FETUS and so stayed
Till later Isidore made
A diphthong of the vowel E
Confusing us and Dr. B.

The FETAL noun you can relate
To the verb *feo* – generate.
Its origin cannot be hung
On the verb *foeto* – bring forth young.
If so, then FOETUS should adorn
The newborn child, not the unborn,
And so in mother's arms we'd see
Our FOETAL physiology.

To other words the diphthong came,
But they've their old form back again
You won't be thanked in '69
To tell your bird she's *foeminine*.
To call the FETUS transatlantic
Will drive the editors quite frantic
Ere Norsemen on Cape Cod were wrecked,
The spelling FETUS was correct.'
*Geoffrey Chamberlain, King's College Hospital,*
*London SE5, Lancet 2 (1309) 1969*

from the moment of birth and, as we will see in later chapters, it must prepare for postnatal life and in particular for the challenge of surviving to reproduce and sustain the species. Central to this last challenge is trying to predict what kind of environment it will be born into, and adapting appropriately.

The environment of the fetus is created at several levels – at one level it is the environment in which the mother finds herself – food plentiful or scarce, high or low altitude, hot or cold, the presence of infectious agents, and so forth. In turn these environmental stimuli determine the physiological and health status of the mother, which thus determines her body temperature, the level of oxygen and nutrients in her blood, and the rate of flow of blood to the placental bed. And, as we shall see in later chapters, some aspects of maternal health and physiology were determined when the mother herself was a fetus! In addition, if the mother absorbs a toxin that can cross the placenta, the fetus is passively exposed to that toxin. When the mother smokes, the level of nicotine and carbon monoxide in her blood rises and both can cross the placenta and enter the fetal blood stream. Effectively the fetus of a smoker is chronically carbon monoxide and nicotine poisoned but cannot cry for help. There are other ways in which smoking can adversely affect the fetus – for example, components of tobacco smoke will interfere with the ability of amino acids and calcium to be transported across the placenta.[7]

Can we say that the fetus is thus 'aware' of its environment? In some aspects we can, and this is a direct awareness. For example, it can sense maternal movements and can hear some sounds through the uterine and abdominal wall. But most of the fetus's sense of the external environment is determined by placental function. The placenta has a major role in being the transducer of the maternal environment to the fetus. The levels of oxygen, glucose, amino acids and other nutrients that enter the fetus are determined by placental function. So if the placenta is not working well and supplies inadequate glucose to the fetus, the fetus assumes that its mother is living in a deprived environment.

The particular challenges the fetus must meet are determined by its absolute dependence on its mother for food, water and particularly oxygen. It is also dependent on her for removal of the waste products of metabolism such as carbon dioxide, urea and heat. All these exchanges occur across the placenta. The key maternal adaptations of pregnancy have been first to change her circulation so that much more blood flows to the uterus (to deliver nutrients and remove waste products), and secondly to alter her metabolism so that more glucose – the most critical metabolic fuel – is available to the fetus. These changes are brought about by hormonal changes induced directly or indirectly by the placenta. The cardiovascular changes are largely induced by oestrogens. In the middle of pregnancy the placenta starts

---

[7] If the reader thinks this is an appeal for responsible motherhood, it is!

**Fetal Supply Line**

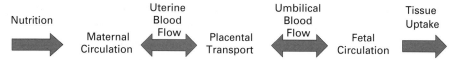

Nutrition  →  Maternal Circulation  ⇄ Uterine Blood Flow  Placental Transport ⇄ Umbilical Blood Flow  Fetal Circulation → Tissue Uptake

Fig. 2.2    Fetal nutrition is not simply a reflection of what the mother eats, because the fetus is at the end of a very long supply line for the nutrients and oxygen that it needs to grow and develop. Significant factors such as maternal and placental metabolism are interposed between what the mother eats and the nutrients that eventually arrive at the fetal tissues. All these processes, and the potential problems that may arise with them, have to be borne in mind when considering fetal nutrition. (Derived from Bloomfield and Harding: *Fetal and Maternal Medicine Reviews*, 1998.)

to make large amounts of oestrogens from precursors produced by the fetus – so in a sense the fetus is telling the mother what to do. The metabolic changes of the mother are largely induced by hormones (placental lactogen and placental growth hormone) made by the placenta and secreted into the mother's blood stream.

## Fetal survival

The placenta has a limited capacity to deliver oxygen, glucose and other nutrients to the fetus. Furthermore the placenta itself is a major consumer of these two key fuels and can use between 40 and 60 per cent of the fuels extracted from the maternal circulation. As the placenta must survive in order for the fetus to survive, the placenta has first call on the nutrients provided by the mother, with a higher priority than the fetus. Because oxygen delivery is determined by the uterine blood flow and because the anatomical details of the two vascular systems have to cooperate to exchange oxygen between the maternal and fetal circulation, the fetus has to live with a blood oxygen tension[8] only 25 per cent of that of the mother. It is as if the fetus is living on top of Mount Everest without oxygen cylinders. Thus during the course of evolution the fetus has had to adapt its style of living to conserving and using this precious resource optimally. Whenever oxygen delivery to the fetus is compromised, and it can be compromised in many ways[9], the fetus must take urgent steps to conserve it.

[8] The oxygen tension is critical to determining the diffusion of oxygen from mother to placenta to fetus. To make this diffusion fast enough, the fetus has a low oxygen tension in its blood. Further, the haemoglobin in fetal blood differs in structure from adult haemoglobin in that it has a higher affinity for oxygen. Thus it can carry more oxygen despite the low tension.

[9] For example maternal disease, placental disease or problems with the umbilical cord.

When the fetus gets short of oxygen it shuts down non-essential functions and shifts blood flow to protect supplies to the most vital organs – the developing brain; the heart, which is essential to pumping blood to the placenta so it can pick up more oxygen; and the placenta itself. The brain also reduces non-essential functions. The fetal brain is very active – it dreams, it controls fetal body movements, it controls the practice of breathing movements.[10] All these energy-consuming activities of the brain stop when the fetus is short of oxygen. If the oxygen shortage continues, as it will in placental failure, then the fetus will stop the most energy-consuming activity of all – growing.

Similarly when placental problems mean a shortage of food in the form of glucose and, to some extent, amino acids, the fetus will stop growing or change its growth pattern to protect brain growth relative to other organs. The fetus has quite clearly evolved to recognise that a properly functioning brain is essential to postnatal survival and invests enormous effort to protect it – this in turn requires protection of heart and placental function.

These various responses give the fetus a range of strategies for surviving in the face of reductions in its nutrient or oxygen supply. We can summarise then as follows: the fetus can reduce its energy requirements – in the short term by changing its behaviour; if this is inadequate, it can slow its growth; if even this fails, it can die. It may seem strange to call this last response a strategy but, from an evolutionary point of view, we can argue that survival in the face of an inadequate fetal–placental–maternal collaboration is not advantageous for the species and is a waste of resources in the short term.

## Maternal–fetal 'conflicts'

From conception, the interests of the mother and her fetus[11] are not always aligned. The fetus and mother are not genetically identical because the fetal genome is an admixture of maternal and paternal genes. These genetic differences create immunological differences between mother and fetus. The hormonal changes in

---

[10] While the fetus is in utero its lungs are not useful and play no role in fetal oxygenation because they are filled with fluid. Nonetheless, the fetus does go through periods of breathing and other body movements, usually lasting about 15 minutes and consuming a substantial amount of energy. So why does the fetus breathe? First, it does so in part to 'practise' because the neural networks that control breathing must be consolidated by activity before birth and, second, because these fetal breathing movements induce growth of the fetal lung. But the fetus can cope for a day or so without breathing movements. Fetal breathing consumes oxygen. When the fetus becomes short of oxygen, e.g. due to maternal uterine contractions, which limit uterine blood flow, or because of placental malfunction such as partial abruption, it rations the oxygen it gets to those functions it cannot live without, such as heart function, and stops unnecessary use such as breathing. One theory is that inappropriate persistence of this response to low oxygen after birth may explain some cases of the sudden infant death syndrome.

[11] At the risk of semantic impurity, we will sometimes use the term fetus to cover the entire period from conception to birth. It will be less tedious than constantly referring to pre-embryo (the favoured term for the preimplantation embryo), embryo and fetus each time.

early pregnancy are thought to stop the mother from rejecting the fetus. In addition the invading trophoblast disguises its immunological differences to prevent invoking an immune response in the mother. Once the placenta forms, it creates another barrier to immunological rejection.

In later gestation the fetus and mother can be in competition over nutritional requirements. If the nutrient supply is very limited there will be a conflict about whether energy should be used to support the mother's needs, placental function or fetal growth. Evolution has solved this problem harshly because the fetus is replaceable in the drive to ensure gene transmission to the next generation. It is preferable (in evolutionary terms) that the mother survives so as to be able to reproduce in future. If the mother were to die, the fetus would die and the mother's gene line would not be preserved. Thus there is a hierarchy of demand created and regulated through pregnancy. If energy is limited, fetal growth is compromised first, followed by the placenta (which must function if the fetus is to survive) and the mother last. In extreme situations it is possible to demonstrate wasting of the fetus in late gestation, as nutrients from the fetus are pulled back to support the placenta.

But there is another potential conflict – that of fetal growth and maternal pelvic size. If the fetus can outgrow the maternal birth canal, then both mother and fetus will die in the associated obstructive labour (in the absence of medical intervention). Thus the mother must have mechanisms to limit fetal development – this phenomenon is termed maternal constraint. In evolutionary terms the mother's interests are therefore best protected by having smaller babies that put her at less risk. But bigger fathers are probably stronger and so any of her babies that possess a big father's genes are more likely to survive as adults. It is common in many species, especially those such as the elephant seal and the antelope where harems are the normal social structure, for the female to be attracted to the biggest and strongest males. The paternal perspective is that he wants his genes passed on as he has invested much (in evolutionary terms) to have a gene-expression pattern favouring dominance in size etc. Thus there are conflicting interests as to fetal size. In the end, however, survival of the species means that this conflict must be resolved to favour maternal survival. We now know a considerable amount about the processes by which the mother's genome takes precedence over the father's in regulating fetal growth. There are several processes by which genes can be 'silenced' to prevent them being unnecessarily transcribed, and they are utilised in resolving the maternal–fetal conflict.

While, for most genes, both alleles are actually expressed, there are exceptions and sometimes one of the alleles is silenced. In females this must happen for one entire X chromosome because the offspring has inherited one X chromosome from her mother and one from her father. The reason that silencing is needed is that while the X chromosome has about 1500 genes, the Y chromosome has less than 50. Thus most genes on the X chromosome have evolved to be optimal in a monoallelic state rather than affected by the potential for heterosis (or heterozygosity). In mice, one X chromosome is silenced 3.5 to 4.5 days after fertilisation, the choice of chromosome usually being random. In humans, X inactivation may start by the eight-cell stage. Similar considerations of gene silencing on one chromosome apply to individual genes on other chromosomes. As each allele comes from a different parent, one can envisage situations where evolution found it advantageous to determine which allele is silenced so that only a maternal or paternal effect can be exerted. This parent-specific silencing of an allele is called imprinting.[12]

The most common mechanisms for gene silencing involve chemical modification by methylation of cytosine nucleotides, within special DNA sequence regions (called CpG islands). This alters gene structure and function drastically and can stop the gene from being transcribed into RNA and thus into protein. DNA methylation is used to determine which of the alleles (maternally- or paternally-derived) of a particular gene will take precedence under given conditions. About 50 to 100 genes show maternal/paternal imprinting and many of them are involved in the regulation of fetal growth and development. The best-described example of genomic imprinting involves a hormone termed 'insulin-like growth factor-2' (usually abbreviated to IGF-2).

The hormone IGF-2 is made in a range of embryonic tissues and is a very important promotor of embryonic growth. It acts on receptors (called IGF type 1 receptors) in the target tissues to promote cell division, differentiation, and hence growth. It turns out that IGF-2 expression is imprinted such that only the paternal allele is expressed. Thus the production of IGF-2 and hence, potentially, embryonic growth are driven more by the paternal than the maternal genome. But we have just suggested that the mother must hold her own in the 'conflict' otherwise the fetus would outgrow her pelvic canal. There is another type of receptor to which the IGF-2 can bind (termed the IGF type-2 receptor), which does not activate cell growth but instead effectively destroys IGF-2 so it cannot act. And the crucial point is that the gene for the type 2 receptor is also imprinted, but this time it is the maternal allele that is active and the paternal allele that is silenced. Thus the mother has a simple and effective way of regulating the amount of active IGF-2 available to the conceptus, and hence of limiting fetal growth. Here is an example of processes we

---

[12] It is unfortunate that some words are used in biology with several different meanings. Cloning is one such word that has very different meanings to reproductive biologists, cell biologists and to botanists. Similarly, imprinting is used to describe two very different processes by two groups of biologists. Molecular biologists use it to describe the genomic imprinting and gene silencing that we are describing here. However, animal ethologists have a quite separate use of the word to describe a biological mechanism – the imprinting of emotional attachment. The most famous example of the latter is the goose of Konrad Lorenz which, because some birds will identify the first animal they sight as their mother, imprinted Lorenz rather than a goose as its mother!

are only just beginning to understand by which balanced competition between the maternal and paternal genomes determines fetal growth.

Another way to promote fetal growth is via placental growth. It would appear, at least in the mouse, that similar mechanisms of genomic imprinting involving the IGF system may also influence placental growth.

The idea of such a competition between our parents (or at least their genomic DNA!) occurring during our fetal existence has been explored by David Haig, a theoretical biologist from Harvard. His thesis is that the competition is based on differing evolutionary pressures acting on the two sexes, with respect to the way in which they respond to the parental drive to pass on their genomic DNA. The pressure on the male is to pass his DNA to an offspring who will grow to be as big and strong as possible – hence the paternally imprinted drive for enhancing fetal growth, for example via the IGF-2 gene. Because males can potentially father large numbers of offspring, the goal of ensuring passage of DNA to future generations is adequately met by the father passing his DNA to one offspring, provided that this offspring grows to reproductive age and is fit to compete with rivals. The evolutionary pressure on the mother is somewhat different. For her, reproduction itself is a risky business and she must ensure that she survives pregnancy to produce more offspring if possible – hence her need to regulate fetal growth according to her body physique. This is a rather simplistic view of the evolutionary forces that may have acted on the primitive mammal in the mists of prehistory, but, as we shall see, the operation of such processes even during contemporary human pregnancy may have important consequences for the health of the offspring in later life.

## Maternal constraint in late gestation

We have described the need for the mother to be able to limit fetal growth so that the fetal head can pass through the birth canal. The concept of maternal–paternal conflict has been introduced. Genomic imprinting is one of the early gestation mechanisms by which the mother can limit fetal growth to match her pelvic size. This however is not the only mechanism and it is critical that there are others operating in late gestation, when the fetus is rapidly growing and putting on weight. This is obviously most important in monotocous species (i.e. those that usually have only one fetus at a time) such as the human, sheep, elephant and horse. They remain poorly understood processes but the sum total of these various mechanisms is termed *maternal constraint*.

Maternal constraint can be defined as the set of mechanisms monotocous species use to limit the growth of the fetus so that pelvic delivery is still possible. As farmers of sheep and cattle know, there is a very narrow margin of safety in this matter, and obstructed labour (dystocia) is quite common if the fetus grows too large.

While dystocia has been selected against in wild populations, in farmed animals (where selection has been done by the breeders to magnify certain characteristics) the risk of dystocia becomes greater. In humans obstructive labour with a large fetus is particularly risky for both mother and fetus, and maternal constraint has been critical for the survival of the hominid species. The degree of human development at birth is a compromise brought about by two differing evolutionary realities – the adoption of an upright posture and the development of a large cerebral cortex to deal with higher processes and language. The latter determines that the mature human must have a large head size. The former determines the pelvic canal must be narrow so as to allow the abdominal contents to stay intra-abdominal! The result is that the human is born in a relatively immature neurological state, and fetal size must be very carefully calibrated by maternal constraint so as to allow vaginal delivery. We propose that maternal constraint has another very important role that will be discussed in chapters 7 and 8.

The genetics of birth size provide further evidence to support the role of maternal factors. The correlation of birth size[13] between twins suggests that about 35 per cent of the variation in the weight of one can be explained (or perhaps better, predicted) by knowing the weight of the other. This might then be seen as the genetic component of variation in growth. A very similar size of effect is seen in siblings with the same mother and father. In half-siblings with the same mother the correlation is still high, but in half-siblings with different mothers but the same father there is no significant correlation. Even when we go to cousins, the same thing applies – maternally-related cousins have more correlation in birth weights than paternally-related cousins. Clearly the paternal genome has less direct influence on birth size and there are important maternal factors, some of which are direct genetic mechanisms but most of which reflect the maternal environment.

Smaller mothers have smaller pelvic canals and thus it is essential that there is some link between maternal size and the capacity of the fetus to grow. It is easy to imagine that if fetal growth was determined solely by paternal and maternal genes that it would be a fatal combination for a slight 148-cm women to bear a child to an ectomorphic (big-framed) 185-cm tall man – yet such matings between tall men and short women are not uncommon. Moreover, postnatal growth is not subject to constraint and is much more genetically determined than is prenatal growth. This results in height in adulthood being largely genetically determined (in the absence of disease in childhood) and adult height of an individual is correlated well with the average height of his or her parents. So we can see how tall men can have

---

[13] Such correlation is usually measured by a correlation coefficient. This is a statistical tool for measuring the strength of a relationship between two variables. In statistical terms the square of the correlation coefficient, expressed as a percentage, gives the fraction of variance in one variable that is explained by the other.

**Correlation between birth
weights of relatives**

| Description of sample | Correlation of birth weights r (n) |
|---|---|
| Maternal half-sibs (adjacent birth rank) | 0.581 (30)[a] |
| Full sibs (adjacent in birth rank, non-consanguinous parents) | 0.523 (367)[a] |
| Full sibs (adjacent in birth rank, parents first cousins) | 0.481 (442)[a] |
| Full sibs (one sib intervening) | 0.425 (654)[a] |
| Full sibs (two sibs intervening) | 0.363 (153)[a] |
| Paternal half-sibs | 0.102 (168)[a] |
| First cousins, maternal sisters | 0.135 (554)[b] |
| First cousins, maternal brothers | 0.015 (288)[b] |

[a]N.E. Morton (1955), *Ann. Hum. Gen.* **20**,125–34; [b]E.B. Robson (1955), *Ann. Hum. Gen.* **19**, 262–8

Fig. 2.3   The correlations between birth weights among relatives show maternal vs. paternal influences on this complex phenotype (birth weight) (*r* is the correlation coefficient, *n* is the number of subjects). Correlations are stronger between siblings sharing the same mother but different fathers than vice versa. The correlation in birth weight between maternal siblings is also diminished as they are separated by one or more siblings in birth rank, suggesting that maternal constraint processes change in magnitude with parity.

relatively tall adult sons even if their partners are short: maternal constraint limits fetal growth to match maternal size, but postnatal growth can still be determined by the paternal genotype.

The most famous demonstration of maternal constraint comes from studies done in the 1930s with horses. Breeders had known that depending on the choice of the stallion and mare, certain characteristics would appear in the foal. So what would happen if a large breed of horse, say a Shire horse of the type used traditionally to pull the plough, was crossed with a diminutive breed such as the Shetland pony? The cross could be done in two ways – a Shetland mare with a Shire stallion or vice versa. This experiment demonstrated dramatically that the size of the foal was very different in each cross even though both crosses had similar genotypes (50 per cent Shire, 50 per cent Shetland). If a Shire stallion was crossed with a Shetland mare (the experiment was first performed using the then relatively new technique of artificial insemination, which solved an obvious practical problem!), then the resulting foal was closer in size at birth to a pure-bred Shetland foal than to a Shire foal. If on the other hand a Shire mare was crossed with a Shetland stallion, then the foal was much

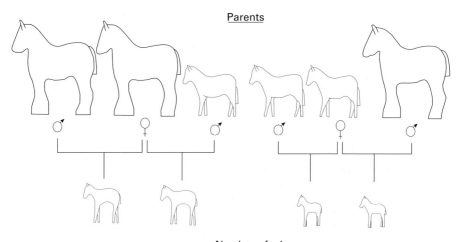

Parents

Newborn foals

Fig. 2.4      Outcome of crosses between the large Shire horse and the tiny Shetland pony, reported by Walton and Hammond in 1938. A Shire mare crossed with a Shetland stallion produces a foal of similar size to a pure-bred Shire foal (left). A Shetland mare crossed with a Shire stallion, on the other hand, produces a much smaller foal similar in size to a pure-bred Shetland foal (right). Maternal size determines the degree of prenatal constraint of fetal growth.

larger and was closer to a Shire foal. These studies strongly suggested the presence of maternal constraint: a Shetland mare in some way limited the growth of a fetus with a genotype that would be too large to deliver through her pelvis. The reciprocal cross also showed that the same genetic composition could lead to a larger fetus if it grew in a larger uterus – this was the first suggestion that mammalian fetal growth is *normally constrained* below its maximal rate by the uterine environment.

We do not fully understand the mechanisms of such maternal constraint. The genomic imprinting of IGF-2 secretion and IGF-2 clearance receptors is one partial explanation. But late in gestation IGF-2 seems less important as a fetal growth regulator – although it may be more important for matching placental transport to fetal demands. Instead, the closely related hormone, IGF-1, becomes the primary regulator of fetal (as opposed to embryonic) growth. IGF-1 is not imprinted but there is preliminary evidence that it too is extracted from the fetal circulation by the placenta, particularly if levels get too high. Thus it may be that the placenta acts as a 'governor', placing a maximum limit on fetal IGF-1 levels. The most favoured explanation however is that uterine size is correlated with pelvic size and maternal stature. The smaller pelvis and uterus thus have a smaller vasculature, which limits the nutrient supply to the placental bed and hence delivery of nutrients to the fetus, and this constrains fetal growth.

The phenomenon of maternal constraint has been shown elegantly in recent years using embryo-transfer techniques in several species – while such studies have eliminated genetic confounders in their interpretation they do not change the conclusions reached. Data is now also available from studying the offspring of human-assisted reproduction. One technique is that of oocyte donation where the egg from one woman is harvested, fertilised with sperm in a test-tube and placed as a fertilised embryo into the uterus of a recipient mother. This would most likely happen where the recipient mother has an inability to make eggs. The birth size of the fetus born in such scenarios correlates with the size of the recipient mother, again showing that the size of the uterus in which the embryo/fetus grows determines birth size more than its genetic origin. Such embryo-transfer experiments also argue against the sole operation of another genomic mechanism that has been suggested for maternal constraint – that is the role of mitochondrial DNA.[14]

In humans, maternal constraint operates in all pregnancies. However, some situations are associated with greater degrees of constraint than others. The most obvious is small maternal size. In populations such as those of India where the combination of genotype plus many generations of poor nutrition, infection and disease have led to small skeletal size in mothers, most babies are subject to serious maternal constraint, and the mean birth size is 25 per cent less than in developed countries. Other major causes of maternal constraint are the first pregnancy and maternal age. Multiple pregnancy is a special form of enhanced maternal constraint, where the limited capacity to deliver nutrients is exaggerated by the greater demand of twins or triplets.

It is well described that the first baby to a mother is on average smaller at birth than her subsequent babies by about 200 grams. It is also true both in humans and in animals that adolescent mothers give birth to smaller fetuses than do mothers who are fully mature. Both of these related situations appear to be examples of increased maternal constraint. The mechanisms are not fully understood, although it may be an erroneous assumption that the mechanisms of primiparous[15] and adolescent maternal constraint are the same as those underpinning maternal constraint associated with limiting the effect of the paternal genome. It is suggested from work in sheep that in adolescent pregnancy the mother competes with the placenta

---

[14] Mitochondria located in special organelles within a cell's cytoplasm are important in cellular energy homeostasis. They carry some DNA of their own, coding for a small number of genes involved in cellular energy homeostasis. When cells divide, the mitochondria split to end up in the daughter cells. Because sperm have no cytoplasm and eggs do, the only mitochondrial DNA in fertilised eggs is of maternal origin. As the fertilised eggs are the progenitors of all cells in the organism, all the mitochondria and thus all mitochondrial DNA is of maternal origin. This is an interesting mechanism because it allows passage of genomic information only down the maternal inheritance line.

[15] Primiparous refers to the first pregnancy, multiparous to subsequent pregnancies.

and fetus for substrates to complete her somatic (i.e. musculo-skeletal) growth. As the placenta produces hormones such as placental growth hormone, which are intended to alter maternal metabolism to favour nutrient supply to the fetus, it may be in these situations that these hormones exert an inappropriate anabolic drive in the mother.

An explanation for the reduced birth size in the first born is the impact of pregnancy on the uterine vascular bed. The blood vessels in the non-pregnant uterus are small and very tortuous, and blood flow is low. In pregnancy, under the impact of oestrogens and prostanoids made by the placenta, these vessels become much more relaxed and dilated to permit more flow. Just as elastic bands are more stretchable after they have been stretched once, the first pregnancy makes the uterine vessels more pliant in the second and subsequent pregnancies. Greater uterine blood flow and better placental bed formation are reflected in better nutrient supply to the fetus.

This phenomenon of primiparous maternal constraint is now of great importance. For example in the Western world, where the number of children born has fallen, over 50 per cent of babies are now from primiparous pregnancies, whereas 100 years ago the proportion would have been under 20 per cent. The impact of changed family practices in China is even more dramatic and may be a time bomb in relation to the changing pattern of disease – we will discuss this in chapter 8. Thus the proportion of babies born where maternal constraint is a major feature has risen, despite the increase in maternal size during this period. The high proportion of teenage pregnancies is an additional contributor in many populations.

Maternal constraint is also seen in polytocous species, and is manifest in the inverse relationship between fetal size and fetal number. For example, in the pig the average size of a piglet in a litter of four is greater than in a litter of twelve. This would suggest that there is a limitation in the supply of nutrients to the multiple fetuses and this is part of the explanation of maternal constraint.

We see this echoed in humans with multiple pregnancy. Even allowing for prematurity, the average size of triplets is less than that of twins, which in turn is less than that of singletons. The rapid increase in multiple pregnancy in developed countries owing to increasing maternal age and, particularly, the increased use of assisted reproductive techniques, needs to be considered.

Maternal constraint is thus a general phenomenon, and in chapter 7 we suggest that its importance in evolutionary terms may be broader than just ensuring a match between maternal size and fetal growth. However it is particularly in the human that it may be of greatest importance as it allowed our ancestors to adopt the upright position by balancing the needs of protecting fetal development against the problem of too wide a pelvic canal, risking our abdominal contents prolapsing! We discuss this in chapter 8.

## Brain growth

Brain growth has quite a distinct pattern of growth from that of other organs. The number of neurons is almost entirely determined in fetal life and is largely completed in mid-gestation. Essentially no neuronal stem cell proliferation occurs after birth, except for a small amount in the area of the brain associated with memory (the hippocampus). Neurons are the cells that carry out brain function but they are supported and nourished by glial cells. These also largely develop in fetal life but the peak of glial cell formation is somewhat later than for neurons, occurring in the last weeks of pregnancy. Brain development is very complex – involving the processes of stem cell proliferation, migration, axon and dendrite formation, differentiation into neurons and glia, then differentiation into the myriad forms of neuron with different neurotransmitters and the formation of billions of connections. There is also a carefully coordinated pattern of cell death as neurons that do not make connections are weeded out. Indeed neurons die at a great rate from fetal life and throughout the rest of life.

This complexity means that the fetal brain is very sensitive to environmental stimuli that might irreversibly damage it. Fortuitously much of brain function is relatively plastic because of the redundant excess of neurons and connections, but nevertheless we now recognise that many neurological and psychiatric diseases may have their origin, in part, in fetal life. For example, autism is likely to be associated with problems in forming connectivity properly in the fetal brain. Some forms of schizophrenia are associated with a small head circumference at birth suggesting that a prenatal factor plays a role in some cases, although whether this is environmental or genetic or both is not entirely clear. The fetal alcohol syndrome is an example of a toxin interfering with the correct migration of brain cells within the developing brain. Also oxygen lack or infection can cause irreversible damage to the brain and lead to conditions such as cerebral palsy.

During fetal life many specific adaptations ensure protection of the blood supply and oxygen delivery to the developing brain.[16] Considered as a proportion of body size and energy consumption, the fetal brain is relatively larger than the adult brain, even though much increase in brain size occurs after birth (largely as myelin – a

---

[16] We now know that there are also mechanisms which 'spare' the developing heart and the liver. Adequate cardiac function is obviously essential for health, but it is only recently that liver sparing has been recognised. The liver is a major source of growth factors and nutrients and it plays a role in determining the blood-lipid profile. In fetal life the liver may also metabolise hormones such as cortisol that have crossed the placenta. Blood returning from the placenta in the umbilical vein can be diverted to the liver, to maintain such functions, or bypass it, which may assist the developing heart and brain. It is likely that such 'liver sparing' occurs when the nutritional challenge is mild but that this is overridden by 'brain and heart sparing' if the challenge becomes greater. But even the liver-sparing response can produce detrimental consequences for later health as will be discussed in chapter 6.

fatty acid substance that helps electrical conduction along the axons of neurons – forms in the brain). Some of these adaptations include the special structural shunts in the liver and heart and great vessels that preferentially send the blood leaving the placenta in the umbilical vein (which is oxygen rich)[17] directly to the brain. For these reasons, when the fetus is born small the reduction in body size is often disproportionate and there is a relative preservation of head growth – this is called asymmetrical fetal growth retardation.

## The physical phenotype at birth

It is the phenotype that interests every parent at birth. In most cases the mother (but not necessarily the father!) knows the full genotype already (i.e. who is the biological mother, who is the biological father). The first questions at birth are the same for every parent – does the baby have ten fingers and toes, is it a boy or girl and how heavy is it? The physical phenotype at birth (e.g. height, weight, head circumference etc.) is a consequence of several factors – the genotype, the maternal environment and the fetal responses to it, and gestational length. Obviously, premature babies are smaller than term babies but, in turn, prematurity is more common in growth-retarded babies.

Fetal and birth size are determined in the normal fetus by the interaction between the genomic drive to grow and develop and the supply of nutrients from mother via the placenta. Normal fetal growth reflects the interaction. In turn this interaction is compounded by many transient variations in the fetal environment. In the sheep fetus we know that just two days of undernutrition of the ewe will send a transient nutritional signal to the fetus to reduce its IGF-1 levels and slow down growth. On re-feeding with glucose, growth starts again. If there is a transient dip in fetal oxygenation this too will transiently reduce IGF-1 levels and have a temporary effect on growth rate. Maternal exercise can affect blood supply to the uterus and so overzealous exercise in late gestation can affect fetal growth. Even how the mother lies in bed in late pregnancy can be important because if she lies supine the weight of her uterus may compress her abdominal vessels and reduce uterine blood flow. What the mother eats can affect placental nutrient transfer. Maternal health status (e.g. infection), her macro-environment (e.g. altitude) and her behaviour (e.g. smoking or drug taking) all impact on the fetal environment and thus on the fetal pattern of growth. Thus in every pregnancy there are many environmental factors that can lead to transient changes in fetal growth and may affect birth size.

---

[17] The umbilical circulation is the one circulation other than the postnatal pulmonary (lung) circulation in which oxygen content is higher in a vein than in an artery.

Abnormally impaired fetal growth generally occurs for one of several reasons.[18] It may occur because of gross genetic abnormalities – for example, a mutation in the IGF-1 gene or its receptor will cause severe fetal growth retardation because IGF-1 is the most important fetal growth factor in the second half of pregnancy. Insulin is the other major fetal growth factor (acting in part by regulating IGF-1) and genetic defects in the insulin receptors or its action can also cause severe fetal growth retardation. Toxins from smoking or toxic infections such as rubella that interfere with the fetus or placenta are major causes of intrauterine growth retardation. In tropical countries malarial infestation of the placenta is of particular concern because it interferes with normal placental function, and the parasite load utilises energy that should otherwise be available for delivery to the fetus. However, most cases of impaired fetal growth are caused by placental interruption of the supply line – poor placental function associated with pre-eclampsia is a very common cause of intrauterine growth failure. Interruption to the supply line can be at many levels, from the maternal blood supply to the uterus (e.g. maternal heart disease) to anatomical problems with the umbilical cord delivering nutrients from the placenta to the fetus.

Finally some small babies are just small because they have small mothers, not because of any specific disease state.

Fetal growth must be seen as an integrated readout of the many gene–environmental interactions that happen during fetal life. Depending on when in pregnancy the fetus changes its growth rate in response to an external cue, the birth-size phenotype might be affected differently – it is generally stated that late in pregnancy, when the fetus has considerable soft tissues (fat, viscera, muscle), fetal undernutrition leads to a thin baby, whereas earlier in gestation undernutrition of the fetus will affect linear growth as well: thus the baby will be shorter and lighter. Head growth is relatively protected because the fetal adaptations of changing regional blood flows attempt to preserve blood supply to the fetal head at the expense of the trunk in adverse situations. In reality this is a gross simplification[19] but it is easy to see how insults or circumstances at different times can interact to give a vast plethora of different birth-size phenotypes – fat or thin, long or short, large or small head, large or small abdomen (reflecting liver growth) etc. If only we could read accurately what the fetus was telling us from the detail of its

---

[18] Birth size must be interpreted relative to gestational age. There are normal standards for various measures of birth size – weight, length and head circumference being the most common. Intrauterine growth retardation (IUGR) is a term used to describe birth size outside the normal range – the alternative term is small for gestational age (SGA). We prefer the latter as IUGR implies that the mechanisms of the reduction in birth size are known and that it is pathological, whereas not all small fetuses are necessarily pathologically growth impaired.

[19] For example recent studies have shown that altered maternal food intake at conception can alter the development of a variety of hormonal systems in the fetus but these only become manifest in late gestation as reduced fetal growth.

birth phenotype, we might know much more about how it had integrated its environmental experiences from conception to birth with the genomic information it inherited at conception.

Birth size can also be increased under some conditions. One way is genetic. For example if there has been a failure of suppression of one of the two copies of the IGF-2 gene by imprinting the maternal copy, then the fetus expresses twice the normal amount of IGF-2: – this is the cause of the rare Beckwith–Weidemann syndrome, which leads to a very big baby at birth with a number of hormonal abnormalities and an increased risk of some forms of childhood cancer. But the commonest cause of big babies is excessive glucose supply to the fetus. This happens either if the mother is diabetic or prediabetic. Because glucose supply to the fetus is so important during pregnancy, the placenta makes hormones that induce some insulin resistance in the mother. She thus primarily uses fat for her own energy needs and gives the glucose to the fetus and placenta. But if the mother has a latent diabetic tendency, this will be exposed by these placental hormonal changes and insulin resistance induced, and thus glucose delivery to the fetus becomes excessive. But bone and muscle growth primarily require amino acids, and the supply of these remains somewhat limiting. High levels of glucose in the fetus make its pancreas secrete more insulin and this, together with high energy availability, promotes storage of the excess energy as fat. Therefore the fetus of a diabetic mother has only a small increase in muscle and bone size (i.e. length) but is rather obese and has a high birth weight. The implications of this are discussed further in chapter 8.

## Developmental plasticity

It will be clear to the reader that the development of the mature organism from a single egg can take multiple paths and lead to a range of phenotypes. These different pathways result from the interaction of the environment with the genome both before and after birth. The mechanisms involved can encompass any of the developmental processes we have already referred to – changes in cell number, in proliferation rate, in differentiation, in gene expression, to name but a few. The capacity of cells, organs and systems to change their function or state is referred to as *plasticity*. Essentially development is all about plasticity as the embryo starts as a single cell and ends up as a mature adult with fully differentiated organs and cell types. This global set of plastic responses is termed *developmental plasticity* but plasticity is not limited solely to development. Some tissues remain plastic throughout life – for example, although muscle cells cannot change in number in adulthood they can change their characteristics and size when subject to repeated exercise, such as in body-builders. Equally such hypertrophied muscles return to a reduced state when not exercised. This is reversible plasticity. A skin wound in adults or older children leaves a scar: the skin proteins and cells that form the scar derive from the same cells that form normal skin and its underlying proteins, so to this degree they are plastic; but the scar, once formed, does not disappear – this is an example of irreversible plasticity.

Developmental plasticity is generally irreversible. At the most obvious level, once a stem cell has been committed to a lineage – say of ectodermal cells (e.g. liver cells) – that is an irreversible commitment of that cell, and its progeny must be liver cells. The basic programme for development from a single cell to a complete organism is obviously entirely located within the genome of the fertilised zygote, so developmental plasticity itself is inherently genomically determined. However it is the capacity of the direction, timing or magnitude of each developmental plastic event to be influenced by the environment that leads to the multitude of phenotypes possible from a single genotype and that is the focus of this book. During early development many environmental influences can act on the programme of embryonic and fetal development to amend or influence plastic change. For example exposure to the male sex steroids at a point in development when the genitalia are forming can lead to permanent changes in their appearance. While we have focused here on structural plasticity, plasticity can be functional, e.g. in the set-point of a physiological process. For example there may be a permanent change in the expression of a gene controlling the number of receptors for a hormone and this will be reflected in altered hormone sensitivity.

Permanent plastic responses of this type play an important role in the developmental origins of adult disease, which we will discuss in chapter 6.

## Critical windows of development

Birth defects and malformations can arise in one of two ways – either there is a genetic defect so that the orchestrated programme of development is defective, or there is an environmental factor (called a teratogen) that somehow affects the genetic programme. Studies of the latter give us insight into an important concept in development – that is of *critical windows*. Thalidomide is an example of a teratogen, and its effect in producing limb and hand abnormalities was critically linked to when in pregnancy the mother ingested it: the earlier in pregnancy the more gross the limb malformation. While most teratogens are drugs or chemicals, infectious agents such as rubella can also be teratogenic leading to malformations of the fetal heart. Although the teratogenic effects of many drugs are clearly understood, there remains much uncertainty about xenobiotics such as pesticide residues etc.

Teratogens act by interfering with the developmental programme at a critical point in time to cause an overt anatomical malformation. This might arise as an acute insult, e.g. from exposure to a drug or chemical for only a short period of time.

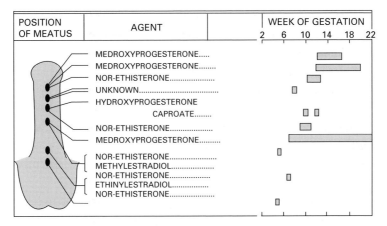

| POSITION OF MEATUS | AGENT | WEEK OF GESTATION |
|---|---|---|

Fig. 2.5    Cases of hypospadias in male offspring related to time of beginning of maternal treatment with various estrogens and progestins. Note that the closer the time of treatment to beginning of penis formation the more severe the hypospadias. Redrawn from Schwarz and Yaffe (1980).

An example of this can be seen in the male fetuses exposed to certain hormonal medications containing forms of progestogenic steroids. Between the seventh and twelfth week of pregnancy the male fetus develops his penis under the influence of a derivative of the male hormone testosterone made by the fetal testis. The urethra is the urinary channel that in the mature penis exits at its tip. As the penis develops, the urethra first opens at the base of the penis and the penis gradually wraps around the urethral tube – so that as the penis matures the urethral opening progresses along its underside until it reaches the tip at about the twelfth week after conception. The progestins act as anti-testosterones and can cross the placenta. If the mother is exposed to such progestins between the seventh and twelfth week[20] then the maturation of penile growth is interfered with and the urethra opens not on the tip but underneath the penis – this is called hypospadias. The degree of hypospadias can be related to when exposure to steroid occurred – the closer to 7 weeks the closer the urethral opening is to the base of the penis, the closer to 12 weeks the closer to the tip of the penis. But after 12 weeks, when the penis is fully formed, progestins and oestrogens have no effect on penile development. Thus the critical window for affecting penile development is 7 to 12 weeks.

Another example of a critical window relates to the sexual behaviour of rats. As in most species, rats have quite distinct patterns of sexual behaviour, with males taking mounting positions and females submissive positions. This behaviour is controlled by a part of the brain known as the hypothalamus. The hypothalamus is crucial for the regulation of reproduction and other hormonal mechanisms such

---

[20]  They used to be prescribed as drugs to reduce the risk of miscarriage.

as the response to stress. In the rat, which has a very immature brain at birth, the development of the hypothalamus largely occurs after birth. If a female rat pup is exposed to the male hormone testosterone between three and ten days after birth, the hypothalamus will develop like a male hypothalamus, and at adulthood the female will show male-like mounting behaviour. Conversely, a male rat pup castrated before this critical period will not develop male behaviour. But if a female is exposed to testosterone before 3 days or after 12 days it will have no effect on her adult sexual behaviour. Obviously there is a critical window in hypothalamic development when exposure to the male hormone will irreversibly produce changes in wiring leading to adult male-like behaviour.

It is much more debatable whether such a window relating to sexual behaviour occurs in humans – if it did it must occur some time in fetal life as the human brain is much more mature at birth than the rat. There have been claims that girls born with adrenogenital syndrome (a genital defect in the way the adrenal gland makes steroid hormones so that it makes more androgens than cortisol) have altered psychosexual development and that this in turn reflects the elevated androgen levels they were exposed to in utero. East German scientists, prior to the destruction of the Berlin wall, presented data to suggest that male fetuses exposed to stress in utero had lower testosterone levels and they claimed this was the biological origin of male homosexuality. This claim may have better suited the ideals of Marxism, but neither observation nor claim has achieved standing in the scientific community.

Two important questions arise from the above discussion. First, are there insults that cause less obvious but nevertheless permanent changes in function if the fetus is exposed to them in utero? Second, are there environmental factors that affect the developmental programme in the later part of pregnancy, after organ formation is largely complete, but while functional development is still occurring? We will primarily address both questions in later chapters but the short answer to both is 'yes'. There are many functional abnormalities that have their origin in environmental factors acting in early development. Furthermore, while gross organ development is achieved in humans in the first half of pregnancy, the finer aspects and functional maturation extend throughout the fetal phase into childhood, and permanent changes in function can be achieved by environmental factors operating throughout this period.

## Prematurity: an alternative strategy

Prematurity has a variety of causes. Some cases are due to infection ascending the cervix and entering the amniotic fluid and membranes. This leads to an inflammatory response causing induction of prostaglandins in the uterine muscle, leading to contractions. Perhaps 40 per cent of cases of premature labour have such a cause.

The origin of the ascending infection is unknown – one study has suggested that intercourse late in pregnancy might be a factor but there is disagreement about this. Most premature labour has an unknown cause although recent studies in sheep raise the possibility that at least in that species it has its origin very early in pregnancy.

Babies who are born premature often seem more mature in some functional aspects than we would expect. This is even more so the case in growth-retarded fetuses born prematurely. This is because the fetal period prior to premature labour may have been associated with higher cortisol levels in the fetal blood than a normal pregnancy at the same postconceptional age. A rise in cortisol (the primary hormone made by the cortex of the adrenal gland) occurs in the blood of the fetus prior to delivery in all mammals. After birth, cortisol is best known as a stress hormone and it plays a major role in regulating blood pressure, fluid balance and blood glucose levels and assisting the body in responding to stress. It also reduces the immune response, hence its powerful medical use as an anti-inflammatory drug.

The rise in fetal cortisol is responsible for the maturation of many organs before birth. Elevated cortisol levels are therefore likely to be the cause of the apparently greater maturity in the prematurely born fetus. In some species such as the sheep, the linkage between maturation and delivery may be quite direct. In these species the rise of fetal cortisol levels is an active part of the cascade of biochemical pathways that leads to the initiation of the uterine contractions and cervical relaxation that constitute labour.

These observations in premature and growth-retarded fetuses reflect the two strategies the fetus has in adverse situations – to grow more slowly (or differently) in order to conserve nutrients, or to accelerate maturation through cortisol release and then deliver prematurely. In reality these two options are a continuum – many growth-retarded fetuses have accelerated maturation of some organs such as the lung owing to the effects of elevated cortisol but still have not delivered prematurely.

## Maternal nutrition

Maternal behaviour can do much to determine fetal outcome. At one level this statement reflects the obvious point of avoiding toxins such as cigarettes and drugs of abuse and promoting maternal health. But it is becoming increasingly clear that at a more subtle level the fetus is constantly responding to signals from its mother that relate to her nutritional status. This brings us to the vexed but critical question of maternal nutrition. Fetal nutrition is not the same thing as maternal nutrition and it is not simply a reflection of maternal nutrition. Maternal nutrient status is but one factor in determining the supply of nutrients to the fetus. But the subtleties of the maternal metabolic state, reflecting in turn her nutritional status, may be the most important signals to the fetus about the environment it is going to be born into.

We still know frustratingly little about the best maternal nutrition for achieving optimal pregnancy outcome. Both micronutrient supply such as the provision of folate and other vitamins, minerals such as iodine and zinc, and the amount of, and balance of, macronutrients (protein, carbohydrates and fats) have a major impact on the outcomes of pregnancy. For example, extreme iodine deficiency in the mother leads to cretinism in the offspring and this is a key reason why salt is iodised. Folate deficiency plays a role in neural tube defects such as spina bifida, and we suspect that micronutrient availability plays an important role in the phenomenon of PARs through much more subtle effects including the regulation of epigenetic changes.

Macronutrient supply is also critical. We are yet to identify the best mix of macronutrients for different periods in pregnancy and possibly for different populations. The evidence is mounting that both the absolute and relative amounts of macronutrients are important. History has taught us this. In a reprisal for the activities of the Dutch resistance in late 1944, the Nazi authorities imposed severe rationing on the population. The mean caloric intake was reduced almost overnight from about 1800 to between 400 and 800 calories per day. The Dutch Hunger Winter, as this episode has been termed, lasted for seven months until the Allied forces liberated Holland in 1945. Food intake was returned to adequate levels almost instantaneously. While famine is sadly not uncommon in many parts of the world, what is unusual about the Dutch Hunger Winter is, first, that the famine was imposed on a previously well-nourished population; second, there was a sudden onset and relief from the famine; and third, in places such as Utrecht, despite the adversities of the wartime occupation, midwives and doctors continued to offer a professional obstetric service and to keep detailed records of birth weights and other relevant data. Subsequently it has been possible to analyse the pregnancy outcomes of women caught in this famine in terms of those who delivered before the famine, who conceived during the famine, or were in early, middle or late pregnancy at the time the famine was imposed. Initial studies suggested that unless the maternal food intake was less than 800 calories per day the fetus could grow adequately and there were no real consequences of mild or moderate maternal undernutrition. As we will discuss in chapter 4 we now suspect this was an incorrect conclusion. Many of those more subtly affected as fetuses have gone on to develop health problems in later life that we now believe are a result of the nutritional stresses they were exposed to before birth.

The first clues that macronutrient balance may also play a role came from studies in food-rationed populations in Scotland after the Second World War. There was a presumption that more protein must be better, and studies were performed of giving supplementary protein in the form of meat. Paradoxically under some

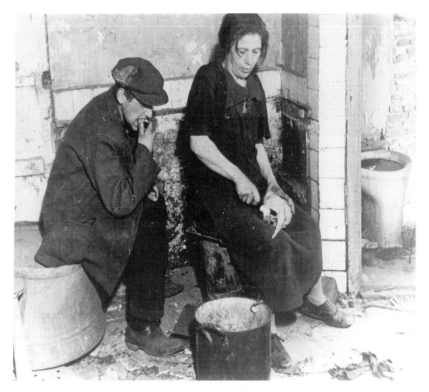

Fig. 2.6     Conditions were extremely harsh for the people of the Netherlands exposed to the near-famine conditions imposed by the Nazis in the winter of 1944/45. The effects of the poor and unbalanced diet of women during pregnancy on their children and grandchildren have been studied in detail. Photograph courtesy of the Dutch Institute for War Documentation.

circumstances this led to smaller, not larger fetuses although in other circumstances it did assist fetal growth. More recent studies from Southampton show that the mix of dairy and meat products and the balance of protein, carbohydrate and micronutrients such as folate can have important influences on the patterns of fetal growth. The reality is that we actually know very little about what is the optimal nutritional mix for a mother at different stages in pregnancy and in different circumstances. A major message of this book is that this is an area needing priority in research. It is a topic we will return to in chapter 10.

## Growth and maturation after birth

After birth, growth continues in several distinct phases. In infancy, it is still largely determined by the mother through either the supply of breast or bottle milk. While maternal constraint has been removed, nutrient availability remains the dominant regulating factor and the hormones primarily involved in regulating infant growth are similar to those involved in prenatal growth – that is insulin and the insulin-like growth factors (IGFs). But as the infant grows into childhood there is a gradual switch in the hormonal regulation of growth. Somewhere between 6 and 12 months after birth, growth hormone (made by the pituitary gland) becomes the dominant regulator of growth and takes over regulation of IGF secretion from the direct effects of nutrition itself. The patterns of growth-hormone secretion between individuals are relatively distinct. They are genetically determined to a degree and it would appear that both maternal and paternal genetic factors are much more important in determining postnatal than prenatal growth. This is why postnatal growth tends to follow a given trajectory for an individual child and, if transiently knocked off that trajectory by illness, the child generally returns to it. Hence final adult height is closely correlated with parental height.

Growth in infancy and childhood remains exquisitely sensitive to environmental factors. Infant diseases such as infection can reversibly impair growth and, if frequent enough or severe enough, infant and childhood illness can lead to irreversible stunting of the child. Emotional stresses can impact on growth-hormone secretion and impair growth. And of course adequate nutrition is essential to normal growth.

A special form of growth is called *catch-up growth* (the opposite being catch-down growth). After an insult, when growth has been transiently impaired, there may be a period of accelerated growth that returns growth to the original trajectory. How this catch-up growth is regulated is poorly understood. Many children who are born small due to a constrained intrauterine environment show catch-up growth in infancy when relieved from the physiological and pathophysiological constraints in utero. Some children who have grown excessively in utero, often because of maternal diabetes, show catch-down (i.e. slower) growth after birth in order to reach their genetically determined growth trajectory.

Relative growth in length and weight do not go in parallel. The change in relative weight for length is reflected in measures such as ponderal index and body mass index[21], which are measures of weight for length. As the size of skeletal muscle in childhood is generally proportional to bone mass and thus length, these measures are somewhat crude measures of relative fatness. Relative fatness varies at birth – low fatness being a major indicator of a sub-optimal fetal environment. Catch-up in fatness and in length do not go in parallel, and the processes regulating these growth patterns are not understood. Generally, fat gain occurs earlier than height gain and the height gain may never be complete: children who are stunted as a result of malnutrition when re-fed often end up with truncal obesity but are still short.

[21] Ponderal index is weight/height$^3$ and body mass index is weight/height$^2$.

For reasons we do not fully understand, humans are the fattest of all species at birth. Perhaps it is to ensure a fuel reserve to protect the high energy demands of the disproportionately large human brain. This places extra demands on maternal nutrient supply to the fetus in late gestation when the fetus is laying down fat. In relative terms, this adiposity decreases over the first 2 to 3 years of life (perhaps because it is used for brain metabolism) but then fat is again deposited during childhood; from then on it is easy to get obese! This 'adiposity rebound', as it is called, varies among individuals and populations, but as we will see later its timing may have important consequences for subsequent health.

In late childhood, additional hormonal changes occur. The adrenal gland starts to make, at least in humans, adrenal male-like hormones (androgens) and then the gonads under hypothalamic control start to make either male or female hormones according to the gender of the individual. This accelerates linear growth but at the same time leads to development of the secondary sexual characteristics (breast development, penile enlargement, pubic and axillary hair). Linear growth occurs at special zones at the ends of the shafts of the long bones, called growth plates. These are made of cartilage and at one side of the plate the cartilage cells multiply to form columns, while at the other end they convert from cartilage to bone, thus elongating the shaft. As sex-steroid levels stay high over time, the growth-plate cartilage cells convert into bone cells and the growth plate disappears; linear growth is then over. This is not universal in all mammals, and some rodents continue to grow, albeit slowly throughout life. Even after linear growth is over in humans, other tissues continue to develop over some years, e.g. muscle continues to increase in bulk by adding protein within the cells for some time. Psychosexual and psychosocial maturation continues through adolescence.

Fat or adipose-tissue proportions also change greatly through development. Both tissues have their cell number largely determined in fetal life, although recent evidence questions this in relation to the regulation of fat-cell number. After birth the relative amount of fat and muscle is largely a matter of how much protein exists within a muscle cell and how much fat exists within a fat cell. Both are very labile tissues and hormones such as insulin, growth hormone and cortisol regulate whether fat is being laid down or mobilised, and whether protein is being laid down in muscle and in the liver or being metabolised. The regulation of this partitioning is essentially how metabolic homeostasis is maintained – that is how blood glucose levels, plasma lipid levels etc. are regulated.[22]

---

[22] Insulin acts mainly on three tissues – liver, fat and muscle – to promote storage of fuels, and in every cell type to promote glucose uptake for energy consumption. Insulin increases the conversion of glucose into glycogen (the storage form of glucose in the liver), enhances fat deposition in fat and amino acid incorporation into proteins in cells. Insulin's actions are counteracted by other hormones so that blood-glucose levels are maintained in a narrow range. When insulin deficiency occurs or insulin resistance is

In this chapter we have seen that development is an extremely dynamic process. It is not simply determined by the genotype, and so does not occur solely in the form of an encapsulated, hardwired developmental 'programme'. Instead, the developmental programme can be influenced by a range of environmental conditions and these interactions can have long-term consequences for later health and disease. We have to be extremely careful not to view body size and shape at birth as measures of developmental outcome, especially in terms of the underlying physiological function. The baby at birth has come a long way, and indeed may have arrived at the same point down one of many paths. The detailed structure of its organs, their function and the homeostatic processes that govern them, are obviously not visible to the naked eye. But already the individual's biological destiny is written in the birth phenotype.

induced, diabetes ensues. Type 1 diabetes mellitus occurs when the pancreatic cells making insulin are damaged by autoimmune processes. Type 2 diabetes occurs when the body's cells become resistant to insulin and the pancreas cannot keep making enough insulin to overcome the resistance. Insulin is a hormone and it binds to receptors on the cell surface. In turn this stimulates a complex chain of events within the cell that ultimately lead to changes in cell function. There are several ways in which insulin resistance can be induced. One element is obesity, because insulin works less well when fat cells are distended with fat. High fatty acid or lipid levels in blood also alter the function of insulin receptors and can cause insulin resistance.

# 3

# Fetal choices

In the previous chapter we described how the fetus responds to environmental change to aid its survival. Many of these responses are transient and functional, that is homeostatic, responses – for example the cessation of fetal breathing movements to conserve oxygen. Others involve changes in developmental trajectories – for example altered fetal growth to conserve nutrients. The latter often involve irreversible developmental plastic changes and thus have potentially long-lasting consequences. We will pursue this theme in this chapter and also introduce another concept: namely that the fetus might make some adaptive responses not for immediate survival advantage, but in expectation of future advantage after it is born, by changing its developmental programme before it is born. This is the concept we have termed predictive adaptive responses.

## Fetal strategies

Fetal development is of course not an end in itself. In evolutionary terms, the sole point of the process of development from embryo to adulthood is to achieve competence to reproduce. The author Samuel Butler made the point well when he phrased the aphorism that the 'chicken is just the egg's strategy for making another egg'. The embryonic and fetal phases of development must be survived, the fetus must attain independent life at birth and the child must pass through puberty – these are the necessary steps on the trail to reproductive competence. But as we have seen, the birth phenotype can be highly affected by the environment of the developing fetus. In turn this can have life-long phenotypic consequences, particularly because many of the plastic changes made during development are irreversible.

Darwin realised that both sexual selection and natural selection gain importance in evolutionary terms through reproduction, because only the selected members of the species reproduce and thereby pass on their characteristics to the next generation. Placed in this context it is possible to understand that evolution might

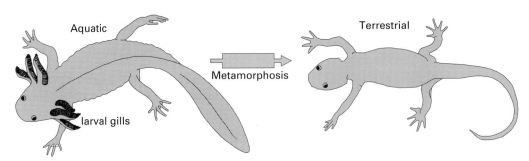

Fig. 3.1     The process of metamorphosis from the aquatic to the terrestrial forms in some amphibians such as the Mexican axolotl (a form of salamander) can be triggered by external environmental influences. Thyroxine applied to the water can do this experimentally. In the wild, such processes (called neoteny in this case) show how developmental plasticity provides an adaptive strategy to cope with environmental challenges, such as a pool drying up. Redrawn from *Principles of Development*, Wolpert *et al.* (eds.). Oxford University Press, 2nd edn.

enable the selection of characteristics by which the embryo or fetus can make strategic choices that would give the adult a greater chance of surviving the rigours of postnatal life, allowing it to achieve reproductive competence. Of course these strategic choices are not conscious, but the use of the word 'choice' is useful because it implies that there may be costs as well as benefits to the option adopted.

This phenomenon is dramatically seen in amphibians and some reptiles. Tadpoles of many species of frogs and toads develop in ponds that are at risk of drying up. For example the spadefoot toad lays its eggs in rainwater puddles in the Texas desert. Clearly if they are still tadpoles when the pond has evaporated, they die. So to survive, these species have evolved the capacity to change the timing of their metamorphosis into the mature form of toad when they sense the pond is drying up. Other species of toad will hasten their metamorphosis if, as tadpoles, they sense they are at higher risk of predation from dragonflies. There is a price to this strategy however, in that the terrestrial forms have a reduced body size that may have a cost later in life. These are examples of adaptive plasticity where there is an obvious advantage to changing the rate of development.

In some salamanders these issues of environmentally induced metamorphosis are even more dramatically demonstrated. Some such as the axolotl may stay in the infantile (non-gilled form) throughout life, and only under situations where they are forced to leave the pond do they undergo metamorphosis to the legged form. Obviously the early environment is acting on the genotype to determine something as striking as whether legs will form or not!

These examples show that the immature organism can indeed make adaptive responses for immediate survival advantage that can also have life-long consequences. The responses occur within the lifetime of the organism and, while genetically determined (in that having the capacity to make the response must have been selected), they are clearly purely environmentally induced. This is in contrast to the rabbit's ears or Darwin's finches that we discussed in chapter 1, where the change happens across generations and thus primarily operates through classical Darwinian selection processes. Unlike amphibians and reptiles, mammals in general appear to have a more limited repertoire of gross morphological change-strategies that they can adopt. But as we shall see, developmental choices about body size and body composition are made early in life in every generation in many mammalian species, including *Homo sapiens*.

In chapter 1, we referred to the effect of season on the coat thickness of newborn voles. But many of these mammalian choices are much more subtle than just external appearance. They may involve being relatively resistant to a hormone such as insulin, to changing the pattern of stress hormone release etc. The central feature is that these are 'strategic choices' that can be made early in life by the fetus. While in some cases, as for the timing of metamorphosis, they have immediate survival advantage, in other situations such as the meadow vole's coat thickness the choices are made in anticipation – that is, in response to *predictions* of the nature of the future environment, so that the organism will maximise its chances of survival in its predicted future environment. Thus the key question becomes, 'How can the embryo or fetus predict its future environment?'

## How can the embryo and fetus predict its future environment?

There are obvious differences between the environment of the mammalian embryo/fetus (echidnas and platypuses excepted) and that of the larval forms of insects and the egg-laying vertebrates.[1] While we can learn from the latter, we shall restrict further consideration to mammalian species because our focus is to understand this biology with reference to the human, and thus its role in the determination of our health and disease.

As detailed in chapter 2, environmental 'perception' by the mammalian embryo/fetus is largely dependent on the mother and the placenta. They act, in series, as two transducers of information about the external environment to the fetus. The crucial point is that the levels of nutrients passing into the fetal blood from the placenta act as vital coded messages about the external environment, which the growing fetus utilises to make strategic adaptive choices. It is intriguing that such choices depend on the levels of nutrients themselves, rather than on a special surrogate signal that has evolved for the purpose. Perhaps this represents an economy in nature – what could be simpler than using nutrient levels to signal one

---

[1] Intriguingly some live-bearing lizards and skinks also have a placenta-like structure by which nutrients are transferred from mother to offspring, suggesting that placentas evolved more than once.

of the most important aspects of the environment: nutrition[2] itself? But we will also see that other non-nutrient signals, especially blood hormone levels, play a part in environmental signalling. As we might expect, they can signal information about many aspects of the environment, including the global nutritional environment in which the mother is living.

The fetus responds to this maternally transduced environmental information, with transient homeostatic responses as were described in chapter 2 or, under some situations, by making some form of developmental plastic response. In turn this response may have immediate adaptive value, like the decision to accelerate parturition if the maternal environment is harmful (for example an infected uterus[3]). Other responses, as we shall see, have less obvious immediate value but have clear longer-term postnatal advantage, provided that the predicted future environment matches the environment as transduced by the mother and placenta to the fetus.

So the fetus/embryo uses this environmental information in two ways – firstly, to make immediate survival-related choices and secondly, to make long-term *predictions* to maximise its advantage postnatally. The postnatal advantage can be defined in Darwinian terms as choosing the best physiological trajectory for development in the predicted postnatal environment to achieve maximal reproductive fitness. This can be illustrated by reference to fetal nutrition and fetal stress. If the fetus is exposed to a long period of reduced nutrient supply, it might expect to be delivered into a world where nutrient supplies are low. Or if it experiences a high blood glucose level constantly, it might anticipate being born into a carbohydrate-rich environment. Or again, if its mother has continuously high blood cortisol levels, then so will the fetus, and it might anticipate being born into a stressful environment. None of this is an active decision-making process. It is the outcome of evolutionary processes that have defined the capacity to adapt as a valuable aspect of the survival of the species: indeed these adaptive mechanisms are present in every species examined. The processes could not occur if it were not for the phenomenon of developmental plasticity. Otherwise there could be no long-term permanent difference in phenotype as a result of transient environmental change acting in fetal life.

Thus how the fetus perceives its environment is critical both to its immediate survival and also for its long-term adaptive advantage in the environment in which

---

[2] It is important to re-emphasise what we mean by 'fetal nutrition'. The fetus primarily uses substrates such as glucose, amino acids and oxygen coming across the placenta from the mother. The fetus does swallow amniotic fluid and can absorb some nutrients from this source but amniotic fluid is in part formed by secretions from the fetal lung and fetal urine; there is no significant nutrient transfer from mother to fetus through this route, although there may be some recycling! Fetal nutrition is thus the sum total of nutrients the fetus receives from the placenta. This is not a direct reflection of maternal nutrition. Nutrients do not cross the placenta with equal efficiency and, as we discussed in the previous chapter, the placenta itself is an active metabolic organ.

[3] This is a common cause of premature labour.

it anticipates living after birth. The mother and placenta act as transducers of aspects of the environment to the fetus. As with any electronic or mechanical transducer – for example a smoke sensor used in a fire-detection system – there is a risk of malfunction. If the mother has diabetes mellitus that is not properly controlled, she will have high blood glucose levels. These will be reflected in high blood glucose levels in the fetus and the fetus will adapt in the expectation of high nutrient availability postnatally. But the mother might very well be living in famine conditions in the Horn of Africa. There would then be a gross mismatch between fetal nutritional expectations and the reality of the environment in which the child will live after birth. Similarly if the mother has heart disease, the fetus might adapt in the expectation of being born into a low-oxygen environment when it is not – a similar thing happens in the infant of a mother who smokes during pregnancy, where her elevated blood carbon monoxide levels produce the same effect as having low blood oxygen levels.

In these examples, the mother is incorrectly signalling information about the environment to her fetus. Similar faulty signals can arise from the placenta, for if it is abnormal, the transduction of the maternal/external environment to the fetus will not be accurate. If the placenta has poor perfusion with maternal blood, then the supply of oxygen and glucose to the fetus will be reduced. This will lead to reduced fetal growth as an immediate adaptive survival response. It will also lead to adaptive responses by the fetus in the expectation of being born into a nutritionally deprived postnatal environment – it is the last of these responses that is *predictive.*

## When to choose

While so far we have focused on the embryonic/fetal period, there is mounting evidence that some predictive responses can be initiated even prior to this, perhaps even as an egg before fertilisation. In rats in which nutrition was altered only for the period prior to conception there were irreversible consequences for the progeny throughout life (see chapter 5). There is increasing evidence that the conditions in which in vitro fertilisation is conducted can have long-term consequences, at least in farm animals.[4] The human correlates of this in modern reproductive technologies are poorly documented but there are data suggesting comparable phenomena. The data show that environmental influences acting in the earliest period of development can have echoes throughout life. Some of these might have immediate adaptive value, although it is extraordinarily difficult to imagine how that can be the case for the egg even before it is fertilised. Indeed it seems probable that

---

[4] The alleged accelerated ageing of Dolly the sheep again suggests that the origin of the embryo (in this case by a unique form of cloning) can have long-term consequences, although Dolly's origin is so bizarre (in biological terms) that we hesitate to use this as a definitive example of the point we are making.

most responses made at this stage are either neutral or are likely to confer future advantage.

Thus the period in which these predictive adaptive responses could be initiated extends from prior to conception, through embryonic life, fetal development and perhaps into early childhood. Obviously as the human embryo develops from a one-cell, multi-potential zygote to an organism with billions of cells, the impact of a given challenge changes. Hippocrates (460 to 377 BC) was the first to draw the analogy between the fetus and a plant, such as a fir tree. If damage occurs to the main stem at the seedling stage, a very deformed tree will develop, one that does not have the beautiful symmetrical shape of a main trunk, with decreasing branch size at each level, culminating in a tip at the top. On the other hand, if the tree is damaged when it is mature, the damage does not affect the basic shape of the tree and its underlying symmetry. We might predict that a challenge occurring at the one-cell embryo stage will have far more widespread effects on the adult organism than one occurring in late adolescence. This is exactly what is found. As will be described in chapter 6, a change in the growth-factor levels in the fluid surrounding the early embryo can affect the DNA of the cells (stem cells) whose progeny will go on to form every organ of the body. But if the change occurs later it may only affect one lineage of cell: for example just the kidney or a specific subset of cells in the brain. The overriding point here is that predictive responses are likely to have more widespread functional and structural consequences if they are induced early rather than later in life.

## The importance of phenotypic change

In chapter 1 we introduced the concept of phenotype. In chapter 2 we illustrated how the phenotype at birth is influenced by interactions between the fetal genome and its environment. We have now suggested that these interactions may not only be important for the immediacy of fetal survival but may have longer-term consequences. As we have discussed, the postnatal phenotype develops in embryonic, fetal and neonatal life in response to how the environment has been perceived. The question is: how important is that phenotypic variation to later life? Our thesis is that it is critical to shaping the biological destiny of individual animals and to the prevalence of health and disease in human populations.

As we progress we must remember that phenotype should not be seen in terms solely of physical dimensions. We insist on the generic use of the term phenotype to describe the biochemical, physiological as well as the physical characteristics of an animal (or person) at the point of observation, even if physical appearance is the easiest to study and describe and many of our examples concern physical phenotype. Moreover, as discussed in chapter 2, the phenotype of 'birth size' is a reflection of the sum total of a wide range of fetal experiences. We can view birth size as the phenotypic result of the interaction between the prenatal environment and the inherited genome, but there are many processes that result in such a phenotype. This diversity means that size at birth is therefore a rather crude integrated measure of many fetal processes, and its scientific usefulness as an absolute measure may be limited. Thus when one finds a correlation between birth size and an outcome, it does not mean that birth size *per se* is the cause of the outcome. Such a correlation is more likely to reflect some intrauterine event that has had independent effects on birth size and *also* had long-term consequences. Using such associations to argue for a causal linkage between low birth-weight and life-long consequences is an important conceptual trap to avoid – and unfortunately many scientists have fallen into it!

So if phenotypic variations at birth are a consequence of earlier developmental influences, do they confer an adaptive advantage postnatally? If they do, then they would be Darwinian adaptations as defined by evolutionary biologists.[5] This seems probable but is not easily provable. If they do not, we might assume that developmental plasticity has little role in shaping our lives. If the genome alone held the key to our phenotypic lives, we would also have to resign ourselves to the slow process of Darwinian evolution, and not expect to see any positive changes in human characteristics (whether they be intellectual, resistance to disease or purely aesthetic) for hundreds or thousands of generations. But it appears probable that Darwinian evolution has largely been halted in the human (see chapter 8) as we have controlled and standardised our environment, generated sufficient food to go round (although of course we know it is not evenly distributed in our world as yet) and intervened as a result of our development of moral and religious values to allow the less fit to survive to reproduce – a process greatly accelerated by the development of medicine.

So let us address the issue of environmental influences on the genome. Our initial focus must be on the environment of the embryo/fetus because we contend it is the interaction between genes and environment at this stage that has the most important consequences. This might sound counter-intuitive because we know that many environmental influences – such as smoking – act on the mature human to induce diseases such as lung cancer and cardiovascular disease. Nor do we ignore the importance of the purely genetic causes of some disease but, as we have already pointed out in chapter 1, even in single-gene diseases environmental influences play an important role (not every one with beta thalassaemia has the same phenotype and there are clearly environmental factors leading to this variation). We know certain

[5]  See footnote on p. 21.

polymorphisms confer an increased risk of diabetes, but the risk will be amplified by obesity, poor diet and lack of exercise. So the genomic make-up can influence how the organism will respond to the immediate environment. Equally, as we shall see, the consequences of predictive responses are affected by the concurrent postnatal environment, and in turn the way in which an adult responds to the environment is conditioned by developmental adaptations.

Let us use a hypothetical example: we know that individuals with obesity of the trunk (especially within the abdomen, as opposed to the hips and thighs) are more likely to get Type 2 (or adult-onset, non-insulin dependent) diabetes. This may be more so in individuals with a certain genetic make-up affecting genes responsible for insulin sensitivity. But truncal obesity is related to bad diet and poor exercise habits. This is a good example of a gene–environment interaction that results in an increased risk of disease. But what if the appetite and metabolic responses to exercise were established early in life, or even before birth? What if the tendency to lay down truncal fat was determined by developmental events that set out a map of how body fat would be deposited, not for fetal advantage but for a predicted postnatal advantage? In this case is the important gene–environment interaction the one happening in adulthood or the one that happened in utero? If the organism had not developed truncal fat in the first place then the risk of diabetes occurring as a result of adult dietary and exercise habits would have been much less. From the disease prevention point of view, it is likely to be the first event that occurred, namely the phenotypic change in utero. It should be obvious that, if this theoretical scenario is correct, then measures aimed at modification of adult lifestyle in order to reduce the risk of diabetes would in the long-term have less effect than a strategy aimed at optimising fetal development so that the right adaptations happened before birth. We have presented this as a hypothetical example, but is it? As we shall see in chapter 8, we believe this to be a real and common scenario and its resolution may have profound importance to preventative medicine.

## Predictive responses and life history

Life-history theory is a biological framework in which the strategies chosen by an organism at one period in its life are considered in terms of the implications for the rest of the organism's life. For example the early maturation of the dung fly, described in chapter 1, in a nutritionally restrained environment is a trade-off between growth and timing of maturation versus the chances of reproductive success. This type of biological theorising has become very popular in the past two decades.

But evolution can only select for biological 'trade-offs', which are advantageous during the reproductive period of life. This was pointed out by Williams as long ago as 1957. He argued that natural selection would favour characteristics that would be of benefit in the reproductive phase of life, even if they were subsequently deleterious to survival. Thus a small mutation or a polymorphism in the genome of a species that produced a better chance of survival to reproductive age, or indeed produced better reproductive function, would be selected even if it also reduced longevity in that species. Extending this idea, we would argue that, while environment could change at any point in the life cycle, and that any adaptive response to such change would be helpful to survival, predictive adaptations made during development would be more likely to be retained by evolutionary selection because they would confer an increased chance of survival to reproductive age.

More recently, Williams' theory of trade-offs has been refined by Tom Kirkwood in what is termed the 'disposable soma' model to explain ageing. This seemingly complicated term refers to the idea that different species have different life spans because they have evolved to invest different amounts of resources in the provision of reproductive processes, as opposed to repair mechanisms to rectify the damage of environmental threats. If members of a species are likely to die because of predation, then it makes sense to evolve assuming a short life span, breed early and invest little in cell repair and maintenance systems. Thus small mammals that are subject to more predation produce more offspring, but live less long, than do large mammals. Furthermore, there is no easy way in which evolution can select for the repair processes that are needed with increasing age, because selection cannot act strongly beyond the peak period of reproduction. Therefore species such as our own are bound to suffer more from conditions such as cancer and arthritis than do mice.

These ideas have usually been considered in terms of genomic mechanisms. However, we can see that they apply equally to the phenotypic changes produced by PARs, which themselves are defined by evolutionary selection (see chapter 7). Thus when choices are made early in life that predict the future, they may be both advantageous in the intermediate term but costly in the longer term: that cost being manifest in humans as a greater risk of disease.

## Environmental responses during development

Before we proceed, it may be useful to recapitulate about the processes of adaptive change occurring during development. Clearly there are two kinds of adaptive change to environmental stimuli that occur, although they overlap. The fetus will make a set of *immediate* adaptive changes that are essential to immediate survival in an acute situation. An example would be the shift in blood flow distribution that occurs during a period of transient oxygen shortage, e.g. when the umbilical cord is kinked. Blood flow is redistributed to the vital organs, and the heart and brain, at the expense of blood supply to the gastrointestinal tract. This blood flow redistribution serves preferentially to supply oxygen to critical tissues. Such acute adaptations are reflections of homeostatic processes.[6] Structural changes may occur if the insult persists – for example the altered body size that occurs secondary to these blood flow changes if there is chronic lack of oxygen caused by placental failure. Under persistently adverse conditions a developmental plastic response may be induced, such as the accelerated maturation of the lung so that the baby is more likely to survive if born prematurely.

These structural changes, with adaptive value, must be distinguished from developmentally disruptive (i.e. teratogenic) effects induced by an environmental factor. It is even possible for nutritional imbalance to induce such developmental disruption. One obvious example would be the neural tube defect induced by folate deficiency.

But we have already suggested that the developing organism has a further set of responses. These we have termed *predictive* adaptive responses, by which the fetus makes a set of changes triggered by the immediate environment specifically to deal with the environment it predicts will exist later in its life, especially during the period leading up to and during the phase of reproductive competence as an adult.

In many cases, such as altered growth rate, these longer-term changes are simply extensions of the immediate responses. The fetus immediately slows its growth rate when it senses reduced nutrient supply from the placenta; but if the period of nutritional deprivation is sufficiently prolonged, the fetus predicts that this will be its life-long nutritional environment and makes irreversible changes in its physiology to adapt. This is an example of PARs superimposed on an immediate homeostatic adaptation.[7] In other cases the PAR leading to permanent physiological change has no obvious relationship to immediate adaptive responses in utero – for example changes in the hormonal receptor pattern in the brain controlling stress responses have no immediate in utero adaptive value but have long-term survival value in a stressful environment.

In general what we are proposing is that the embryonic/fetal responses to an environmental cue are two-fold – first, short-term adaptive responses for immediate survival and second, predictive responses required to ensure postnatal survival to reproductive age. These two processes may often start with overlapping physiology (e.g. a change in growth rate following maternal undernutrition) but must then

---

[6] *Homeostasis* refers to the myriad of mechanisms, first proposed by Claude Bernard (1818–78), by which the body makes constant physiological adaptations to try and preserve its internal milieu.

[7] There are analogies to a concept that has been termed homeorhesis. In contrast to homeostasis, which reflects physiological changes that occur on an immediate and short-term basis, there are mechanisms where the adaptations occur over a longer-term basis and where the required physiological change persists over weeks or months. An example are the changes in insulin sensitivity that occur in pregnancy in the mother, to ensure glucose supply to the fetus. However, such homeorhetic processes, in contrast to PARs, are reversible if the environment changes again.

diverge. The former are generally reversible, the latter are not. As we have already pointed out, essentially the only way the fetus knows about its immediate and future environments is through maternal cues transduced by the placenta. These cues must drive both immediate adaptive responses and predictive responses. The cue inducing both types of adaptive response may be the same, but the consequences are different, especially if the cue is perceived as having a long time-base or is frequently repeated leading the fetus to reinforce its prediction of its future environment. For example maternal stress leads to a rise in cortisol that in isolation has immediate effects on the fetus to hasten its maturation, in case premature birth is the only possible survival response. In addition maternal stress leads to predictive adaptive changes in the offspring that alter stress hormonal responses, an appropriate adaptation to living in a postnatally stressed environment.

In general, PARs may not be obvious in the fetus whereas immediate adaptive responses should be obvious in utero or at birth. It was fortuitous to the discovery of the role of PARs in the origin of human disease that birth size is the integrated sum of fetal experience; thus fetuses who have been subject to many environmental cues suggesting a deprived postnatal environment are likely to be smaller because of the net effect of their immediate adaptive responses. As we will see in chapter 4, it was this correlation between evidence of fetal environmental miscues and postnatal pathophysiology that led to the epidemiological discoveries from which our current thinking arose.

## Predictive responses as a survival strategy

Our thesis is that early-life plastic responses occur in a single generation to increase the chance of survival of the individual to reproductive fitness.[8] These changes occur early in development when the individual is most plastic, and in mammalian species this period is primarily in embryonic and fetal life. Accordingly we presume the phenotype that develops in this period is that which the fetus has 'chosen', based on its perception of its future environment. But before we can make that deductive leap, we must first show that it is possible for phenotypic change to be made in expectation of the future environment.

Once again, we will choose examples from comparative biology so that we can develop a theoretical framework that we can then extrapolate to the human situation. In such circumstances the most telling examples often come from unusual or superficially bizarre species or ecological situations – this is because they represent extreme cases of what we believe to be a common biological solution to the

---

[8] Fitness is the life-time reproductive performance – because of transgenerational effects, it is best determined by studying the number (and 'quality') of grandchildren.

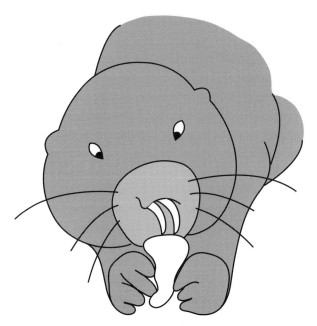

Fig. 3.2     A naked mole rat (*Heterocephalus glaber*). These extraordinary-looking animals have a complex and unusual social structure that illustrates how developmental processes, involving not only body size and shape but also behaviour, can be initiated by environmental cues such as population density.

essential evolutionary problem – how to ensure species survival and preferential passage of the common gene pool to the next generation. The danger of adopting this approach is that one can always find some example in biology that can be interpreted to support a position. We hope we have avoided this trap and that our position is validated by the detail of the human and experimental data given in the following chapters.

So let us consider an animal with the wonderful name of the naked mole rat. This animal lives underground in the barren and arid countryside of the Eastern part of the Horn of Africa. These animals are bizarre both in appearance and in their social structure. They look like a rat without hair, have loose skin hanging in folds, and they possess giant incisor teeth. All of these devices assist in their adaptations to living underground most of the time and for burrowing long distances. But the individual phenotypes of the animals vary considerably and they throw light on the model we are developing.

Mole rats have a complex social structure – they live in subterranean colonies of about 80 animals, usually located about 1 km apart. As in a well-ordered society, every animal knows its place. Somewhat like a termite or bee colony, all the breeding is performed by a single queen mole rat – the other females being sterile workers assisting in maintaining the colony. The number of breeding males is also small. There is much variation in body size and shape between individuals within the colony and this is put to good use – the smaller mole rats being responsible for burrow maintenance (rather as children were used as chimney sweeps in Victorian England) and the larger animals for defence of the burrows (perhaps like the bouncers outside a club). The variations in size are not purely genetically driven – they arise from a complex interplay between the environment and mole rat development. In this case the environment is largely determined by the size of the colony and the availability of food.

That these phenotypic differences are not purely genetic can be easily demonstrated. First-born litters in a new colony tend to grow fast, but they remain non-reproducing. Hence they can play a key role in colonising, defending and digging at an early age, without squandering valuable energy resources on reproduction. In contrast, their siblings from subsequent litters grow more slowly; they become reproductively active but use relatively less in the way of resources. In fact, despite considerable homogeneity in the gene pool of the colony (given that in each generation they all have the same mother), reproductively competent and incompetent females show quite different phenotypes. The reproducers grow fast, and have a permanent elongation of the bones of their spines (vertebrae), which fits them for bearing offspring. They are as different from their non-reproducing female colleagues as are queen bees from worker bees.

The breeding males are also larger than non-breeding males. Following the death of a breeding male, other male rats show an accelerated growth in adulthood (rodents, unlike humans, do not fuse their growth plates and continue to grow, albeit slowly, throughout life). Here is a classic demonstration that phenotype is not solely genetically determined but can be influenced over a sustained period of continued growth by environmental factors (in this case by the social environment).

But the story does not end there. Once the mole-rat colony reaches a critical size, which is dependent on the ratio between colony size and the supply of their principal food – a tuber that is more spaced out when there is drought – something dramatic occurs. A new male phenotype emerges called the 'disperser'. This rat is fat, uses minimal energy and is sexually primed by high levels of luteinising hormone in its bloodstream. It is most interested in mating with foreign mole rats[9] and so in time it will use its greater energy reserves to assist it in the trek to an adjacent colony, sometimes more than a mile away. Here of course its advances may be

---

[9] In neoDarwinist theory, it would be apparent that survival of this animal's genes is more likely if he moves to a less nutritionally stressed colony.

rebuffed, if the population there is thriving and the defenders are up to the mark. But the disperser may find that its adopted colony is in need of some reproductive assistance, in which case he will help to swell the population, and of course add a new source of biodiversity to it because his gene pool will be different.

The naked mole rat therefore provides a clear example of the way in which environmental cues, in this case population density and food supply, can determine a phenotype that is desirable for some future time. The phenotypic changes are manifest in adult life and determine whether each individual will remain in the colony as a thin, burrow-maintaining and relatively non-reproductive member of the species, or become the fat, reproductively active disperser phenotype. Many of these phenotypic changes are cued early in development although exactly when has not been established. At the start of the chapter we highlighted the need to focus on *development* as the period in the life cycle likely to be the most efficient time for gene–environment interactions. The phenotypic determination in the mole rats appears to occur early in their lives although there are consequential effects, e.g. the vertebral elongation in reproductively active females, which occurs after puberty.

Remaining with the environmental stimulus of population density, let us look for an example that such predictive gene–environment interactions can occur even during *fetal* life. In 1831 the manager of one of the Hudson Bay Company outposts wrote to his company in London to explain the recent decline in the number of fur pelts that he was sending. The Ojibwa Indians he used as trappers were starving, and they were forced to spend more time fishing than trapping. He attributed the predicament of the Indians to the lack of 'rabbits', which gave them a ready source of food during good years. The rabbits to which the manager referred were actually snowshoe hares. In fact, the population of hares shows a pronounced fluctuation in the form of a 10-year cycle.

There has been much research into this intriguing population cycle which, as can be guessed, not only affects the snowshoe hares but also the lynxes, for declining hare numbers were not only bad news for the Indian trappers, but also for other species such as the lynxes, which predate the hares. Records of the Hudson Bay Company also show a similar cycle in the number of lynx pelts harvested – over 65 000 at the peak of the cycle, falling to less than 2 000 at its trough. The decline in lynx numbers appears to follow the decline in hare numbers. So the poor lynx-pelt returns during the bad years of the cycle were not only because the Indians had to fish rather than spending their time trapping, but also because the low hare number had drastically reduced the lynx population and so fewer were trapped.

When food for the snowshoe hares is scarce, for example after a late spring that gives little growth of the vegetation they eat, the population of hares declines, as many die of starvation. This poses an additional threat to the remaining members of the population, because the fewer hares there are the more likely any individual hare

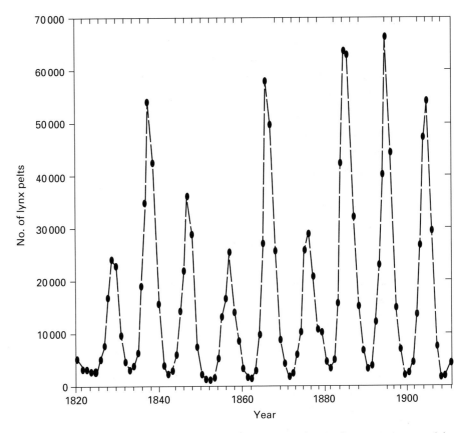

Fig. 3.3    Graph showing the number of lynx-fur pelts returned from the Northern Department of the Hudson Bay Company from 1821 to 1910. The cyclical changes have a period of 9.6 years. Such changes are driven not only by economic factors affecting the trappers, but also by the cyclical population changes in the prey for the lynx, especially the snowshoe hare. Cyclical changes in the behaviour (e.g. alertness, driven by stress hormone levels) of both predator and prey will occur with a similar timescale, and these may be in part initiated prenatally by predictive adaptive responses. Data from C. Elton and M. Nicholson. *Journal of Animal Ecology* (1942).

is to be picked off by their natural predators, the lynx and coyote but also raptors such as hawks and owls. The remaining hares must be extremely vigilant. Because the female hares are stressed, they have high cortisol levels during pregnancy.[10] This cortisol is transmitted across the placenta to the fetal hares. As we noted in chapter 2,

---

[10] Cortisol is the effector hormone of the hypothalamic–pituitary–adrenal axis (HPA) and is a vital part of the body's defences. It is made by the adrenal gland and plays a critical role in maintaining blood glucose, blood pressure and the stress response. It will also change both the alertness and the anxiety level in the animal. The stress could be in the form of the low oxygen encountered on ascending to altitude, a period of cold or starvation, or the stress on the appearance of a hungry-looking predator. The adrenal gland is under the control of the pituitary gland, which makes the hormone ACTH, which in turn stimulates the

cortisol has the additional role in utero of enhancing the maturation of certain organ systems and preparing the fetus for birth and the rigours of postnatal life. If the fetus is exposed to a disordered pattern of cortisol exposure, then the genetic machinery regulating gene expression is affected and the subsequent development of the animal may be altered permanently.

In the case of the snowshoe hare this abnormal exposure to cortisol in utero alters the sensitivity of the hypothalamic–pituitary–adrenal (HPA) axis so that it is more hyper-responsive (that is more cortisol is released for a given stress) after birth. This makes the offspring more jumpy as they grow up, more aware of the greater threat from potential predators. They are more likely to survive until food supplies improve and population numbers can increase. It also appears that fecundity in these animals is increased (presumably because of parallel changes in the hormonal axes controlling ovulation, which are not dissimilar in involving the hypothalamic–pituitary control of the gonads) in that they become fertile even as small juveniles. This is unusual, as the opposite effect is found in many other small mammals where stress such as poor diet reduces fecundity. In the snowshoe hare it has the consequence of increasing population numbers as rapidly as possible. The immediately following generations of hares will be less stressed as they are more numerous and the risk of predation is correspondingly less in each individual. They will have fewer litters and fewer leverets per litter.

Hard times for the hares will also mean hard times for the lynxes and predatory birds that eat them, and these species will also show a population decline. When the predator numbers decline and/or the supply of vegetation improves, the hares can relax, so to speak. Nutrition is now relatively plentiful in relation to the population numbers. The pregnant does are less stressed, and so their offspring are adapted to be less stressed; they do not need to be so vigilant because the chance of being taken by predators is less. But of course more hares bring the predators back; they will thrive and their population numbers will increase. The cycle of life, with its fluctuating population numbers, is repeated.

This example provides evidence that environmental influences happening early in development can have life-long consequences. The maternal stress led to changes in the maturation of the fetal HPA axis, which persisted through life and allowed the progeny to have an altered biochemical/hormonal phenotype that made them more likely to survive and reproduce. As we will see, this phenomenon, by which developmental environmental influences set up permanent changes in the phenotype, is very common.

adrenal gland to make and release cortisol. The pituitary gland is under the control of the hypothalamus. Within the HPA axis are a number of feedback loops (for example cortisol feeds back on the pituitary gland to reduce ACTH release) – the sensitivity of these negative feedback loops can be changed and this is one way of regulating the body's stress responses.

## Maternal Influences

In giving attention to the developing offspring, however, we must not forget the mother. We must remember that our thesis is that the environmental effects that determine the phenotype of the offspring are transmitted (or transduced) through her. So we must be careful here in our use of the term 'environment'. While in the case of the snowshoe hare the environmental influence was transmitted through the placenta, in some cases the mother herself *is* the environmental influence. For example we know that rat pups born to dams that groom their pups more while they are suckling grow into adults with different HPA axis set-points and behavioural responses from those born to dams that groom their pups less. Recently it has been shown that this environmental change is mediated by changes in methylation in a non-imprinted gene coding for a hormone receptor within one region of the brain, which alters the capacity of a transcriptional factor to regulate this receptor – and while this sounds very complex, it serves to illustrate that such adaptive changes in the offspring have a definable structural basis.

Returning to the snowshoe hare it is the mother that is in a position to sense the environment into which her offspring will soon be born – monitoring the plentifulness of food, the population density etc. This initiates a physiological change in her. However, these effects do not (necessarily) produce phenotypic effects on her, but rather send a signal to the embryo or fetus, which will then be translated into developmental adaptive responses reflected in altered phenotype. In addition there may be changes in placental function, including its nutrient transport, metabolism and hormone production, which will also have downstream effects on the fetus.

As discussed in chapter 2, there are many ways and levels in which maternal physiology can profoundly influence the development of the offspring. These influences can occur even under normal situations – that is, independently of signals from the external environment or arising from disease. This is the situation of physiological maternal constraint where the presence of twins, low parity or maternal size can influence fetal nutrient supply. Alternatively the maternal cues to the fetus can arise from extreme external or pathophysiological internal (disease) environmental factors. These influences can occur at any stage in development but increasingly our focus is on the earliest phases when, as discussed earlier, the capacity for plastic responses is greatest. It is important to realise that the change in phenotype need not be immediately apparent at birth – by definition a change in phenotype may only be manifest when the offspring are adult, depending on when the genes that have been affected by the gene–environment interaction are transcribed. They might, for example only be transcribed when the offspring becomes sexually active, or when it is itself challenged in postnatal life. The latter was of course exactly what was observed for the offspring of the snowshoe hare, because the change in the

HPA axis responsiveness only becomes apparent under conditions when the hares might be nervous of predators: kept in a safe environment, such differences would not be evident.

## The fidelity of the prediction

So we have seen how gene–environment interactions can programme long-term phenotype and that this may not be manifest until adulthood; and we have seen that this can be biologically important, at least in animals, in determining the survival of individuals and the maintenance of the population. But our discussion has progressed on the assumption that the choice is made by the fetus and that the fidelity of the information transfer about the environment has been high and that the fetus therefore makes the right choices. But as we discussed, the fidelity of information transfer is not always high – maternal disease can suggest to the fetus that the environment it is going to be born into may be enriched, when it is in fact poor. More frequently the problem occurs the other way round, e.g. because the placenta has malfunctioned the fetus chooses a phenotype appropriate for a poor postnatal environment and yet is born into an enriched environment.

A short-eared rabbit in a hot environment clearly shows how a mismatch can occur between the phenotype and the environment. The same can be true for predictive adaptive responses – the wrong HPA phenotype in the snowshoe hare will reduce the probability of survival, and a naked mole rat that does not have the appropriate energy stores could not survive the long trek to the next colony as a disperser.

## A general model

This leads us to a general model that we will now state and that we will expand in chapter 7. Such models are helpful as ways of encapsulating and summarising large amounts of data. And they are also invaluable when they serve to highlight observations that do not fit the theory and thus lead to new hypotheses, then new studies and thence to new theory.

We can envisage that there might be two forms of predictive adaptive response. In the first the information transmitted from the mother to the developing offspring (as egg, embryo, fetus or neonate) is an accurate predictor of the future environment, and the phenotype resulting is thus one that will aid survival to reproduction. We will call this form of predictive adaptation, *appropriate prediction*. In the other form, because of maternal or placental factors the embryo/fetus misreads its future environment and makes a phenotypic choice that turns out not to be advantageous, or may even be harmful (e.g. a snowshoe hare with a suppressed HPA axis at a time when population density is low is more likely to be eaten). We will term this form of response, *inappropriate prediction.* Clearly the distinction between the two is only possible in retrospect. Our thesis is that the fetus makes its prediction based on the totality of the information it has about its future environment. In general it gets it right and the result is an appropriate PAR. If the environment shifts or if the information it receives has been faulty then an inappropriate PAR will result, even though at the time the choice was made the fetus must assume that its prediction will be appropriate.

Our concept, which we will expand upon in chapter 7, is that PARs are a critical element in determining the survival of a species and thus of a particular gene pool. They are a common element in explaining many aspects of developmental biology. That is why the various strategies of PARs have been preserved across diverse species and through evolutionary time.

In most species we do not consider inappropriate adaptations in much detail because they are likely to be lost to the gene pool early and can be seen in simple Darwinian terms as the losers in the battle for the 'survival of the fittest'. But when we turn to human biology the story is different. Humans have the capacity to adjust to their environment in multiple ways, ranging from complex social structures through to building houses and wearing clothing. Thus, unlike other members of the animal kingdom, a human with inappropriate adaptation is not lost and is likely to be reproductively competent. But, as we shall discuss in chapter 4, such individuals are at a higher risk of disease. This is further accentuated because humans now live long beyond the reproductive phase, and evolutionary selection pressures for appropriate adaptation are much weaker once the reproductive period is over. Thus the consequences of inappropriate prediction are likely to be manifest in middle and old age in the human population, and indeed that is the case. This important component of biology was not recognised or understood until some critical studies were made in humans. And that is the focus of the next chapter.

# 4

# Predictive adaptive responses and human disease

The previous chapter introduced the concept that PARs are a general phenomenon that have evolved because they confer some protective functions in postnatal life. We will return to these questions later, but first can we demonstrate these phenomena exist in humans and, if so, what is their significance? This is the issue that, above all the others, led us to write this book. If PARs exist in humans, they might give us tremendously important insights into human health and indeed human evolution; moreover, they may have extremely important medical implications, for inappropriate PARs might lead to increased risk of disease in later life. The next two chapters present the evidence that this is indeed the case and begin to explore the implications.

## Focusing on populations

Epidemiology is the study of disease patterns in whole populations, and epidemiologists look for correlations and associations that might suggest causal and risk factors. Epidemiology's power is in taking a population-based perspective. This hides individual variation by averaging it out. On the one hand, it will suggest factors that, on average, are likely to contribute to the causal pattern of disease. On the other hand, individual life histories focus on the individual risk of disease. These two very different perspectives must be kept in mind as we consider the role of PARs in the origin of human disease.

One of the most extraordinary facts about our human life expectancy is that it is influenced by the month of our birth. If you are born in the Northern hemisphere in spring you are statistically more likely to live longer than if you are born in autumn. The difference is not great – about 6 months was reported in a study in Austria – but the difference is real. The month of birth that confers greatest longevity is the converse in Australia, which of course has reverse seasons. So if you are an Australian it is good to be born in November and if you are Austrian it is good to be born in May. But if you are Austrian and move to Australia you carry the likelihood associated with the time and place where you were born, not of the place you moved to. These observations were made on very large populations and the epidemiologists who performed them have made sure that they removed from the analysis such confounding[1] variables as the effects of gender, social difference in the season of birth, or greater infant mortality associated with a greater risk of infection in those born at certain times of the year. The analysis is restricted to those who had already reached 50 years of age. The only conclusion that can come from these studies is that there is some set of factors that arise in utero or perhaps in very early infancy that are seasonally influenced and that determine susceptibility to disease in later life. Indeed we know that children born in spring are slightly longer and heavier at birth than those born at other times of year. This simple but surprising observation is very clear evidence that something about early existence does determine the risk of disease in adult life. As will be obvious from our emphasis, we see this as clear evidence that PARs play a role in the origin of disease in humans. Because the major cause of death in people over 50 is heart disease, let us now focus on this.

## Heart disease

For much of the past 30 years medical research in the USA, UK and other Western nations has been focused on the causes of cardiovascular disease. This is not surprising as in such societies over 40 per cent of deaths are caused by heart attacks (myocardial infarction), heart failure and hypertension or stroke – all manifestations of a spectrum of disease that involves loss of distensibility in the arteries and the build-up of fatty and inflammatory deposits in blood vessel walls (atheromatous plaque formation). Such plaques can grow slowly in the blood vessels for many years or decades. They are normally covered by the cells that line the inner surface of the blood vessels, and so do not constitute a problem until they become so large that they obstruct blood flow. The problem is usually picked up from the consequences of poor flow to the heart or brain. However, these atheromatous lesions have a tendency to rupture, for reasons only partly understood, and when this occurs they provide a focus for triggering local blood clotting. Such clots can become detached and are carried downstream to jam in the small arteries. If this occurs in the coronary arteries supplying the heart, a myocardial infarct will occur; if it occurs in

---

[1] Confounding variables are a nightmare for epidemiologists who study population data and try to draw conclusions about risk. Such variables are aspects of the population that are associated with, for example, an increased risk of disease but that are not measured or allowed for in the analysis being made. Ignoring these factors will 'confound' the analysis being undertaken and make any conclusions drawn insecure. If, like the social scientists working in Victorian England, we were to note the link between low social class in cities and disease, we might draw the conclusion that the poorer classes in Britain were of 'poorer genetic stock' – clearly wrong, and partly so because we ignored the confounding effects of poorer diet, overcrowded living conditions and exposure to industrial pollution, which each increase the risk of disease.

the blood vessels to the brain, a stroke will result. Lesser degrees of the build-up of plaque (also termed arteriosclerosis) in other vessels lead to increased resistance to blood flow and high blood pressure (hypertension). Heart failure is frequently the outcome of multiple small ischaemic episodes to the heart or the end result of hypertension overloading the heart's capacity to pump blood.

Increasingly we recognise that cardiovascular disease is accompanied by disorders of blood lipids (fats) and indeed it has been popular to blame cholesterol as the primary cause of vascular disease. However, the problem is much more complex than that, because the cholesterol and other lipids in the blood are associated with specific proteins called lipoproteins, and it is the proportion of lipids associated with each of these kinds of protein that actually determines risk of atheroma. One of the success stories in modern medicine is the use of drugs such as fibrates and statins to lower the levels of dangerous lipids in the blood. This treatment can be life-saving in people who have already had cardiovascular disease and there is compelling evidence that, across the whole population, reducing cholesterol levels with statins confers benefit. Clearly, having high cholesterol is a proximate risk factor[2] for heart disease. However, perhaps it is possible to prevent the development of factors that create a risk of heart disease: for example, truncal obesity (the abdominal fat distribution typical of middle-aged men) or the altered metabolism that gives rise to the high fat levels. Increasingly this causes us to focus not on the adult environment but on the environment of early life.

In the 1980s there was intense interest in identifying the causes of cardiovascular disease. The belief was that this was a so-called 'lifestyle' disease because it seemed to afflict the more affluent societies and it was believed that, by identifying causes, public health measures could be taken to reduce its incidence. Smoking, high cholesterol and a sedentary lifestyle were all identified as risk factors and as potential causative factors. But whatever the explanation, it had to be compatible with the known epidemiology. The problems with the 'lifestyle' concept arose when the risks in populations were examined more closely. Then it was seen that some populations had more cardiovascular disease than others. For example the French appeared to have a low incidence despite having a lifestyle that should lead to more – a fat-rich diet and being relatively sedentary. Indeed the French pattern was so strange it became known as the 'French paradox'. More recently it has been suggested that wine consumption may explain the apparent contradiction but there are other possible explanations – we shall return to these later. It was also clear that non-affluent populations in transition had rapidly rising incidences of heart

---

[2] It is important to separate risk and cause – they are not the same thing. If high blood cholesterol was the *cause* of heart disease, everyone, or nearly everyone, with high cholesterol would get heart disease. High cholesterol is a *risk* factor because having high cholesterol makes it more likely, but not inevitable, that one will get heart disease.

disease or other components of the metabolic syndrome.[3] For example Polynesian migrants to New Zealand had much higher risks once living in New Zealand than they did in Polynesia. The large shifts in population from rural to urban environments in the Indian sub-continent are associated with an increase in cardiovascular disease and the metabolic syndrome of epidemic proportions. Similar trends are being seen in China.

## Shifting the focus from adult to fetus

Perinatal epidemiology had its origins in the 1950s and1960s when epidemiologists started to focus on the factors that influenced maternal and perinatal mortality, and in particular those that influenced birth weight. The latter was used because it is the most reliable measurement taken at birth and because it is known that smaller babies tend to do less well. Some of the conclusions drawn were not surprising – for example smoking reduces birth weight, first babies are smaller than second babies, very young mothers give birth to smaller babies, older mothers have a greater risk of the baby having Down's syndrome, and so on.

But in the late 1980s a new perinatal epidemiological focus arose from quite a different epidemiological origin – the study of the patterns of heart disease in old age. This discovery, its interpretation and its significance, is the subject of this chapter. It will allow us to apply our understanding of PARs to generate new insights into the origins of human disease such as cardiovascular disease and the metabolic syndrome. It will also link the concepts of appropriate and inappropriate responses that we have developed to new ideas about evolutionary biology. It changes our perspective on health policy in both the developed and developing world. We shall return to these themes in later chapters. But it is also an extraordinary story in the history of science. It demonstrates the problems of trying to challenge established dogma and vested interest. It shows the importance of adopting an integrated scientific approach. It is an instructive story and this is why we will tell it in some detail.

## Lifestyle and genes

In the West, the incidence of coronary heart disease rose steeply at the beginning of the twentieth century and it rapidly became the most common cause of death. Its incidence is now rising in other parts of the world, for example in India, China

---

[3] The metabolic syndrome or Syndrome X is the clustering of hypertension or cardiovascular disease, insulin resistance or Type 2 diabetes mellitus, high blood lipid dyslipidaemia and altered blood-clotting factors in a single patient. It is a concerning association suggesting linked causes and is discussed in greater detail in chapter 5.

and South America. The usual explanation for this is the arrival of affluence and considerable improvements in lifestyle for all but the poorest members of the population. This occurred in Western Europe earlier in the twentieth century, with similar trends appearing in developing countries in recent years. Lifestyle factors were therefore invoked to explain the increase in disease. In particular, attention has been focused on the consumption of diets high in saturated fat, smoking, lack of exercise, exposure to environmental pollutants and the 'stress' of modern life. Evidence to support these ideas has grown steadily but it turns out that these factors do not adequately explain the patterns of incidence of heart disease.

Faced with this outcome after very large amounts of research, doctors and scientists have turned to an alternative view, namely that the origins of cardiovascular disease and Type 2 diabetes – another major disease of affluence – are in fact genetic. In other words, that those who develop heart disease carry genes that put them at particular risk. It is of course true that some forms of cardiovascular disease, particularly specific types of congenital heart disease and of high blood-lipid levels have a genetic (i.e. heritable) basis. However they are relatively rare and cannot explain why cardiovascular disease will kill roughly half of the population in the UK at the present time. Nor could a purely genetic origin explain how the incidence of such disease can increase substantially within a generation, as appears to be occurring in India. This is not to say that certain genes do not play a role in determining the predisposition to cardiovascular disease or diabetes – indeed as we shall see some polymorphisms certainly play a role in the development of risk factors such as insulin resistance. But genetics cannot give the whole story.

Perhaps the first clues that the origins of cardiovascular disease might lie earlier in life than previously thought came from the work of Forsdahl in the 1970s, who examined the influence of living conditions in childhood on the incidence of cardiovascular disease in adults living in Finnmark, the most northerly part of Norway where such disease had been lamentably common. Forsdahl found that poor living conditions in childhood were associated with later disease. Many researchers and public health planners have cited these studies, arguing that prevention of poverty in childhood will have far-reaching consequences in society: we shall return to these studies in chapter 9.

But now we need to pursue further the story of the discovery of an early origin to these diseases. The crucial clues came from looking in detail at maps.

## Clues from maps

In the early 1980s David Barker, an epidemiologist from Southampton, and his colleagues were investigating the rates of mortality for coronary heart disease and other vascular diseases in England and Wales over the previous decade (1968–78).

They noticed an extraordinary thing, which was that the highest rates of mortality did not occur in the areas of greatest contemporary affluence, in the South East of Britain for example. In fact the highest rates occurred in the North West and South Wales and in parts of Scotland, areas associated with relatively high unemployment, poor social conditions etc. The fact was alarming because the North/South divide in Britain was widening under a new Conservative government and the rise in cost of health care by the National Health Service made it imperative to target resources effectively. They pondered why a so-called disease of affluence such as coronary heart disease did not seem to occur most frequently in the currently most affluent areas of the country.

A number of possibilities were considered but rejected – including, for example, regional differences in the calcium content of tap water, because calcium was known to be part of the atherotic plaque. However, the rates of heart disease *were* closely associated with the past distribution of infant mortality rates over the country. The association was not with contemporary infant mortality rates, but with this mortality in the early part of the century – at the period when the people, now dying of heart disease, were born. Infant mortality is a sensitive indicator of the general health of the population, particularly of course its young women and children, because mortality level is usually related to the number of infants dying from infection, malnutrition and poor environmental conditions. Barker suggested that this correlation, spanning events over 70 years apart in time, might be causal – that is heart disease might have a partial origin in early life.

Was it that people born in relatively poor conditions around the turn of the century were at greater risk of heart disease – the disease of affluence – in later life regardless of the level of affluence that they had actually achieved as adults? Could it possibly be true that the risk of a disease that usually affects older members of the population was in fact determined by what had happened to those people much earlier in their lives? It was a question that had to be pursued further, if only because the geographical data for differences in mortality ratio for coronary heart disease revealed that the differences were large – greater than those produced by smoking, high salt intake etc. Geography seemed much more important than lifestyle.

How could this question be pursued? The observed association was so remote, and it was so likely to be influenced by confounding factors that were not quantifiable. The next step was to move from gross correlations over integrated populations and across time to a specific population where individuals could be studied. What was needed was a set of records about the growth and development of children in the early part of the century that could be linked specifically to the causes of death in later life. With the assistance of an archivist, Barker and his colleagues scoured Britain for records about birth and infancy, dating from the early part of the century. They of course found many such records, but most were incomplete or scanty in

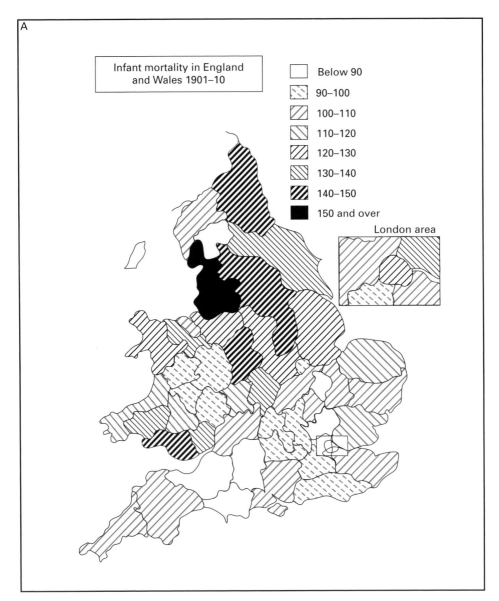

Fig. 4.1    Maps of the UK showing infant mortality rates from 1901 to 1910 (A) and the incidence of coronary heart disease (CHD) from 1968 to 1978 (B), as used by Barker and coworkers in formulating the fetal origins of adult disease hypothesis. Note that the areas of highest incidence of CHD are not in the areas currently most affluent, such as the South East, but in areas such as the North West, which had high infant mortality in the early years of the twentieth century. Data from Registrar General's Statistical, Review of England and Wales and from M. J. Gardner *et al. Atlas of Mortality from Selected Diseases in England and Wales 1968–78* (1984), John Wiley, Chichester. Figures redrawn from D. J. P. Barker, 1998.

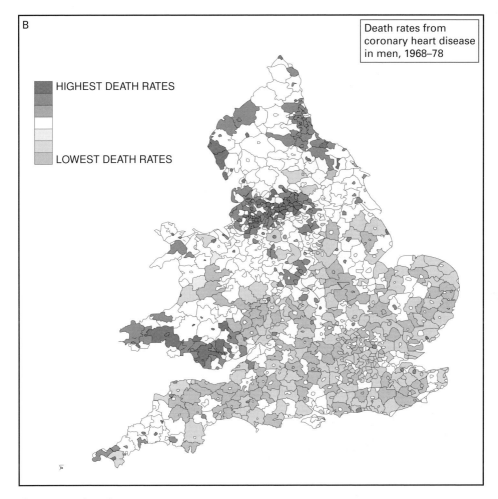

Fig. 4.1 (cont.)

detail and many had been stored in conditions such as sheds or basements where they had deteriorated.

The largest set of records that were found related to the county of Hertfordshire. These included weight at birth, weight at one year of age and whether the baby was weaned at one year. The ledgers were maintained from 1911 to 1945. Barker and his colleagues used the National Health Service Central Register at Southport to trace approximately 16 000 men and women born in Hertfordshire between 1911 and 1930, and to determine their cause of death. The results – first published in 1989 – were astonishing and caused furore and controversy within the medical community. What they had found, for both men and women, was that risk of death from heart disease was doubled in individuals born with a weight of less than 5.5 lb(2.5 kg) compared to those born with a weight of more than 9.5 lb(4.0 kg).

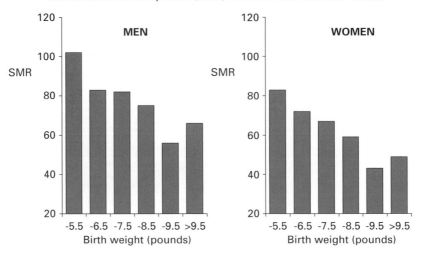

**Coronary heart disease**

Standardised mortality ratios (SMR) in 10 141 men and 5585 women

Fig. 4.2     Bar graphs showing the incidence of coronary heart disease in adults born in Hertfordshire in the early/mid twentieth century, in relation to their birth weight. The risk of heart disease increases in a graded manner across the normal range of birth weights in both men and women. Redrawn from C. Osmond *et al.*, *British Medical Journal* (1993) **307**: 1519–24.

The interesting thing is that the results were graded across the birth-weight range. In other words, they were not simply caused by strong effects produced by overweight babies at one extreme or underweight babies at the other – there was a continuum of changed risk across all birth weights. In fact the data did not really relate to pathologically small or pathologically large babies as these were relatively few in number in the sample:[4] more than 95 per cent of all the births fell within the range 5.5–9.5 lb. In other words, these were healthy and apparently normal infants but those weighing 8 lb at birth had a lower risk of heart disease than those apparently healthy babies born weighing 7.5 lb, who had a lower risk than those born weighing only 7 lb, and so on down the birth-weight scale. The graded nature of the effect provides an important clue. It suggests that whatever causes the high risk of future heart disease, it is in some way related to the choices the fetus had made in setting its growth trajectory. The more severe or the more long-lasting the set of environmental influences have been in utero, the greater the degree of shift in birth size. If in some way heart disease is related to the degree of this shift, then we would expect birth weight (or other measures of the fetal environment) to be related to the risk of heart disease in a continuous way. If however the relationship

---

[4] See chapter 6 for further comment.

was only owing to some severe pathology, e.g. to a gene defect or exposure to a toxic agent, we would expect the relationship only to be present in those individuals showing the extreme patterns of fetal growth: this is not what was found.

The Hertfordshire studies did not stop simply with birth weight, because there was also information about placental size at birth. Since it has been known for many years that the placenta can increase its growth in a compensatory way, for example in animals and humans living at high altitude where the air is thinner and oxygen supply is lower, it was of interest to look at placental size in Hertfordshire. Putting this together with birth weight made the links with adult disease even stronger – because it was those men and women who were relatively small at birth *and* who had relatively large placentas who were at greater risk. It appeared as if the story of reduced fetal growth (coupled with an attempt by the placenta to compensate) and an increased risk of disease in later life were all coming together.

The first publications from this study were not met with enthusiasm by those who believed that the origins of cardiovascular disease, diabetes and the metabolic syndrome lay in lifestyle factors such as diet, exercise and even socio-economic status. The fact that Barker and his colleagues found that, even allowing for such confounding factors, the association between small size at birth and high risk of heart disease in later life persisted, did not alter the situation. The studies were criticised as flawed, as implausible and as not giving sufficient recognition to widely accepted current dogma. The antagonism between Barker's group and other cardiovascular epidemiologists who were committed to adult lifestyle-focused explanations was intense. The fact that Barker did not deny a role for lifestyle factors was irrelevant – indeed from the outset his studies had demonstrated an interaction between prenatal and postnatal factors, in that those born small who later became obese were at greatest risk, while in those who remained thin the risk was reduced. The matter was exacerbated when further studies demonstrated that it was not just the incidence of heart disease that was related inversely to birth weight but that so was the incidence of Type 2 diabetes, high blood lipids and the metabolic syndrome. This extension of the relationship to other diseases rang of implausibility to the critics.

## The founding hypothesis

Barker did not attempt to define the biological basis of the relationship – indeed such definitions are not possible from retrospective epidemiological studies – but he concluded that a poor fetal experience altered development in such a way that, on one hand, growth was affected and, on the other, the propensity to develop disease in later life was changed. He adopted the term 'programming'[5], which had been coined by Alan Lucas to reflect the later consequences of altering infant nutrition. Subsequently, in association with Nick Hales of Cambridge, Barker developed a teleological argument that became known as the 'thrifty phenotype' hypothesis to explain this phenomenon.[6] This hypothesis is in many ways the forerunner of the ideas presented in this book. The concept was that in some way the programme of development had been altered and that, once altered, this determined the individual's risk of disease in later life. The thrifty phenotype argument was uni-directional, in that it suggested that the fetus adjusts its biology in response to the poor nutritional signals from mother so that it is best equipped to live in a relatively poor postnatal nutritional environment. This was the starting point for our own thinking, but as we shall see it is only one perspective, a subset of the much broader biological phenomenon of PARs.

Barker's group looked at other populations but there were few data sets where long-term disease outcome could be related to birth size. So they turned to relating birth size to measurement in younger people of blood pressure, as a surrogate marker of the future development of potential hypertension and heart disease. Many studies were then performed by them and other groups, showing relationships between blood pressure and birth weight, and again these showed a continuum across all birth weights. However it is important to note that blood pressure is not the same as hypertension. Hypertension is a pathological state requiring therapy and it eventually became clear that the major statistical relationships were between birth weight and disease states, and less so with the intermediate measures such as blood pressure. The failure of some subsequent commentators to appreciate this distinction unfortunately led to confusion and uninformed criticism.

The same sets of studies soon showed comparable relationships between birth size and the risks of Type 2 or adult onset diabetes or its precursor, insulin resistance. In contrast to the insulin-dependent diabetes of childhood, in which the pancreatic islet cells are injured by an anti-immune response leading to a shortage of insulin, Type 2 diabetes is caused by the tissues (fat, muscle and liver) where insulin acts becoming insulin resistant. This generally starts to occur in middle age and is compounded by obesity and, at some point, altered control of blood glucose. There are many possible explanations for the linkage between insulin resistance and cardiovascular disease: indeed insulin resistance is commonly associated with hypertension. The clustered association of insulin resistance (or Type 2 diabetes)

---

[5] See footnote 26 in chapter 1.

[6] It was so-named to contrast with the concept of the 'thrifty genotype' first proposed by J. V. Neel in 1962. This hypothesis suggested that adult-onset diabetes had a primarily genetic origin. It had evolved by differential selection to favour populations who were capable of living in a thrifty environment. We return to this concept in more detail in chapter 5.

and hypertension (or cardiovascular disease) is common and is called Syndrome X or the metabolic syndrome.

There were additional problems. In the growing number of confirmatory epidemiological studies, a range of measures of birth size was examined, including length of the baby and other body dimensions. These variables appeared to be associated in different populations with different pathological conditions in adult life, and this raised further questions. It is worth noting some of them, in order to help us understand the nature of the problem. Why did long, lean babies have a different outcome to short, fat babies? Did babies with a small head in relation to overall body size have a different risk of later disease from those with appropriately proportioned heads? Why was it that in one study higher blood pressure was associated with lower birth weight, and in another with altered length? Did things such as ponderal index (ratio of weight to length – a measure of obesity) or placental weight matter? To the sceptics the plethora of relationships that were emerging appeared to be the result of a well-known statistical phenomenon by which, if many comparisons are made, they will inevitably lead to some significant associations being found. Could valid conclusions be drawn, and did the range of relationships reveal something about the nature and timing of the intrauterine insult? Was poor fetal growth itself somehow the cause of the high blood pressure in adulthood, or was it that fetal biology was altered by some event, or by some genes, such that birth size was affected on one hand and, independently, physiology was altered on the other, leading to conditions such as high blood pressure in adults?

There was no way of answering questions such as these from the epidemiological data alone. Studies were needed to test this novel idea experimentally, and this would have to be done in animals, as it would not be ethical in humans. To a large extent, animals do not suffer from the same chronic diseases as humans, e.g. heart disease or diabetes. But if it could be shown that fetal adversity was linked to hypertension or glucose intolerance/insulin resistance in animal experiments, then the epidemiological associations could not so easily be dismissed as spurious.

## Proof in animals

As it turned out, this challenge to the experimental biologists came at an opportune time. Developmental and fetal physiology was in the doldrums in the late 1980s and early 1990s. The methods employed were expensive and labour intensive and, even more important, involved taking a multidisciplinary approach to the subject. Few fetal physiologists, for example, worked only on one body system: whether their prime interest was neural development or cardiovascular function, they had also to be endocrinologists, behaviouralists, metabolic biochemists, and so on. This integrative approach to science was at increasing odds with the 'reductionist methodology' that was becoming the norm for most science following the revolution in molecular and cellular biology, and funding bodies were increasingly unwilling to provide support for such integrative studies. In addition, the prospect of decoding the genome had led to claims that all developmental processes could be described in terms of the genetic programme and that fetal physiology was passé. The distinction between genotype and phenotype was seldom made, and the consequences of this narrow focus were little appreciated. Many developmental physiologists were therefore finding it hard to maintain their research groups. It is easy to see why they so readily took up the challenge of determining whether the 'programming' processes could also be seen in experimental animals.

Their first question was what kind of prenatal disturbance should be used experimentally to try and induce programming. The physiologists knew that any effect on birth size usually had its origin in some disturbance to the supply of nutrients to the fetus, be it because of maternal undernutrition, maternal disease or placental dysfunction. To the experimentalist, the fetus might perceive any of these insults as a reduced supply of nutrients, so an approach that achieved reduced nutrient supply would be appropriate. The most obvious starting point would be nutritional manipulation of the mother.

The initial studies were performed in rats. If the rat fetus was undernourished in utero, simply because the pregnant dam was fed a reduced caloric or just an unbalanced (e.g. a low-protein) diet, it grew up to become hypertensive as an adult. These adult rats were also shown to have insulin resistance and to live less long than those whose mothers had been fed a balanced diet in pregnancy.[7] The effect was magnified if the rat was placed on a high-fat diet after birth – echoing the human data and demonstrating that the interaction between the fetal and postnatal environments determined outcome. Other studies showed that the maternal cue did not need to be nutritional – exposing mothers to a high dose of a glucocorticoid (a cortisol-like drug) produced similar effects on the offspring.

But rats were somewhat problematic animals to focus on. For one thing they could not be studied as fetuses, and a key question that needed to be answered was the nature of the fetal response to the altered maternal environment. This meant studying the fetal response to a known stimulus, as well as following up the offspring postnatally. Measuring fetal responses was only technically feasible in a large animal such as the sheep, and expertise in this physiology was becoming a rarity. Nonetheless the crucial observations were made: dietary imbalance during pregnancy in the ewe resulted in fetal sheep with altered blood pressure, endothelial function and stress responses in late gestation, and higher blood pressure after birth. Some of these features could be reproduced by reduction of placental size, which mimicked

---

[7] Further studies from the authors' groups in Southampton and Auckland have shown that these rat offspring have many of the features of the metabolic syndrome: they have vascular endothelial dysfunction, obesity and altered appetite. The possible mechanistic basis for these phenomena are discussed later.

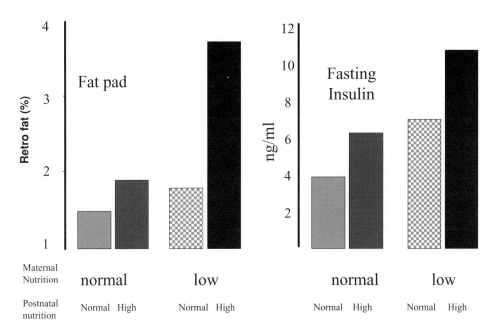

Fig. 4.3    Experimental evidence of the induction of the programming of obesity and insulin resistance (measured as higher fasting insulin levels) in rats. Half the mothers were subjected to undernutrition while pregnant, and half were fed a normal diet; the offspring of both groups were then fed a normal diet or a high-fat diet after weaning. Both-undernutrition in utero and a high-fat diet after birth gave a degree of obesity in the adult offspring; the combination had a far greater effect (left panel). Similar effects were seen when fasting blood-insulin levels were measured (right panel). Prenatal induction leads to sensitisation of the postnatal gene–environmental interaction. Very similar results were seen for blood pressure measurements. Data redrawn from Vickers *et al.* 2000.

the reduced nutrition of altered maternal diet, or by giving the pregnant ewe stress hormones for a short period in early gestation. Thus the fetal physiologists produced data in which various forms and timing of nutritional or hormonal manipulation in the pregnant ewe altered fetal biology, with respect to control of blood pressure, glucose metabolism or stress responses. Physiologists really wanted to show that as adults these animals went on to have pathological changes that were reminiscent of the metabolic syndrome in humans, but this meant keeping the animals for years after birth, which made getting funding for the experiments difficult, although eventually enough long-term data were obtained to be convincing.[8]

Gradually the scientific community began to recognise that the 'programming' phenomenon was real and could be observed in a variety of species including

---

[8] These were indeed complex and expensive experiments. They involved many animals, as only singleton fetuses could be studied (twins and singletons grow along different trajectories) and each gender needed to be considered separately. One of our groups (PDG) started talking about the sheep as the 'golden sheep' – we reckoned the experimental protocol meant they had cost their weight in gold!

sheep, pigs, guinea pigs, rats and mice. Something else also began to emerge from these studies. This was the realisation that, even though the experimentalists had started out by trying to show that reduced birth weight in lambs was associated with altered fetal and postnatal cardiovascular and metabolic function, in reality such effects could be achieved by *mild* prenatal nutritional challenges that did not always reduce birth weight. This strengthened the interpretation of epidemiological observations in humans still further, because it became clear that birth size itself was not necessarily on the causal pathway for later pathophysiology.

The experimentalists were now convinced that their data were entirely compatible with the human data. This was close to formal proof of the existence of a link between the fetal environment and postnatal environmental adaptation. Because the phenomenon could be reproduced in several species and, in each case, within narrowly confined populations with little genetic variation, then the inference was clear – this was a general biological phenomenon and it was likely to be as true for humans as for other mammals. Such studies did not attempt to show that nutritional insults were the only basis of the human phenomenon but clearly the crucial question had been answered – a biological phenomenon existed. The next step was to establish the fundamental mechanisms underlying the phenomenon, to address issues of whether diverse stimuli acted via final common pathways and to define the nature of the critical window for the responses. This new phase of research is still very much ongoing – we will return to it in chapter 5.

## Further epidemiological studies

There were soon a large number of studies published by many independent groups that confirmed the founding epidemiological observation. All over the world, populations with birth records that could now be studied were found. The number of studies published grew to over a hundred. Most showed a relationship between birth weight and the development of hypertension, heart disease or diabetes in the adult population, but some negative studies were also reported. Virtually all of these negative studies had limitations – many had used either prematurity or multiple pregnancy or extremes in birth weight in drawing their associations, or had involved very small groups of subjects – all confounding influences that had to be carefully handled.

But two very important sets of positive data came to the fore – one from Finland, and some very large studies from the USA. Finland has currently one of the highest rates of death from coronary heart disease and other forms of cardiovascular disease and a high rate of adult-onset diabetes mellitus. There were a superb set of data in Finland, dating back to before the Second World War, since for many years people in Scandinavian countries have been issued with social security numbers that are linked to records about their birth, their growth in childhood, their schooling and of course their subsequent health and disease. As these data relate essentially to the whole population, the analyses that can be conducted are very sensitive, and even small effects, which might not be present in smaller samples, become clear in such large populations. As it turned out however, the data from Finland did not show small effects at all. Indeed they demonstrated very large effects. Importantly they showed that the blood pressure–birth weight relationship, while present, was even stronger when restricted to those individuals with clinical hypertension.

But for those working in medical research outside the USA, it sometimes appears that nothing in medical science becomes properly accepted until it has been Americanised. American medical research is so dominant that until similar data are found in North America, it is unlikely to be accepted as mainstream. One problem was that perinatal science and the fetal origins field had been dominated by non-Americans. Then in 1998, a study was published involving an analysis of the health of some 100 000 American nurses. It turned out that blood pressure in nurses was predicted by birth weight: the world's biggest powerhouse of medical research could no longer ignore the phenomenon.

So much for 'Western' countries where the 'diseases of affluence' such as coronary heart disease are relatively common. What about looking at the problem the other way round – to examine the story in countries where birth weight itself is low? Since these countries are usually relatively poor, the incidence of coronary heart disease will be low, although it is rising where the countries are undergoing rapid transition to a Western diet. Do the ideas about developmental origins of disease still apply? Studies were therefore conducted in the Indian sub-continent. Here the average birth weight is almost a kilogram lighter than in the UK. Nonetheless the association between low birth weight and risk of coronary heart disease was found. In addition, links with low maternal weight during pregnancy also emerged. Similar observations have been made in other Third World countries such as China, parts of the West Indies and in South America.

## An experiment of history

Barker had been impressed by the experimentalists' ability to mimic the human epidemiological observations by manipulating the nutrition of animals during pregnancy, and he looked for examples in recent human history where there had been exposure to undernutrition in pregnancy. The rationale was that if the imposition of a severe insult on a population produced consequences on the next generation, then it would be very difficult to view the effect purely in terms of a genetic effect. The telling example was the so-called Dutch Hunger Winter of 1944/45 which we referred to in chapter 2. In November 1944 the Nazi occupiers of Holland had imposed severe rationing on the Western Netherlands population in reprisal for resistance activity. The mean caloric intake, which had been relatively good (1800–2000 calories per day) prior to the imposition of severe rationing, fell to below 800 calories per day. The rationing restrictions were to last seven months and were only relieved when the Allies liberated Holland. Despite the rigours of war, many Dutch hospitals continued to maintain good birth records. They were later to analyse the data and show that those mothers who had been undernourished late in pregnancy gave birth to smaller babies; those whose mothers were undernourished in early pregnancy were of normal size at birth, although as we shall see they were not protected from the consequences of in utero famine exposure. While the numbers followed up were relatively small, relationships appeared that gave strength to the general developmental origins of disease model. Fetuses undernourished early in pregnancy were more likely to develop insulin resistance and obesity although there was a greater risk from being undernourished at any time in pregnancy. Yet those who were undernourished during the first part of pregnancy did not have a reduced birth weight, showing that it was the environmental miscue acting early in pregnancy, rather than fetal growth itself, that was associated with later disease. While it is tempting to conclude that this proves the point about the role of nutrition, there are confounding influences – war is a time of great stress, and steroid hormone levels in the mothers must frequently have been very high.

## Clinical proof

One criticism of Barker's work and of other epidemiological studies was that they had been *retrospective* studies. Such studies have inherent limitations in that they can only consider data that were collected many years ago, without regard to the present investigation. In contrast, *prospective* studies are designed to answer a specific question – this is the preferred scientific method.

All sorts of biases can creep into retrospective studies and for this reason they are viewed with extreme caution. They can suggest answers, but usually all they do is to point to a direction that prospective studies could follow. An analogy is a 5-year-old car. If you have owned a car from new you know everything about it; but if you buy it secondhand, you can never be absolutely certain about some important things: whether it has been regularly serviced, whether it has been in an accident, whether it has been poorly driven etc. You infer answers to these questions from inspecting the car and assessing the person who sells it to you, but you will never be 100 per cent certain. Some biological questions can only be considered retrospectively – for example evolution is largely a matter of retrospective analysis of the fossil record, and prospective data, while supportive, cannot revisit biological history. Obviously it was not going to be possible to perform prospective clinical studies on birth size in a new cohort of individuals who would be followed for 60 or 70 years to see if they developed hypertension or heart disease. But it was possible to prospectively study groups of children to see whether they had any early evidence of cardiovascular or metabolic dysfunction related to birth size.

A variety of studies were performed. In one study[9] children who had been born small and who were now 6–8 years old were compared to children who were born of normal size. For statistical validity there was careful matching of the two groups of children for height, weight, age and relative obesity. Sophisticated measures of insulin sensitivity were used, and the results were dramatic. All the children born small were insulin resistant and none of those of normal birth size were. The degree of insulin resistance related to the degree of fetal growth retardation. Other studies conducted in Italy and France led to very similar conclusions.

But these studies were performed in children who were born abnormally small and this might also be a problem. It was not certain that children born at the extreme of birth weights, primarily as a result of maternal or placental disease, and children with birth weights within the normal range represented a biological continuum. Could it be that the former represented the consequences of a pathological intrauterine environment with outcomes that contrasted with those born within the normal birth range? This distinction was important because Barker's conclusions were based on data sets of children born largely within the normal birth size range. This was because very small babies (caused by either prematurity or intrauterine growth retardation) had a poor survival rate in the early twentieth century, the period in which the Hertfordshire and Preston babies on whom Barker had data were born. Similarly there had been historical shifts in the survival of infants of diabetic mothers – the source of most large babies at birth. It was therefore vital to bring the epidemiological observations into a contemporary context, and this meant performing prospective studies.

Several prospective studies of cohorts of children were initiated in England and India. Data were collected from before birth and the offspring were studied through childhood. India was particularly interesting as the incidence of Type 2 diabetes was very high and it occurred at a young age. Maternal undernutrition and fetal growth restriction were commonplace. Indeed the mean birth weight of the population in villages in southern India was only about 2500 gm (30 per cent less than in Europe) and women often weighed less that 45 kg when pregnant. Nonetheless these prospective studies showed very similar relationships between birth size and subsequent measures of blood pressure control and carbohydrate metabolism and those that Barker had reported in his retrospective studies. Now the evidence was not only retrospective but also prospective and consistent – something about fetal

---

[9]  Performed in PDG's laboratory

life that was reflected in birth size influenced cardiovascular and metabolic status after birth and thus linked fetal development to disease risk in adult life.

## Gene–environment interactions

At the same time other researchers were less enamoured with the concept that environmental factors could have such a dominant influence on disease patterns. This was the era of the gene and surely any prenatal effects were likely to be the product of genetic variation. They argued that it was not a 'thrifty phenotype' but a 'thrifty genotype' that mattered. They suggested that natural selection had been at work and had selected polymorphisms that would be reflected *both* in reduced birth size *and* in a greater risk of disease. This was untenable to the experimentalists who had shown effects in one generation of animals independent of genetic variation.

Such a conclusion does not rule out a possible role for the 'thrifty genotype' concept. Indeed given the various genetic bottlenecks that humans have passed through since they migrated out of Africa about 65 000 years ago, it is inevitable that some genetic alleles will have been selected that favour thrift in a poor environment. As we shall discuss in chapter 8, an uncertain nutritional environment has been the norm through much of our evolutionary history. Obviously for prehominids to have survived and evolved, selection must have favoured retention of genes that assist in such environments.

Two points need to be reiterated. First, genes do not work in isolation from the current environment and, while we cannot do anything about our genes, we can do much about our environment. Second, the point which is the focus of this book is that gene–environment interactions early in development induce PARs that, in turn, determine the nature of the postnatal gene–environment interaction. These two interactions are the proximate cause of interest and such PAR mechanisms operate on any genotype, although particular genotypes may influence the degree and nature of the particular interaction. Indeed evidence was soon found that polymorphisms could alter the individual sensitivity of a fetus to its prenatal environment or affect the magnitude of the PAR made. The finding of such relationships gave strong support to the emerging theory that environmental influences before birth have long-term consequences.

As we have already suggested and shall detail in the next chapter, the relationship that had been found between birth weight and risk of adult heart disease had also been found for risk of Type 2 diabetes. Insulin was also known to be involved in the regulation of fetal growth. In a study from Finland it was found that certain polymorphisms determined whether the relationship between birth size and the risk of diabetes in later life was weak or strong. A gene was found that coded for a protein called peroxisome proliferator-activated receptor (PPAR) gamma 2, involved in a pathway determining insulin's action inside a cell[10], and which itself could be considered a 'thrifty gene'. When the incidence of PPAR polymorphism was analysed using samples of the DNA from the Finnish cohort, it was found (as expected) that the polymorphism was associated with higher levels of fasting blood insulin in the subjects, an indicator of Type 2 diabetes. It was also found, again as expected, that lower birth weight was associated with higher fasting blood insulin levels. But the really striking observation was that the specific genotype determined the nature of the interaction, namely that the effect of having been smaller at birth on the level of blood insulin in adult life was only seen in the subjects with the PPAR polymorphism. The other subjects, without the polymorphism, did not show a relationship between their birth weight and adult insulin level.

Here then was the definitive evidence that gene–environment interactions occur in the programming of disease in humans, as was predicted from studies in animals. The studies showed that, in the presence of a gene polymorphism that made insulin resistance more likely, the birth size–insulin relationship was apparent. In the absence of that polymorphism there was no such relationship. This made sense because environmental factors do not act in isolation from genetic factors – indeed environmental factors operate by interacting with the genome. It was clear that, at least in this population, whatever was the adverse fetal event causing a reduction in birth weight, its effect in leading to insulin resistance was magnified by the genetic polymorphism. Thus it appears that, with respect to the risk of human disease, the early-life environmental effects may be magnified or reduced by individual genotype.

## The role of the postnatal environment

From the outset of this research, the importance of the interaction between birth size and current weight was recognised. The incidence of diabetes and heart disease was much higher in those born small who become fat than in those who stayed thin. Being born large (provided it was not owing to gestational diabetes – see chapter 8) appeared to be associated with a lower risk of developing diabetes or hypertension even if one became relatively fat as an adult. Studies in both India and England showed that, even in children, the highest blood pressures were seen in children who were born small and were now growing the fastest. During the 1990s the discussion increasingly focused on the issue of whether the important precursor to disease was the intrauterine environment as evidenced by being born smaller,

---

[10] Peroxisome proliferator-activated receptor (PPAR) gamma-2 is involved in the way cells respond to fatty acids and to local hormones. This is important in regulating lipid metabolism and insulin sensitivity in many cells, especially fat cells and skeletal muscle. One form of the PPARγ-2 position 12 polymorphism is associated with a high risk of Type 2 diabetes in adults but only if born small.

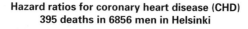

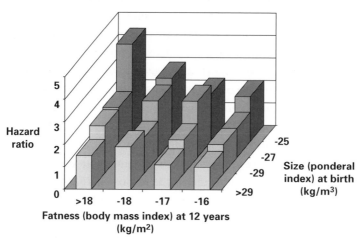

Fig. 4.4     Data from the Finnish epidemiology study showing that risk of CHD is increased both with small size at birth and with greater fatness in childhood. Displayed in this way, the data also show that these factors interact – the highest risk of heart disease occurs in those people who were small at birth *and* then became relatively fat in childhood. Data drawn from J. G. Eriksson *et al.*, *British Medical Journal* (2001) **323**, 572–3.

or whether it was the catch-up growth that generally followed lower birth weight. At the very least it appeared that growing fast or becoming fat after birth was an aggravating factor. This was an important point because this observation would bring compatibility with the traditional view that postnatal dietary and other lifestyle factors were important elements in the development of heart disease and diabetes.

Experimental studies provided the proof. Using rats, we (PDG) demonstrated the role of both an antenatal challenge and postnatal amplification. If fetal rats were exposed to maternal undernutrition, as adults they developed insulin resistance and hypertension. But if after weaning they were also exposed to a high-fat diet the level of hypertension and insulin resistance was much greater. Indeed as we will see we went further to suggest that the full spectrum of the 'couch potato' syndrome[11] could be explained by a combination of an antenatal event coupled with postnatal amplification.

The rationale behind these observations will be discussed in chapters 7 and 8. The observations supported the general model that was evolving. The fetal adaptations made in response to the altered maternal environment were such that the fetus anticipated living after birth in a deprived environment. Accordingly it expected to

---

[11] The only part of the syndrome that escaped us was that we could not demonstrate that the rats had a preference for a TV remote control!

stay small and had adapted its development to match. However, if it was born into a nutritionally bountiful environment it might accelerate its growth and become obese. In either case a mismatch would be set up between fetal expectations and postnatal reality. This predisposed for so-called 'lifestyle' diseases to be exhibited.

It is important to reiterate that this phenomenon occurred in humans across the full range of birth sizes. It was not just a phenomenon of the extremes. While it is easier to describe the phenomenon in terms of smallness at birth, the reality is that a neonate weighing 4.0 kg at birth, who should have been 4.2 kg but for the impact of adverse intrauterine circumstances, is just as likely to be affected as a neonate destined to be 3.0 kg but born weighing 2.8 kg. The only difference is that more babies born weighing 2.8 kg are growth restricted than are those born weighing 4 kg. Nevertheless that is partially why the relationship holds across the full range of birth sizes. The remainder of the explanation is detailed in chapter 8.

The Finnish studies referred to above revealed some other interesting aspects – especially that the pattern of childhood growth mattered. All children have a distinct pattern of fat development – they become relatively fat in the first year (unless malnourished) then become relatively thin between 2 and 4 years of life. They then again start to put on fat before puberty – a phenomenon known as *adiposity rebound*. The earlier and the faster this rebound occurs the greater the risk of disease. As we will discuss in chapter 6 we speculate that these patterns themselves may have their origin before birth.

## Dealing with controversy

By the time we wrote this book, the field of developmental origins of adult disease research had grown extensively – nearly 500 scientists attended the first international congress on the subject held in Mumbai, India in 2001 and over 650 attended the second in Brighton, UK in 2003. Yet despite overwhelming evidence to support a role for early-life environmental effects, scepticism remained. This was most evident in the approaches of two leading medical journals, the *British Medical Journal* and *The Lancet*. The former appeared to encourage papers about developmental origins of disease research and the latter did not. In turn their editorials reflected these attitudes. Unfortunately no forum was really created to allow an objective discussion to take place. *The Lancet* enunciated a sceptical if not outright negative view but did not encourage a robust intellectual debate through its correspondence columns. There were those who wondered whether medical objectivity was being replaced by the journalistic imperative. A negative paper in the *Lancet* largely ignored the substantive epidemiological data, the prospective clinical data and the extensive experimental data. The evolutionary perspective was totally overlooked. Indeed the criticism had failed to appreciate the significance of what had been observed.

The major criticism in that paper was epidemiological, and it was suggested that the epidemiologists had over-interpreted their data. Surprisingly, however, the data referred to were not the core observations between early life experience, as reflected in birth size, and the risk of adult disease, but the relationship between birth weight and later blood pressure. The critical *Lancet* paper flagged up the small size of the effect of low birth weight on adult blood pressure – about 1 mm Hg per kg decrease in birth weight. As we have already noted, elevated blood pressure may indicate some underlying cardiovascular disease, but it is not the disease *itself*. Indeed in the studies emphasised in the *Lancet* paper, that point was obvious. In a study of over 22 000 American males in middle age, there was a very weak relationship between birth size and absolute blood pressure, but there was a very strong increase in the risk of hypertension and diabetes with decreasing birth weight. The majority of the studies examining the relation between birth weight and later blood pressure studied people below middle age. Blood pressure increases along a curve throughout life, and more steeply so in people with overt hypertension. But a single point measurement in young middle age will not allow us to discriminate between people who will remain normotensive and those who will become hypertensive – this is of course why doctors are so keen on measuring blood pressure repeatedly in their patients.

We have already discussed the point that birth weight is not a very good measure of fetal growth, still less of the fetal predictive adaptive responses to a prenatal challenge. This is because many such adaptations can occur without a change in growth, and also because birth weight is determined more by growth in late gestation, while the challenges that the offspring must face are often manifest in the embryonic period. Birth weight is even more unreliable in historical cohorts, which were the mainstay of the epidemiological studies criticised. For example, one charge was that the relation between birth weight and later blood pressure, if a real phenomenon, should become statistically stronger the larger the size of the cohort examined – the larger the number of people studied, the smaller the overall error etc. Unfortunately, however, this argument ignored the fact that birth weight in the largest studies was self-reported (i.e. remembered by the adult subjects),[12] while in the smaller ones it had actually been recorded at the time of birth. Taking all these points together it is clear that we cannot infer very much from the size of the relation between birth weight and later blood pressure. In fact we remain surprised that any significant relation could be found between birth size and disease risk. It is fortuitous that it was, or else an important biological phenomenon may never have been recognised. That the relationship exists at all indicates that the underlying biological phenomenon must be very strong.

---

[12]  And there is objective evidence that people remember their birth weight quite erroneously.

The other commonly expressed criticism of the developmental origins of disease theory was that studies of twins failed to demonstrate the association between lower birth weight and later disease. Twin studies are often used in developmental biology because both twins are argued to have similar experiences in utero and postnatally. Twin studies are therefore used to discriminate factors that are genetic from those that are environmental by examining the difference between identical and non-identical twins. However in this case the critics suggested that, because the lighter twin did not have a higher incidence of hypertension, the theory was wrong. This shows a misunderstanding of the processes controlling fetal growth, because both fetuses will inevitably have been constrained in their shared environment, and more so than for a singleton fetus. Indeed, data have just been published showing that both twins are induced to have insulin resistance in childhood, with the associated risk of later disease, irrespective of their birth weights. Again this makes the point that it is the fetal experience, not the birth weight, that is important.

We believe that the concept of the developmental origins of disease, which started with Lucas' view of programming in infants and almost simultaneously with Barker's hypothesis of the fetal origins of adult disease, and which is now encapsulated in the theory of PARs, has stood the test of time, of experimental verification and of hostile criticism. The overwhelming strength of the experimental, clinical, epidemiological and comparative data mean that it can no longer be ignored as a major determinant of health and disease.

## The theoretical basis

The earliest observations were accompanied by attempts to place them into a meaningful or teleological context. The thrifty phenotype hypothesis provided a first answer to the question of why processes might exist by which a fetally deprived organism might have an altered biology best suited for a postnatally deprived environment. But the argument did not extend to more general components of the relationship. It also implied a uni-directional mechanism. But as we considered the scope of the experimental and clinical data and explored the insights from comparative biology, it became clear to us that the observations first made by Barker and his colleagues were one demonstration of a much broader set of general biological principles, which we have termed PARs.

Early in life-be it in embryonic, fetal or perhaps neonatal-anticipatory changes in phenotype can be induced by the interaction between the genome and the environment. If the prediction is right, this phenotype develops to allow the animal/human to grow and develop optimally (in reproductive terms) after birth. If the fetal prediction of the future environment is wrong, either because of maternal/placental factors (often reflected in poor fetal growth) or if the postnatal environment is grossly different from that anticipated, then the risk of the offspring being unable to meet the challenges of that environment is increased.

This is not an all-or-nothing phenomenon and indeed it can operate in either direction. It becomes a major factor in determining the risk of disease, particularly in the post-reproductive phase when evolutionary pressures cannot generate additional protective mechanisms. The latter part of this book will focus on these broader principles, but before we do so, we should consider other diseases that might arise from such processes.

# 5

# Obesity, diabetes and other diseases

The previous chapter focused on the early-life antecedents of hypertension and heart disease. First, this was where the epidemiological story started and as a result most clinical and experimental work derived from these initial observations. Second, it also drew attention to the central role of nutrition as a signal to the fetus of its potential future environment. Thirdly, it drew attention to the role of postnatal nutrition and obesity in the progression of the PARs cascade.

The role of nutrition as a key postnatal environmental determinant for reaching reproductive competence is easy to understand. There is, for example, clear evidence that nutrition and reproductive competence are linked: fecundity is influenced by nutritional status at mating in many species.[1] In all mammals, humans included, the passage of the genome from one generation to the next can be preserved despite a slow growth rate in a poor environment, so long as reproductive competence is achieved. Thus adaptive responses that include insulin resistance, associated with small muscle mass and lower capillary density in many tissues, give an appropriate survival route (for the genotype) if the organism expects to live in a deprived postnatal environment. Conversely if that predictive choice has been made, but the environment turns out to be enriched, then it is easy to see how this will become manifest as a greater risk of hypertension and diabetes. The latter scenario will not necessarily compromise reproductive performance, so the genotype will be passed on to the next generation, even though the risk of disease in later life is greater. But as we saw in chapter 1, phenotype is a very broad term. So, are there other phenotypes that can be developmentally determined and that have consequences for disease arising from inappropriate prediction – in other words, how wide-reaching is the PARs phenomenon?

There is an increasing body of literature relating size at birth to the risk of adult diseases, ranging from diabetes and osteoporosis through to impaired cognitive

---

[1] In some species such as the stoat, populations use altered fecundity in response to periconceptional nutrition as the primary strategy to match population size to the available food resources.

function. The assumption in much of this work is that the altered birth size is a surrogate measure for the quality of the fetal environment: the smaller the fetus the greater the degree of adversity it has faced prenatally. In itself this may be a reasonable assumption but other explanations remain possible. For example a genetic defect or polymorphism affecting fetal growth might also be the same genetic defect that leads to or alters the propensity to disease. Examples of both have been identified but, to date, purely genetic causes seem relatively rare. As we shall describe below, genotype does affect the sensitivity to prenatal environment and thus the PAR. As in the case of the hypertension/heart disease story, epidemiological studies must be supported by animal experiments, as they provide mechanistic data and rule out primary genetic causes, and where possible by prospective clinical study.

While a teleological or theoretical argument can only ever be supportive rather than definitive, (and we will return to this in chapter 8) the argument in support of inappropriate prediction as a cause of a particular disease is made stronger if it can be placed both in a mechanistic and evolutionary perspective. The ultimate proof, as will be discussed in later chapters, is a virtual impossibility: it would require an intervention that changes the fetal environment to ensure it matches the postnatal environment and then showing a consequent reduction in disease incidence. This would be a complex 70-plus-years experiment and that would still depend on knowing the correct intervention!

In the discussion that follows we will briefly review those disease conditions where inappropriate prediction may play a role and try to give our assessment of the quality of the supporting evidence. In our view, the evidence is compelling for diabetes and the metabolic syndrome and for two other major diseases, obesity and osteoporosis. Indeed the evidence relating to obesity adds much to the evolutionary arguments we are developing in this book.

## Type 2 diabetes mellitus and the metabolic syndrome

Throughout the previous chapter we frequently alluded to Type 2 diabetes because the same data sets that showed relationships between birth size and heart disease generally showed parallel relationships between birth size and Type 2 diabetes or insulin resistance. This was also the case in the animal studies.

Type 2 diabetes is due to the tissues becoming resistant to insulin – more insulin needs to be made by the pancreatic islet cells in an attempt to overcome this resistance and maintain glucose and amino acid entry into the cells. Eventually the combination of resistance and pancreatic exhaustion means blood sugar levels can no longer be kept under control, they rise and need treatment. It is generally a disease of middle age and is associated with truncal obesity. The obesity is both a cause and an effect. Insulin acts on fat cells to cause them to store fat so if the food intake is high in the prediabetic stage, the insulin will drive the excess energy into fat. But as fat cells become distended they become more resistant[2] to insulin, insulin deprivation occurs and the excess glucose stays in the circulation. Another tissue where insulin has important actions is the liver, where it inhibits glucose production and promotes glucose storage in the form of glycogen. Fatty acids released from omental fat appear to make the liver resistant to insulin and fat becomes deposited in the liver. Insulin acts on muscle to allow glucose to be taken up to fuel its contractions. Muscle is also a site of glucose storage in the form of glycogen. In virtually every tissue, insulin plays a role in promoting amino acid and glucose transport from the outside to the inside of the cell. The pathway by which insulin acts is a complex cascade of intracellular actions initiated by its binding to the insulin receptor and culminating in glucose transporters being sent to the cell surface to bring glucose into the cell. Insulin resistance appears to involve problems with any one of or many of these steps.

There is also human evidence that changes in neonatal nutrition in the neonatal period can alter the risk of later insulin resistance. Alan Lucas, who originally introduced the term 'programming', has found that premature infants who were fed different milk formulas for only a few weeks had biochemical changes in insulin secretion measurable as adolescents. It would appear that a diet promoting more rapid growth also induced insulin resistance, whereas those babies fed a milk formula that did not promote such rapid neonatal growth did not develop insulin resistance. If these data are confirmed it would be strong evidence that, in humans as in the rat, the window of opportunity for PARs to operate extends beyond birth.

The evidence that Type 2 diabetes has some prenatal factors contributing to its origin is convincing. The epidemiological data are as strong as for cardiovascular disease and the prospective clinical data (detailed in the previous chapter) and experimental data are also very strong. Teleologically it is easy to understand why a fetus would adapt its physiology towards insulin resistance if it expected to live in a deprived postnatal environment. It would then have less drive to put glucose into its tissues and would have smaller energy demands. Because insulin is important to muscle development, muscle mass would be less and the higher insulin levels might assist fat storage (see next section).

For reasons that are not fully understood there is a close relationship between high insulin levels, Type 2 diabetes and heart disease. This cluster is sometimes called the metabolic syndrome or Syndrome X. It includes other elements as well – in particular high cholesterol and fatty acid levels in blood. The relationship is so strong that the high insulin levels have been seen as a potential causative factor in

---

[2] Resistance to a hormone is rarely absolute. Except in some very rare genetic diseases, provided there is enough insulin, the resistance can be overcome. That is why adult-onset diabetes can be treated with insulin.

hypertension, and many mechanisms for the linkage have been speculated upon. This is a major cause of 'lifestyle' diseases. It has generally been assumed that this linkage is either genetic (although no single genetic complex can explain the relationship) or is simply the result of obesity and low energy expenditure in adulthood, leading to both heart disease and diabetes. This has not been a satisfactory explanation. It is possible, if not probable, that PARs may provide the missing link. Both insulin resistance and the various adaptive mechanisms that lead to high blood pressure (see chapter 6) are appropriate responses for a fetus to make if it predicts it will live in a poor postnatal environment. If it then finds itself in an enriched environment then the effects of the insulin resistance and the altered cardiovascular control will become apparent. In humans, with our long life span, this becomes manifest as disease.

## Obesity

There has been an explosive rise in the incidence of obesity in both children and adults in recent years. This rise and its consequences have been so marked that some critics have argued that there is no role for prenatal factors in the aetiology of cardiovascular disease and Type 2 diabetes – all we need do is to focus on the rise in obesity. We hope we have convinced the reader that this cannot be true. Certainly, the rise in the incidence of obesity has been so rapid, so dramatic and so universal in all but the poorest societies that no genetic explanation is feasible. In part it is obviously dependent on changing fashion and greater availability of fast foods, foods with high fat and carbohydrate content, a more sedentary lifestyle etc. We all live in a nutritional environment in rapid transition. The rise in the incidence of obesity occurs in an environment where genetic selection operates very little, if at all. But is there a deeper explanation – is this response to the nutritional environment exaggerated by inappropriate PARs? We think so.

Perhaps the first clue came from studies of infants in Southern India who had an average birth size of only about 2.6 kg, an effect largely owing to small maternal size (see chapter 8). To everyone's surprise it turned out that, unlike children after birth who are stunted and remain thin, these children had, in proportionate terms, as much body fat as normal-sized children at birth, born in the UK. This surprising result suggests that even in an intrauterine environment of limited nutrient availability, fat will be conserved at the expense of other substrates prior to birth. It is suggested that obesity might have its origins before rather than after birth. Similarly, the fetal survivors of the Dutch Hunger Winter were more likely to get obese as adults. Studies in the UK showed that the measures of truncal (abdominal) obesity in adolescent girls were related to their size at birth. In France, children who were born small were shown to be more likely to get truncal obesity as young adults. Thus around the world it appeared that the phenotype of obesity in childhood might be established prenatally. One particularly intriguing study of children in Scotland showed that first-born children were more likely to develop childhood obesity than were second and subsequent children. First-born children are smaller because of a greater degree of maternal constraint. This is an important clue to the theory we will develop in chapters 7 and 8 that maternal constraint is of primary importance in ensuring we are programmed towards what we will call the survival phenotype.

In addition, experimental data are overwhelmingly supportive of the idea that central or truncal fat mass is prenatally induced and that obesity itself is in part prenatally determined. Laboratory rats will consume a junk food diet with great gusto, and it is not surprising that they then become obese. What is surprising, however, is that if rats are undernourished in utero by undernourishing their mothers and then after birth are placed on a high-fat diet after weaning, they get particularly obese compared to those who were not undernourished in utero, even if they were on the same high-fat diet after birth. Indeed the rat pups undernourished in utero get relatively fat even if they are kept on a *normal* diet after birth! Intriguingly, at least three mechanisms are involved. Firstly, it is clear that there are alterations in the hypothalamic control of appetite and, just like many humans with Syndrome X, the rats have 'browsing' eating behaviours – they eat between meals! Secondly, they have reduced muscle mass and a reduced propensity to exercise. We are not yet certain whether this reduced willingness to exercise is a consequence of the reduced muscle mass or whether the brain centres that drive activity are abnormal – we suspect that both are involved. Thirdly, it would appear that they have altered hormonal profiles that favour fat deposition at the expense of muscle growth. These multiple mechanisms suggest that evolution has selected the development of a propensity to deposit fat as a core survival mechanism whenever the offspring predicts a postnatal environment poor in nutrition.

The fat involved is largely that within the abdomen. The major store is in the omentum, which is a membranous structure connecting the intestines to the abdominal wall. Omental fat puts humans most at risk in terms of heart disease and contributes to the 'pot belly' of middle age. Such intra-abdominal fat is different in some ways to subcutaneous fat. It is the most metabolically important fat and the most labile – it is the first to be laid down when calorific intake exceeds demand and the first to be mobilised during undernutrition. We think of this fat as an emergency fuel reserve: we normally first metabolise glucose that is stored in the form of glycogen, but when we need more energy than glycogen can provide we burn fat. At night, when we undergo a fast during sleep, we tend to use up small amounts of omental fat and in the day we lay it down again. This fat has a different pattern of gene expression and its regulation has important differences from that of subcutaneous fat.

Specialised fat stores are not unique to humans. Perhaps the most obvious example is the camel. Contrary to popular belief the camel's hump is not a water reservoir – it is a fat reservoir. The camel carries its labile fat supply in its hump and has evolved and then been bred[3] for this special organ. The hump permits the camel to survive periodic starvation, where it uses up its hump, then to rapidly restock its reserve supply when it has access to food.

Teleologically such a strategy makes sense in the human too – if we anticipate being born into a deprived nutritional environment then we want to have features like a camel – when food is available we need to lay down fat as a high-energy store, to use when food may be less plentiful. Fat per gram stores twice as much energy as carbohydrate or protein. Because hepatic insulin resistance is largely achieved by fatty acids released from omental abdominal fat interfering with the liver's insulin receptors, having more omental fat is an advantage in reducing hepatic insulin sensitivity in a nutritionally compromised environment. Thus it would appear that truncal obesity itself is a developmentally induced phenomenon. If the nutritionally deprived fetus is born into a nutritionally deprived environment then it has an advantage if it has a tendency to preserve fat: this is an appropriate adaptive response. If it is born into a nutritionally enriched environment then the response becomes inappropriate, and the degree of obesity that develops becomes a factor in enhancing the risks of insulin resistance, and thus heart disease and Type 2 diabetes.

If being thin was our natural state then why, we wonder, did we not evolve to stay thin? The answer is that we probably evolved anticipating a relatively lean basal state but coevolved a labile fat store for dealing with an uneven food supply. The risks of obesity we now face in the twenty-first century are a price we have paid because our environment is now very different from that we evolved for, but the mechanisms of the past remain with us. Evolution has ensured that we are programmed to a default position, which is to lay down fat when we can; fail-safe PARs are a central part of the process of ensuring this is so.

The control of reproductive function and fat biology are linked. Leptin is a hormone made by fat, especially abdominal fat. Leptin levels are normally high when fat mass is high and leptin acts on the brain to suppress appetite.[4] Among the other things that high leptin levels do is to allow the reproductive hormonal axis to function normally. Thus the logic in developing insulin resistance so as to

---

[3] To the evolutionary biologists, such breeding is a faster form of imposed and directed selection.

[4] In some grossly obese people, there are genetic mutations of the leptin system so that this suppression does not occur, and there have been animal models developed that mimic these conditions. Such people may have a reduced leptin secretion, or a reduction in the sensitivity or number of leptin receptors.

retain fat, invest less energy in growth and optimise reproductive performance is a short-term survival strategy for a species. Conversely in anorexia nervosa, there is very little body fat, low leptin levels and reproductive hormonal function is grossly disturbed.[5]

The argument can be extended further without losing credibility. The transition in nutritional status between those who are now parents and their children, both in developed and many developing societies, has been enormous. The balance of foods eaten by children is very different from that of their parents. Consider a healthy normal human pregnancy. Placental function has evolved to constrain fetal growth, yet provide nutrition to the fetus on the assumption that the optimal postnatal environment is one of balanced food intake and largely unrefined foods. But essentially the postnatal environment of the twenty-first century is unlike the evolutionarily determined, optimal fetal diet – so clearly prenatal PARs are bound to be inappropriate. Within the developing world the implications are obvious, because there the potential for rapid nutritional change is even more rapid.

Truncal obesity is part of Syndrome X. It is often called the 'couch-potato syndrome' because it is so frequently associated with lethargy and a tendency to browsing eating behaviour. Public health interventions have focused on promoting exercise and diet – but these interventions have been very disappointing for those most at need. Perhaps the reality is that the evolutionary survival of hominids depended on the PAR leading to this phenotype. If that is the case then the brains of such 'couch potatoes' may be wired not to want to exercise and not to be able to exercise. Perhaps it is not surprising that the 'human camel' within us is so hard to treat!

## Osteoporosis

Osteoporosis is a disease particularly of post-menopausal women although it also occurs in men. It is due to insufficient maintenance of bone mineral and the supporting matrix in bone. It is complex because bone mineral and matrix are constantly being laid down and mobilised in a recycling process, and osteoporosis is essentially a disease of imbalance in this recycling. There is now good evidence that there is a relationship between a low birth weight and the development of osteoporosis. Because osteoporosis is poorly understood it is difficult to be precise about a mechanistic explanation. However it may reflect on several aspects of the hormonal changes associated with a PAR. We know that the fetus born small or subject to an intrauterine nutritional or environmental (hormonal) stress is born

---

[5]  We should note however that more severe obesity is also associated with diminished reproductive function in humans.

with an altered hypothalamic–pituitary–adrenal (HPA) axis. These offspring secrete more cortisol in a given situation because negative feedback by the hypothalamic and pituitary neurones is reduced. Indeed the biochemical basis of this is precisely known – it is due to a reduction in glucocorticoid (cortisol) receptors in critical parts of the brain – the amygdala and hypothalamus. Every day as children and adults we experience many situations that raise our blood cortisol levels – minor stresses such as an angry interpersonal interchange, pain from a minor accident, stress in a traffic jam, anger with our spouse or child, a letter from the taxman, and so on. If negative feedback is deficient then we will tend to keep our cortisol levels higher for longer than will those people who do not have defective feedback. Recall the snowshoe-hare story – the offspring of a mother in a low-population-density environment was jumpy and alert to avoid being eaten by a predator – in turn this induced her offspring to be similar by changing the sensitivity of their HPA axis.

Such developmental effects have persisted through evolution. Consider the human when the mother is stressed. She releases more cortisol, which crosses the placenta. Normally the placenta has an enzyme that converts cortisol to inactive cortisone but part of the adaptation to maternal stress (which may be nutritional or environmental, e.g. illness) is to reduce the levels of this enzyme (which has the cumbersome name of 11 $\beta$ hydroxysteroid dehydrogenase type 2) allowing more cortisol to reach the fetus. In turn this fetal exposure to cortisol changes the density of glucocorticoid receptors in the neural network that provides negative feedback, which is then reduced. This accelerates fetal maturation allowing earlier delivery, an appropriate adaptation to get the fetus out of a hostile uterine environment, but in turn the offspring develops a different responsiveness of its HPA axis. This makes sense because it ensures a better stress response in what the fetus predicts to be a stressful postnatal environment. It does not stop the offspring reaching adulthood – although it does have effects on fat deposition, muscle mass and reproductive competence as noted above. But chronic exposure to cortisol changes the balance between bone mineral deposition and its mobilisation. Normally this effect is small compared to the powerful bone building-effect of oestrogen, but when oestrogen levels fall after the menopause the effect of the chronic mild hypercortisolaemia becomes apparent as increased bone loss.

We must emphasise that this is an over-simplification because cortisol is only one of many hormones involved in bone deposition and mobilisation. Two of these are growth hormone and insulin-like growth factor-1 (IGF-1, see chapter 3). After birth musculo-skeletal growth is primarily controlled by pituitary growth hormone acting on the liver and other tissues to make IGF-1. In turn IGF-1 promotes cell proliferation and the uptake of amino acids and glucose into tissues; it also reduces protein breakdown. In addition it activates vitamin D, because this vitamin is normally absorbed from the gut or made by sunlight in the skin in an inactive form and has to be converted by an IGF-dependent enzyme in the kidney to its active form. Vitamin D is essential for bone deposition. We know that children (and rats) born small have relative resistance to IGF-1 in muscle, and probably in other tissues. This makes sense in our PAR model because if one expects to be born into a deprived environment one wants to minimise the use of nutrients for growth, and would rather get to sexual maturation at the expense of growth. A degree of growth hormone and IGF-1 resistance would help this. But IGF-1 resistance, both directly and through its effects on vitamin D, will reduce bone mineral and matrix. Together with the effects of oestrogen loss after the menopause, osteoporosis becomes more likely. With age there is also a significant decline in growth hormone and IGF-1 secretion. Interestingly IGF-1 is very closely related to insulin and both have similar receptors. Insulin can substitute for IGF in some situations and vice versa. This may be another reason why insulin and IGF-1 resistance seem to have evolved in parallel as adaptive strategies.

Fetal growth retardation is often associated with placental dysfunction. Bone development necessitates transplacental passage of calcium and this can be compromised by a dysfunctional placenta. This happens in mothers who smoke in pregnancy, because the metal cadmium in the smoke builds up in the placenta and limits calcium transport. Further there may be a genetic interaction in that there are polymorphisms in the vitamin D receptor. This is another example of the gene–environment interactions we saw in relation to diabetes and the PPAR$\gamma$ polymorphism (chapter 4), because the effect of inheriting the vitamin-D-receptor polymorphism on the risk of osteoporosis is exacerbated if the individual's birth weight is low.

The above discussion shows that the explanation of osteoporosis in terms of an inappropriate PAR is more complex than it was for obesity. However it is nonetheless possible to see the interplay of multiple mechanisms whereby the fetus makes a choice for its developmental strategy, based on its perception of a 'stressed' in utero environment. It predicts that this will extend postnatally and so has changed its biochemical phenotype accordingly. This becomes of significance in older life once growth hormone and, in females, oestrogen levels fall; the consequence is adult-onset osteoporosis.

## Polycystic ovary syndrome

Polycystic ovary syndrome comprises a cluster of ovarian dysfunction, obesity and hirsuitism (male-like hairiness), and is a common cause of infertility or sub-fertility in women. It generally appears in adolescent girls with a relatively early appearance of pubic hair (adrenarche) followed by irregular cycles following menarche and gradual onset of obesity. It is called the polycystic ovary syndrome because the ovaries are fibrotic and contain many follicular cysts that mark the sites where ovulation has failed. Studies, particularly from Barcelona, show quite clearly that children born small are more likely to get this syndrome. It seems probable that this is an example of an inappropriate PAR.

What appears to have happened in the polycystic ovary syndrome is a consequence of the insulin resistance that we discussed earlier in relationship to the origins of Syndrome X. Insulin resistance leads to high circulating levels of insulin. The polycystic ovary syndrome appears to result from the changing profile of hormones being secreted by the ovary in the presence of high insulin levels. One result is that the ovary makes more androgens (male sex hormones, which are secreted in some measure even in females) than it normally does. The symptoms of this syndrome can largely be explained in terms of insulin resistance and high androgen levels. Interestingly, it may be more obvious in some populations of women such as those from the Mediterranean, because they have a higher frequency of polymorphisms in their androgen receptors that make them more sensitive to those hormones – another example of the interaction between genes and environment, i.e. between PARs and genotype.

## Psychological disorders and cognitive function

It has been observed that those who are diagnosed with schizophrenia tend to have a smaller head circumference at birth. This suggests that there has been an intrauterine precursor affecting brain development. In at least one study it has been suggested that schizophrenia is more common in the offspring of women who had influenza-like illnesses at a critical period in fetal brain development in midgestation. While this suggests a fetal origin of psychotic disorders in some cases, whether or not this represents an example of inappropriate induction or some developmentally disruptive effect on brain development, which does not become manifest until later in life, is unclear.

There are other studies that suggest relationships between depression and emotive disorders and birth size. Again the snowshoe hare and the desert mole rat examples might suggest evolutionary echoes if such observations are indeed substantiated. In animals the data is much clearer and so we do not think it unreasonable to envisage persistence at some level of these phenomena into the human; but, on the other hand, the evidence in humans is not yet strong.

If pregnant rats are undernourished, their offspring are less likely to spend time in daylight than in darkness as adults. Psychologists interpret such observations as showing that the rats have less exploratory behaviour and higher anxiety levels. Put into the context of PARs, these rats have developed in utero in an environment of poor nutrition. Could it be that this is the appropriate adaptive response:

expecting to be born into a hostile environment, to be less adventurous, and to invest in reaching sexual maturation and mating at a smaller size? Remember these same animals have enhanced HPA responses making them more 'scared' and ready to move away from a perceived threat.

Even more compelling is work from Michael Meaney in Montreal. We referred to this work briefly in chapter 3. He has studied the licking and grooming habits of rat mothers with their pups and observed that there are mothers who groom their pups a lot, and those who do not. The pups of 'high grooming' mothers grow up with a low responsiveness of the HPA axis; and those of 'low grooming' mothers grow up with a high responsiveness of the HPA axis – that is they have a greater stress response. Rat pups are born with extremely immature and plastic brains, more akin to a mid-gestational human brain. What we see here is that high grooming in this critical period of brain development has programmed the rat to grow up prepared for a placid environment, as exemplified by a calm and caring mother; conversely, low grooming predicts a dangerous environment. Meaney has now performed behavioural tests on these pups and found that the pups that had received more grooming grew up to be apparently less afraid of exploring their environment. To show that it was the grooming and not some other factor such as a constituent of the mother's milk, he reared rats artificially, grooming them with either a high or a low intensity by handling them and stroking them with a paintbrush. The same effect of (now artificial) grooming was observed. He went further to show that the origin of this changed behaviour was caused by changes in glucocorticoid receptors in the amygdala and in the activity of various neurotransmitters in the brain. His most recent work demonstrates that the effects are associated with changes in DNA methylation patterns in the promoter regions of the genes for these receptors in the brain, linking the story back to the dietary and epigenetic effects we discussed earlier.

With such compelling evidence from this example it is not unreasonable to make extrapolations to the human situation. Studies from the USA have been able to relate the incidence of child abuse or other markers of deprivation to permanent resetting to a hyper-responsive HPA axis. It seems likely that fetal and early life experiences change the biochemistry of the brain in ways that influence later emotional behaviour, anxiety levels and the incidence of clinical depression.

## Cognitive decline

As the percentage of elderly people in developed societies increases, so too does the burden of coping with the inevitable processes of cognitive decline. Recent studies have shown that such decline is less in those with larger heads (which seems intuitively unsurprising, but which raises all sorts of other questions). Because so much neuronal development occurs in utero, the question arises of how much such neural function is also determined prenatally, perhaps as an aspect of PARs. It turns out, however, that it is the changes in brain weight in infancy and early childhood that relate to cognitive decline in later life: such developmental plasticity at this time of life offers considerable scope for educational or environmental interventions such as improved nutrition.

## Other diseases

We want to end this section by mentioning some even more provocative observations. Two studies, one in Finland and one in the UK, have shown that men born small have a higher incidence of remaining unmarried! This might suggest that aspects of the socialisation of individuals born small as a result of abnormal fetal environment are different, (perhaps echoing the rat experiments), and making them less likely in the context of modern western society to marry. It also turns out that the method of suicide is influenced by the month of birth – those born in spring are more likely to commit suicide by hanging, compared to those born in winter who are more likely to use an overdose of drugs. It even appears that temperament and personality characteristics are influenced by the month of birth: women born in spring in Scandinavia are more likely to be impulsive than those born in winter, and so on. As the season of birth cannot be genetically determined (unless one is an astrologist), this must say that something about either the fetal or infant environmental influences in different seasons affect brain development in such a way as to influence adult personality.

There are many seasonal differences in hormonal profile – for example the melatonin rhythm in both mother and child are different in winter and summer as this hormone is regulated by light exposure. Melatonin crosses the placenta and therefore the fetus knows roughly the light cycle its mother is exposed to.

Finally, there is evidence that birth weight is correlated with income in adult life, suggesting perhaps that intellectual ability and educational attainment are dependent on aspects of prenatal development. All this evidence needs to be confirmed by further studies. Until it is, we cannot speculate about the predictive adaptive nature of such possible effects. We mention them to show how far-reaching the investigations in this field have become in recent years.

Much other research is currently underway in relation to a broader set of diseases. These include the allergic diseases, sensitivity to infection, asthma, chronic lung disease and some cancers. For none of these is there a set of strong epidemiological data supported by experimental data. We do not wish to mislead the reader by extending beyond areas where we, as informed scientists, have some degree of confidence and therefore we will not discuss these possibilities further. However there is no inherent reason why PARs theory may not have further consequences and different dimensions – we hope that research to explore these possibilities will be extended.

## Transgenerational effects

It is doubtful if the Swedish statistician Hellstenius envisaged the long-term consequences when he published a paper in 1871 on harvests in his country and their effects on the population. His data formed part of a study of the parish of Overkalix in Northern Sweden in which the medical history of those born in 1890, 1905 and 1920 was traced. The main focus was on death associated with cardiovascular disease and diabetes. The results were, however, quite unexpected. What the study showed was that the risk of death from diabetes increased in the subjects if food had been plentiful during the youth of their grandfathers. The period when food supply appeared to be particularly important was when the grandfather was growing slowly, just before the growth spurt of adolescence. Exactly how such effects come about we do not know, and of course we cannot tell underlying biological mechanisms in any case from such population-based studies. However it is clear that predictive adaptation can extend across generations and this has important implications.

Similarly, one of the surprises from the Dutch Hunger Winter studies has been the finding that the grandchildren of the women pregnant during the famine still show effects of the famine. The pregnancies affected were those where the fetus was exposed to the famine in the first trimester. The female fetuses born were of normal size but when they themselves became adults their offspring had reduced body size. Clearly the effects of an abnormal intrauterine life can echo beyond one generation.

Similar evidence has also been accumulating in animals. Some studies of Stewart over 30 years ago suggested that it took many generations in the rat for the effects of a sustained period of undernutrition to be reversed in terms of birth weight. Specific effects on brain growth extending beyond one generation have also been demonstrated. After a period of malnutrition on a single generation of pregnant rats, the DNA content of the brains of their grandchildren was reduced. Our (MAH) recent observations in undernourished rats using the maternal low-protein model show that the grandchildren have perturbed vascular function. This is particularly striking because in such experiments we were able to ensure that the first generation of female pups were not exposed to any further nutritional challenge, so the effect seems to be able to cross generations without the need for a reinforcing stimulus.

These are challenging observations, because they demonstrate that some environmental influences can have multigenerational effects, independent of genetic inheritance. Of course the concept of PARs has inherent within it a component of transgenerational transmission. This is what lies behind the idea that the pregnant mammal can pass information to her developing offspring, triggering their adaptive processes. But the examples we have shown demonstrate that the process goes further than that: once the programmed female offspring of a particular mother become pregnant, they pass on the signal to their offspring in turn, i.e. the grandchildren of the original female. How might this be achieved?

One obvious mechanism has been demonstrated in studies in children born small in Barcelona. It shows that those born small and who then develop insulin resistance have also developed a small uterus, and thus will have less capacity to sustain the growth of the next generation of fetuses. When these girls are pregnant they are more likely to exert greater maternal constraint on the fetus. A related possibility is that the circulatory responses that the 'programmed' girls make to pregnancy are altered in some way. There is experimental evidence in the rat that this is the case in relation to the way that the uterine arteries relax during pregnancy.

An alternative set of explanations may involve consideration of the germ lines. Females do not make new eggs throughout their lifetimes, because the eggs in a woman's ovaries are formed and start developing when she is still a fetus. They then go into hibernation to be reactivated after puberty, and usually one egg completes its maturation in every menstrual cycle. No new eggs are formed after birth and after puberty the ovarian follicles mature sequentially. Now these eggs, formed when the woman is herself a fetus, will contain the maternal DNA, which will be passed on to her children. Thus the eggs that will form the third generation develop in a female fetus who is influenced by the maternal environment of her grandmother. We have, at one stroke, a highly effective means of transmitting a signal from grandmother to grandchildren. And if the signal involves DNA methylation, a key mechanism for silencing genes, the size of the effect will be influenced by the supply of the 1-carbon methyl groups needed for this methylation. This supply depends in turn on dietary glycine and folate intake during pregnancy, on maternal metabolism and placental glycine synthesis and transport. These are important components of the signalling pathway from mother to fetus. It is tempting to speculate that the rather odd confinement of egg formation to the prenatal period may have evolved precisely to facilitate the exposure of the grandchildren's DNA, specifically that inherited down the maternal line, to environmental stimuli. But at present this is just speculation.

There is, however, a final piece of evidence that we ought to flag up in relation to maternal transmission of the cues for PARs, and that involves the possible role of mitochondrial DNA, which we mentioned in chapter 2. This simple DNA is responsible for making some of the proteins essential for the energy maintenance of all cells. The theory goes that mitochondria may have originally been microscopic invaders into cells, probably as simple bacteria, many millions of years ago. By providing a source of energy to the cells they invaded, they were useful parasites, and so the host evolved to tolerate them. Further, the generation of energy within cells superseded the need to pick it up entirely from the environment by diffusion: so the theory may explain how larger, multicellular organisms could evolve. As they got bigger, they developed internal transport systems – the cardiovascular systems – to deliver the fuel and oxygen substrates to the cells, and the mitochondria got on with the job of energy production. In return, the mitochondrial invaders became immortal, because they were copied every time the cells divided, and passed on from generation to generation.

There are several reasons why this theory is particularly relevant to our thinking here. First, the passage of mitochondrial DNA from one generation to the next is solely down the maternal line – from the mitochondria in the egg, and not via the sperm. So they fit the bill of DNA that is transmitted directly from grandmother to granddaughter. Second, the metabolic capacity of the grandchildren's cells is precisely the type of process that will be valuable to alter as part of PARs. The grandchildren may not be able to control the availability of food in their environment, but they can be induced to alter their metabolism, especially their energy production, to make the best use of it. And finally, the latest evidence shows that the availability of folate in early pregnancy has important effects on the mitochondrial DNA – so we see a potential role for this dietary component as a trigger of the programming processes. And indeed there are experimental data suggesting that the number of mitochondria in mature cells is permanently influenced by the prenatal environment.

Paternal effects also exist, as demonstrated in the anecdote about Hellstenius that started this section. Paternal effects are more difficult to understand as sperm are newly made throughout life but they are derived from germline cells, which do develop in fetal life and this may be the clue. Could germ-cell gene expression be altered by DNA methylation in the earliest stages of fetal life, and then be preserved during spermatogenesis when the fetus becomes an adult? If so these gene-methylation changes in the sperm may reflect effects in the fertilised pre-embryo. We need to know much more about these processes, but it is certain that novel discoveries in this area will throw up exciting possibilities about how and when PARs operate in humans.

# 6

# The biology of predictive adaptive responses

The combination of experimental, clinical and epidemiological data relating an adverse perinatal environment to long-term outcome has one particularly striking feature. That is, despite the variety of models examined, there is a remarkable consistency in the phenotype that emerges in adulthood. The common features include a tendency to insulin resistance, increased blood pressure, vascular endothelial dysfunction, altered lipid and carbohydrate metabolism, a tendency to obesity and small muscle mass. We have termed this the *survival phenotype* for reasons that are discussed below.

This raises two important questions. First, why is it so easy to produce a consistent phenotype from such a variety of prenatal environments? Second, what is the biological basis for the development of this phenotype? The answers to these questions need to apply to both humans and animals because the PARs theory applies across species. In turn this leads to the more general question of the fundamental biological mechanisms underpinning PARs. These fundamental mechanisms must be independent of whether the PARs that are induced in utero are subsequently appropriate or inappropriate. They are also likely to be independent of the specific intrauterine situation in which they arose. These questions are the focus of this chapter.

Such questions can be asked at several levels. At one level there are a set of issues about the nature of the environmental cues that the embryo and fetus respond to, and secondly about when in development these cues act. On another level there are questions about what fundamental mechanisms can lead to permanent changes in physiology. At a third level, we want to ask about the effector mechanisms that lead to the induction of the metabolic syndrome and other postnatal phenomena. And finally we have to think about the relative roles of the primary prenatal adaptive event and what role amplification factors such as postnatal growth play later in life. We will discuss these issues by focusing primarily on the metabolic syndrome and its components, including obesity, as this is where the best evidence is available.

A word of caution: throughout the discussion we will repeatedly refer to reductions in fetal growth as a part of PARs but, as we have already made clear, alterations in fetal growth are not essential in the development of responses. It is clear that PARs occur independently of fetal size and within the normal range of birth size. It is merely a consequence of the magnitude of the effects that any relationships at all are seen with birth size. The continuum in the relationship between birth size and the risk of the long-term consequences of inappropriate PARs demonstrates this. Fetal growth is merely a surrogate for the sum of a number of fetal experiences that can impact on growth – but nonetheless it is true that fetal growth is one of the most sensitive components of the fetal response to an adverse environment because growth is readily sacrificed for survival.

## The survival phenotype

The epidemiological data considered one particular set of relationships, namely the relationship between measures of early-life adverse events, as reflected in birth size, and a set of outcomes involving metabolic and cardiovascular parameters. Overlapping clinical phenotypes could be identified for the outcome of children born small (intrauterine growth retarded), for gradients of growth across the normal population, for those born to pregnancies with severe maternal constraint and indeed for unusual events occurring early or late in pregnancy such as in the Dutch famine. Similar experimental outcomes were observed in rats, irrespective of whether they were subject to protein undernutrition, caloric undernutrition, high-fat exposure or glucocorticoid hormone exposure in utero. In guinea pigs and pigs similar outcomes occurred in spontaneously small or experimentally growth-retarded animals. In sheep, nutritional and placental impairment and glucocorticoid challenges produced not dissimilar outcomes in the offspring. While the precise details of the resulting phenotypes differ in each situation, there are sufficient similarities to suggest common underlying mechanisms.

This extraordinarily wide range of approaches, all leading to a similar phenotype – defined at least in terms of insulin resistance and alterations in blood pressure control – suggests that the phenotype has been conserved through evolution because it conferred a particular survival advantage. It does not however imply that a common pathway leads to that phenotype. In fact we know that this cannot be the case: events acting very early in development and those acting in late development must have a different biological basis, and this argument will be developed further below. What the range of data does suggest is that evolution has protected the development of this 'survival phenotype' when early life experiences predict a deprived future environment. The phenotype does not affect reproductive performance itself but is designed to safeguard the individual's survival in that deprived environment in order to reproduce. There is no a priori reason why a single common mechanism should be involved. Indeed, as will be discussed, multiple and overlapping underlying mechanisms have been shown to be involved even within the same experiment. A focus of our argument is that it is the capacity to induce PARs that evolution has preserved. Various mechanisms have therefore been amplified, according to both the species and the situation that led to the PAR. This has the implication that scientists should not spend time debating the relative merits of one experimental model or another – an activity that it is easy to fall into (and of course one that the peer-review system for appraising grant applications and papers for publication readily tends itself to).

## Common phenotypes and common pathways

Common phenotypes do not imply common pathways in evolution or in biological process. For example there are many ways in which pathological hypertension can develop – a tumour of the adrenal gland producing too much aldosterone (a fluid-retaining hormone), diseases of the kidney affecting another hormone called renin, persistent stress acting on the autonomic nervous system, some brain tumours, insulin resistance and obesity, as well as the common form of hypertension that involves changes in vascular reactivity. Evolutionary biology can provide many examples where quite different routes to a final phenotype have evolved separately. The most well-known example is the eye, which has evolved several times independently in different (cladistic) lines of speciation. The insect eye and the mammalian eye have quite different evolutionary histories. Obviously a visually responsive organ is a highly desirable survival characteristic and thus the visually aware phenotype has had a real evolutionary advantage. Hence there is a common phenotype (possessing an eye) but there are many pathways to achieving it.[1] This phenomenon is called convergent evolution. Another example is colour vision, which has been adopted by a range of species, from insects to birds and mammals, but the photoreceptor mechanisms used are different. Or again, the placenta, which evolved separately in some reptiles and in all mammals (other than the monotremes).

Thus, whenever a phenotype is so well preserved through such a broad range of situations, we need to reflect on the advantage conferred. This will be discussed in detail in chapter 7. We only need to reiterate here that the survival phenotype would have an advantage if the PAR had been appropriate – that is there had been a match between the fetal and postnatal environment, the fetus had been properly informed and had made the correct prediction.

---

[1] For an excellent discussion on the evolution of the eye, the reader is referred to Richard Dawkins' book, *The Blind Watchmaker: Why the Evidence of Evolution Reveals a Universe without Design*. The significance of the story of the evolution of the eye is much broader because of the complexity of the eye: the dispute about whether it was so complex that it needed divine guidance to have arisen is one of the classic arguments between evolutionists and creationists, and is well told by Dawkins.

There is an obvious advantage in response to a deprived environment in having peripheral insulin resistance (i.e. in muscles) however it arises, because it ensures that energy is not wasted unnecessarily on muscle growth or metabolism. Indeed muscle mass is reduced in adults with Syndrome X, in growth-retarded children and in the multitude of experimental models we have discussed. A tendency to lay down truncal fat creates an emergency fuel reserve. The altered HPA-mediated anxiety levels allow the individual a greater chance of survival in a nutrient-deprived and therefore predator-rich environment. But what could possibly be the advantage of cardiovascular changes?

Several mechanisms are involved in the PAR-mediated generation of hypertension and thus in establishing the path towards heart disease. As yet we do not fully understand the relative importance of each. The most critical phenotypic response to a future nutritionally deprived environment is to have small lean body mass – why invest protein and other fuels in growth when the critical evolutionary pressure is to survive to reproduce? Therefore it appears that the fetus has evolved a number of adaptive responses in the expectation of small lean body mass postnatally. These include a reduced number of capillaries in tissues such as muscle and in the gut. There is a reduced renal mass with a reduced number of nephrons because the kidney is a major consumer of energy and demands a high blood flow, and it would be a luxury to maintain a larger kidney than necessary. Similarly the HPA axis adapts to be hyper-responsive, and elevated cortisol levels drive a higher blood pressure. Reduced capillary density leads to increased vascular resistance, as does reduced renal mass. If postnatally the system is challenged by greater nutritional availability, then such a programmed fetus is inevitably predisposed to hypertension and arteriosclerosis.

Again, because this is usually manifest after the peak phase of reproductive competence there has been no evolutionary selection pressure to minimise risk. This scenario is easy to demonstrate in animals where a combination of poor fetal growth and postnatal catch-up growth predisposes to hypertension, insulin resistance and in guinea pigs (which have a similar cholesterol metabolism to humans), to atheroma formation.

## The nature of the cues

The available evidence is that the developing organism is responding to cues that tell it about the nutritional and/or stress environment into which it will be born. As has been discussed there are several mechanisms by which the placenta can transmit such information to the fetus. They are not unrelated: for example undernutrition can influence the placental enzyme that converts cortisol to its inactive metabolite and so with maternal undernutrition the fetus is also exposed to more cortisol. Conversely, high doses of cortisol can interfere with the placental and cellular transport of glucose and perhaps amino acids, leading effectively to tissue undernutrition.

## Nutritional cues

The greatest amount of experimental data relates to nutritional cues. Most of the studies have been performed in rats or mice, and the most widely used challenge is to reduce the dietary protein of the maternal diet by about 50 per cent. This may not be as dramatic as it seems because laboratory rats are normally much better nourished than wild rats. The challenge produces a variable effect on the growth of the fetuses, and while the experimental laboratory rats are usually somewhat smaller at birth, this is not invariably the case. As adults, the offspring show elevated blood pressure, reduced responses of their small arteries to the natural stimuli that relax them, and insulin resistance. All these processes will contribute to the development of cardiovascular disease, but rodents do not usually die of stroke or heart attacks, so we have to remember that we are trying to understand fundamental biological processes, rather than to produce human disease in animals. Overall reduction of the total diet, not just the protein content alone, in the mother can produce similar effects in the offspring to those described above. This raises the question of whether there is a specific dietary component that triggers the response if it is deficient. Much attention here has focused on the amino acid glycine. Glycine is not an essential amino acid in adult life, because the body can synthesise it if it is low in the diet. But the fetal requirements for it in late gestation are much greater than any other amino acid, including the essential ones. Hence if maternal glycine consumption, or its synthesis by the mother or the placenta, is inadequate, then the fetus may be short of it. Studies have shown that adding glycine to the diet of otherwise protein-restricted pregnant rats abolishes the effect on their offspring.

An equally important role as potential dietary triggers is played by micronutrients, especially vitamins. Current research has concentrated on folic acid. As is well known, folate deficiency has been shown to increase the risk of spina bifida substantially and women are recommended to take 400 mg of folate per day for the first half of pregnancy. Folate in fact is involved in aspects of glycine metabolism, and its absence would be expected to impair placental synthesis of glycine, synthesis of protein and DNA by the fetus, and the build-up of toxic compounds such as homocysteine in the fetal body. Folate supplementation of the diet can offset the programming effects of a low-protein diet in the rat. Discussion is now underway as to whether it is appropriate to add folic acid to foodstuffs such as flour: at present the data are very preliminary, and there are many examples of such interventions doing more harm than good if unexpected side effects occur. Clearly, adequate folate intake is essential in all women prior to and during pregnancy – but 'adequate' and

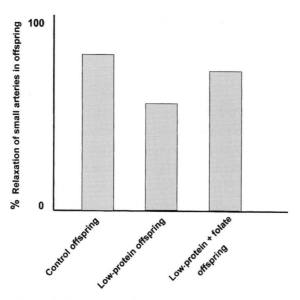

Fig. 6.1     Effects of a low-protein diet in pregnancy on function of small arteries in offspring of the rat. The ability of these arteries to relax to the vasodilator acetylcholine, which acts via the endothelium, is reduced in the offspring of protein-restricted dams compared to controls. This may contribute to other effects such as increased blood pressure in this model. The effect is significantly reduced if folic acid is added to the diet of the protein-restricted dams, supporting the idea that changes in DNA synthesis or methylation and homocysteine metabolism, to name only some, may be important underlying mechanisms. Data courtesy of Dr C. Torrens and Dr L. Brawley.

'excess' are not the same. Similar considerations apply to vitamins C, E, $B_6$ and $B_{12}$ – all of which have been implicated in physiological adaptations to pregnancy.

It is worth reiterating that fetal nutrition in humans can be influenced in many ways – it is not just a reflection of maternal nutrition. Obviously if maternal nutrition is insufficient this will directly affect the fetus. This is common in the developing world, and there is evidence in India for example that the intake of some foods (especially green leafy vegetables containing iron and folate) in pregnancy influences the outcome for the infant. But it has been debated whether maternal nutrition within the normal range can affect the fetus. However, we think the data showing that it can are compelling. There are now several reports that maternal nutritional status and body composition, as measured by subcutaneous fat, correlates with the occurrence of PARs in the offspring. Those mothers with a lower body fat, and who consume a less prudent diet before pregnancy, are more likely to have fetuses who make cardiovascular adaptive changes in late pregnancy, especially alterations to liver blood flow. The possible consequences of this for later health were discussed in chapter 5. These studies were conducted in the UK, so clearly we should not be complacent that the normal range of diets in the developed world provides adequate nutrition for the fetus.

Equally there is increasing evidence that it is the balance of the diet that matters. A high protein diet will, in the absence of adequate folate intake, lead to fetal growth retardation because under these circumstances amino acids become toxic to the mother and fetus. This was best shown in following up the offspring from a 1950s trial from Motherwell in Scotland where it was believed that pregnancy outcomes would be improved by high protein intakes (see also chapter 2): one doctor strongly advised consumption of a pound of meat per day to his pregnant patients – this in a time of post-war rationing! His advice was to snack on corned beef rather than biscuits or scones! Subsequent analysis has revealed that this dietary imbalance was a cue for PARs, and the blood pressure of the offspring was higher than normal. The effect was influenced by the vegetable consumption of these women. Recent data from Southampton suggest that the balance of food types has a major influence on the pattern of fetal growth across the whole of pregnancy. Much more work is needed to know the precise details of an appropriate dietary intake for women before and during pregnancy and during lactation. Indeed it is likely that optimal fetal development will depend on different nutritional intakes at different times across development.

The other way in which fetal nutrition can be disturbed is via abnormalities in the supply line. The fetus is at the end of a long line consisting of the mother's intestines, her own metabolic state, supply of nutrients through the uterine arteries, uptake by the placenta, placental metabolism,[2] uptake by the fetus and distribution to the key fetal tissues. There are many opportunities for disturbed signalling along this pathway and each can lead to the fetus perceiving its future environment to be deprived, which may not be correct. Examples of how the supply line can be disturbed include maternal heart disease, which will reduce oxygen delivery and blood flow to the uterus; pre-eclampsia, which reduces both uterine blood flow and placental transfer; maternal diabetes in which high glucose levels exist; placental infarction reducing transfer capacity; and maternal smoking, which interferes with placental transfer and has many other effects. A feature of these various 'nutritional' (or pseudo-nutritional) cues is that they are likely to act over a long period of development and therefore impact on multiple fetal processes. We should remember that the most common of all these 'nutritional' triggers is maternal constraint, which operates in all pregnancies, but particularly in adolescent and first pregnancies, to

---

[2] The placenta itself consumes 40–60 per cent of the nutrients taken out of the maternal circulation, leaving the remainder for use by the fetus. This means that the regulation of placental metabolism is a major determinant of fetal nutrition. The mechanisms are very poorly understood although recent data from one of our laboratories (PDG) show that both maternal and fetal hormones can regulate this step. This may be a point at which a major opportunity exists for intervention to prevent later disease.

limit nutrient supply to the fetus and the level of growth-promoting hormones in the fetal circulation.

## Hormonal cues

Other stimuli may act over a shorter period. For example maternal illness and stress will both elevate maternal cortisol levels. In experimental animals, exposure during pregnancy to a single dose of powerful cortisol-like drugs will programme the fetus to develop hypertension and insulin resistance after birth. This is particularly evident when the exposure is relatively early in development. Whether this is because of the induction of PARs or because the very high doses of glucocorticoids act to produce development disruption is unclear. The issue of exposure to glucocorticoids such as cortisol remains important. Administration of steroids to the mother with threatened preterm labour is a critical part of the management of the preterm infant, as the treatment helps to mature its lungs and reduce the risk of the fatal lung disease seen in premature neonates. The jury is out as to whether there may be long-term consequences, but evidence is accumulating that this may be so. High-dose steroids often have to be used in critically ill newborn babies and there is evidence that this may be at an unavoidable price for preserving life, particularly with respect to neural development.

There is much overlap between nutritional and hormonal cues. For example, acute stress is generally associated with altered appetite. Cortisol can inhibit glucose uptake into tissues, including possibly the placenta. But intriguingly, undernutrition can affect the amount of mother's cortisol that reaches the fetus. Normally the placenta uses an enzyme to inhibit the transfer of active cortisol from mother to fetus, and this is sensible because cortisol does many things to the fetus including controlling its rate of maturation. The fetus needs to be in control of its own destiny in this regard, and so until close to birth this enzymatic barrier is very tight. But under conditions of undernutrition the barrier becomes leaky and maternal cortisol is not metabolised by the placenta but is transferred to the fetus. This has a logic: the increased cortisol transfer slows down fetal growth and helps to match it to the available food supplies, but also accelerates maturation. In other words the mother is signalling to the fetus 'accelerate your maturation because I may not be able to support you much longer – get ready to leave'. Thus cortisol is an alternative signal to nutrition in signalling aspects of the maternal environment.

## Other cues

We should remember that not all environmental cues need be nutritional or hormonal. In chapter 1 we showed that the neonatal thermal environment clearly programmes the development of the number of active sweat glands. In sheep the thermal stress of life in outback Australia, produces detrimental effects on placental function and fetal growth.

## Timing of the cue

The issue of when in development a PAR is initiated is critical. It is clear that the potential critical window can extend throughout embryonic and fetal life, and probably both back into the preconceptual period and forward after birth. Experimentally there is now a wealth of evidence that the period around conception is one when effects can be powerfully induced and at that time they are likely to have more profound effects than later. Much data come from those researchers involved in aspects of experimental in vitro fertilisation. The glucose, insulin and IGF-1 concentrations in which the embryo is cultured influence its development, as does the length of time it is cultured. Ironically very little is known about these factors with respect to human IVF – an area which is difficult to research for obvious ethical reasons. However Louise Brown, the first 'test tube baby' is now 25 years old, and we can expect that follow-up studies of the thousands of subsequent IVF pregnancies will be published in the next decade.

Undernutrition in the rat just for the period prior to implantation of the blastocyst leads to the development of hypertension in the offspring (see chapter 4). Recent studies by both our research groups show that moderate undernutrition in sheep restricted to the period around conception leads to reduced fetal growth late in gestation, which may reflect insulin resistance, altered patterns of release of growth-related hormones and indeed an increased risk of premature labour. Interestingly, if the challenge is a milder one, gestational length is actually extended, as if to provide an additional period for fetal growth to occur. The implications of such findings are important and challenging – they suggest that maternal nutritional status prior to and at conception may be critical for optimal outcome. One of the features of these studies is that subsequent placental function may have been set by the periconceptional undernutrition and remained altered throughout pregnancy. This confirms the idea that the placenta itself is a changeable organ and that the trajectory of placental growth in early gestation is an early step in the development of PARs in the fetus later. Thus changes in the placenta induced early in pregnancy may programme placental transport capacity, which creates an environmental cue to the fetus later in gestation. Despite its obvious importance, the placenta remains a poorly understood organ – some would say the 'Cinderella' of prenatal life.

It is clear from this discussion that the mother's diet and body condition at the start of pregnancy influences the risk of predictive responses in her fetus later. The characteristic 'pear-shaped' deposition of fat around the hips and thighs in women is thought to be the result of evolutionary pressures to maintain reserves for growing the fetus during pregnancy and for breastfeeding the infant. Such fat deposits produce less of the hormone leptin, which suppresses appetite, than does the abdominal 'apple-shaped' fat deposition that occurs in men, and which we saw confers greater risk of cardiovascular disease. Greater body fat in the woman is likely to programme a faster rate of fetal growth. Clearly then maternal energy stores at the beginning of pregnancy may be critical in determining the outcome for the fetus. The issue is how to transmit this message to women of reproductive age, given that their diet and body composition need to be set *prior* to when they know they are pregnant. We badly need to establish the optimal body composition ranges for young women – clearly both too thin and too fat are bad – and this will have to be expressed simply, e.g. in terms of fat depth in relation to height. Then the problem will arise of how to get the advice adopted, given the pressures of advertising, the fashion industry and culturally induced prejudices.

But induction may occur after birth as well. Certainly this is the case in rats that are born in a very immature state, and it appears to be true for behavioural induction as well. Could this happen in humans? Recent data suggest that PARs may be initiated in human infants born prematurely. In a study performed in children born between 15 and 8 weeks prematurely it was found that by 8 years of age they had profound insulin resistance, similar in magnitude to those born small. These children have developed a programmed phenotype – the issue is why. Premature infants are on a very different diet to a fetus of the same gestational age in utero – they are given a much higher fat intake and have relative difficulty in ensuring adequate protein intake; additionally their hormonal milieu is very different as they are no longer exposed to placental hormones. But being born premature also exposes them to a different pattern of cortisol exposure in the period before and after birth, and we know this is a cue for PARs. A final possibility is that something early in gestation occurred leading both to induction of insulin resistance and to premature labour. Given the growing number of premature babies surviving, the consequences of prematurity require more research.

## Multiple pathways

In attempting to summarise our knowledge on mechanisms of PAR induction for the non-specialist reader we have already suggested that we will not find just one underlying basic mechanism. Perhaps the PARs process is too important for survival of the species to be left to chance: if a single mechanism had evolved, it might only take a harmful mutation in one gene central to the process to eliminate it. In addition, our knowledge is still at the stage where we are relating surrogate measures such as birth weight – which we know to be multifactorial in origin – to later phenotype. And of course phenotype itself is multifactorial in nature. So, before we turn our attention to current ideas about the mechanisms underlying PARs, we should stress that we do not expect to find just one single pathway or cause-and-effect operating. Nor, when we consider the detrimental effects of inappropriate PARs do we expect that there will be a single pathway to disease.

## Fundamental mechanisms

At a fundamental biological level several mechanisms can be involved in the induction of different pathways during early development. These include processes affecting the development of the number of cells in the embryo, alterations in tissue differentiation, or changes in gene expression. Evidence for all three exists. The first two become effectively irreversible because critical windows limit the capacity of the developing embryo to change the development path already induced once the window of opportunity has passed. For example once the period in which kidney nephron number is determined is over, it is not possible to initiate further nephron development. One difficulty is that distinguishing between those effects of an environmental cue that disrupt development from the effects that induce the fetus to make a response for immediate or predictive advantage. There is always a risk of falsely assigning adaptive value to a purely disruptive event. Formal proof is not easy, nor is the distinction necessarily absolute.

## Cell number and cell differentiation

Experiments in early bovine and mouse embryos cultured in vitro show that the number of cells committed to become a fetus or the placenta can be influenced by the milieu created by the culture medium. This suggests that embryonic environmental effects can lead to alterations in embryonic and placental cell number, which in turn determine the potential growth of the fetus. Cells also normally die as part of the developmental process by apoptosis.[3] For example in the insulin-making cells of the pancreatic islets, the first population of cells in the fetal rat largely dies off in the period around birth, to be replaced by a population that is differently regulated by glucose and more appropriate for postnatal existence. If rats are undernourished in utero, they will show increased rates of cell death in the pancreatic islet cells and this will put them at earlier risk of Type 2 diabetes as adults.

From undifferentiated stem cells in the early embryo, lineages of cells gradually differentiate under complex regulation by transcription factors, until the hundreds of types of specific cells, ranging from neurones to skin cells, differentiate. Some,

---

[3] See footnote 5 in chapter 2.

once differentiated, lose the capacity to reproduce (e.g. in the brain and muscle, but see footnote 4 in chapter 2) whereas many cell types can continue to form new cells throughout life (e.g. skin cells). Cellular differentiation is accompanied by tissue differentiation and matrix reorganisation leading to specific organ development; and organs, once formed, generally cannot change their structure. There is much evidence that structural and cell number change are part of the mechanisms underpinning PARs. If the appropriate survival mechanism is to be a smaller animal, more able to invest energy in reproduction rather than growth, then reduced size of organs such as the kidney is an appropriate adjustment. Another example of such an adjustment is the reduced capillary blood-vessel density in the gut and pancreas of rats that were undernourished in utero. The response is predictive because it assumes that less food will be absorbed and less insulin will need to be secreted. In the same animals, blood-vessel density is also reduced in the brain: this may limit growth and energy requirements of this metabolically active organ, but it may also increase the risk of stroke, especially if the PAR is inappropriate and leads to hypertension. In both humans and rats the number of glomeruli (the functional filtering unit of the kidney) is reduced by impaired fetal growth, and in humans this has been implicated in increasing the risk of hypertension. These structural changes are caused by an alteration in the programme of tissue differentiation. In growth-retarded rats, guinea pigs and sheep there are reductions in cell number in some brain areas and this may explain some of the neuropsychiatric abnormalities that occur in growth-retarded humans and may play a role in the determination of cognitive function.

We should not leave these developmental processes without noting that effects can also be manifest at the other end of life, namely in senescence. Apart from the programmed cell death, even tissues in which cells normally divide become senescent as the individual ages. This is in part owing to the shortening of components at the end of the DNA strands[4] that makes the DNA more susceptible to the damaging processes of ageing. Such shortening has been described in the DNA obtained from the kidneys of adult rats whose dams were protein deprived in utero.

## Gene expression and epigenetics

Alterations in gene expression can operate at many levels. Early in development they can operate to regulate stem-cell replication and tissue differentiation, as we have noted. Later in development they can permanently reset the levels of activity of many homeostatic mechanisms and indeed, in terms of final effector mechanisms, it is these changes that are most likely to explain the insulin resistance, leptin

---

[4] Called telomeres.

resistance and hormonal and cardiovascular control changes that are reflected in the final phenotype. About 5 per cent of the genes in the human genome are imprinted, and many of these are involved in growth and development. Imprinting, as detailed in chapter 2, involves the silencing of an allele of either maternal or paternal origin. This silencing occurs soon after fertilisation and involves changes in DNA methylation of one of the alleles. Methylation is dependent on the supply of methyl groups, which primarily comes from glycine; glycine is a dietary constituent but is also formed from the amino acid serine in the presence of folate. Could it therefore be that imprinting can be influenced by the environmental status of the embryo?

Recent data show that indeed this is the case. In sheep embryos placed in culture for lengthy periods before reimplantation (a very abnormal environment), the expression of the IGF-2 growth-factor receptor is affected significantly. The degree of imprinting is reduced, leading to increased IGF-2 production and thus to enhanced fetal growth. Another example concerns the 'agouti' gene in mice. If present it causes the expression of large quantities of agouti-related protein in the mouse. This produces a yellow coloration of the fur, but is also associated with the animals being obese and hyper-insulinaemic. As well as having these signs of the metabolic syndrome they have an increased risk of cancer and a reduced life span. It turns out that the gene for agouti protein is partially imprinted, and the degree of imprinting is strongly affected by the diet of the mother at the time of conception. If the mothers periconceptional diet is rich in folic acid / methyl donors, which favour DNA methylation, the offspring have a different coat appearance, live longer and do not have the high risk of cancer or diabetes.

Gene expression is controlled by levels of a range of proteins such as transcription factors. Because the manufacture of these proteins themselves will be under the control of other genes, the regulation of these latter genes can be all-important. These factors act by binding to promoter regions on DNA and these can be methylated, thus blocking the binding of the transcription factor. This is what has been found in the brains of rat pups exposed to high- or low-grooming mothers (see chapter 5). The change in methylation is very specific – at one site within the glucocorticoid-receptor gene expressed in one particular part of the brain – and it is sufficient to cause altered control of behaviour in these offspring. This gene is not an imprinted gene and so this example demonstrates that while imprinted genes may be favoured candidates for being influenced by environmental factors in an irreversible manner, other non-imprinted genes may be affected as well. We do not know how such specificity is achieved but we now suspect these epigenetic changes are a very important part of the basic mechanisms underlying PARs.

## Secondary effector mechanisms

These various generic mechanisms – cell-cycle effects, differentiation effects and alterations of gene expression allow for multiple and overlapping pathways to pre-natal induction of PARs and can be regarded as the primary effector mechanisms. Such primary effector mechanisms are translated into secondary processes that become manifest as the survival phenotype if the prediction is accurate, and as the disease phenotype in the case of inappropriate prediction. Many organs are involved and we suspect that in different situations – depending on the nature and timing of the cue – different balances of the primary processes and therefore of the effector mechanisms will be involved. These secondary effector mechanisms will be discussed in the remainder of this chapter.

**Pancreas**

The pancreas is a complex gland that lies between the liver and the duodenum, and it secretes into the intestine a component of the juice needed to digest food. But within the 'exocrine' pancreas are islets of cells that secrete several vitally impor-tant hormones into the bloodstream. The most well known of these hormones is insulin, made by the beta cells of these pancreatic islets. In the offspring of animals with inappropriate PARs, evidence for both insulin resistance and defective insulin release exists. In the offspring of rats fed a low-protein diet in pregnancy, glucose intolerance[5] arises because the islets have either not developed sufficiently or there has been excessive islet cell death – the number of beta cells is low and so is the blood supply to the islets. But as these rats age they also develop insulin resistance.

Two theories have grown over the last decade to explain the links between poor fetal growth and such Type 2 diabetes in later life. One is purely genetic, the 'thrifty genotype hypothesis', and proposes that a genetically produced insulin resistance in the offspring will not only produce reduced fetal growth, but also Type 2 diabetes in later life. There is evidence to support the theory, because insulin is an important driver of fetal growth, so resistance to it in the tissues is bound to impair such growth. Furthermore, a genetically inherited defect in the gene that encodes for the enzyme glucokinase does indeed produce in the offspring the combination of reduced birth weight and a form of Type 2 diabetes in the adult. The hypothesis proposes that through hominid evolution, genes have been selected that assist survival through poor nutritional environments. Indeed this appears likely to be the case and may explain in part why different populations have different propensities to obesity and hypertension. However, while this in general explains why we have the genetic

---

[5] Glucose intolerance is a term referring to high blood glucose, either because of reduced insulin levels or relative resistance to its glucose-lowering effects at the level of tissues such as skeletal muscle.

machinery to develop the survival phenotype, it cannot explain the very rapid increase in the incidence of diabetes in some societies. Such changes, within a generation or two and involving millions of people, cannot occur via purely genetic mechanisms. Most convincingly, the animal experiments rule out purely genetic explanations. However, the genotype is the blueprint on which the environment acts before birth to induce PARs. If the postnatal environment is poor then no disease will occur because the prediction was appropriate. Conversely, as is more often the case in modern times, if the postnatal environment is rich then the disease phenotype of obesity, hypertension and insulin resistance is more likely to appear.

For these reasons we must conclude that inappropriate PARs underlie the changing environment of Type 2 diabetes. We have previously suggested reasons why the insulin-resistant phenotype has survival advantage in a deprived environment (p. 121). It involves a range of mechanisms, including the pancreatic production of insulin, tissue sensitivity to the hormone and other changes in metabolic control. Reduced skeletal muscle mass may be a major cause because skeletal muscle is the principal site of peripheral insulin action. Once omental fat starts to develop, it increases the resistance to the actions of insulin in the other key target organ, the liver. Whenever omental fat is mobilised (as occurs every night during sleep), the released fatty acids travel through the portal system to the liver and change the sensitivity of the liver to insulin.[6] Overall, such adaptive responses will favour the use of high energy-producing substrates (fat) at times of dearth of food.

This is why the 'thrifty phenotype' (see chapter 4) is the logical outcome of PARs operating in a species such as the human where maternal constraint is nearly always operative (see chapter 8). Such adaptive responses will be disadvantageous at times of plentiful food, and will lead to obesity and Type 2 diabetes.

## Fat and muscle

Fat and muscle are major targets for the actions of insulin and we have already discussed how these are both affected in the survival phenotype: fat mass is increased and muscle mass is reduced. Both may be the consequence of insulin resistance but there may be far more fundamental mechanisms in the regulation of tissue differentiation involved – this is a fertile area for research. Fat cell number is largely determined before birth but much less is known about its regulation during development. Muscle cell number is also determined in fetal life because muscle cells have multiple nuclei and cannot divide further once formed. They form from uninucleate precursor cells and it may be this conversion, or the number of precursor cells, that is affected.

---

[6] Indeed drugs that limit omental fat mobilisation are used in the management of Type 2 diabetes.

## Liver

This organ plays a vital role in the metabolic responses of the body. The liver is able to synthesise glucose to meet metabolic needs at times when food is restricted, and this is under the control of another hormone produced by the pancreas, glucagon. The liver can also store glucose in the form of glycogen when glucose is in excess. Storage is promoted by the action of insulin. These functions are inducible. Both adults who suffer from Type 2 diabetes and the offspring of rats fed a low-protein diet in pregnancy show altered responses of the liver to insulin, and they may even secrete extra glucose rather than reducing glucose output as expected. As we have noted, this combines with the insulin resistance in tissues such as skeletal muscle to keep plasma glucose levels high.

There are also changes in the overall structure of the liver so that more glucose-producing and fewer glucose-consuming cells are formed. The liver also plays a role in fat metabolism and controls the levels of lipids in the bloodstream, and it manufactures binding proteins for IGFs and other hormones such as cortisol. It is highly active metabolically and can inactivate cortisol returning from the placenta before the hormone gains access to the fetal bloodstream. We can see from this brief summary that the liver must be a prime candidate for the induction of PARs.

During late gestation and at birth, the abdominal circumference is primarily determined by the size of the liver, so it is perhaps no surprise that this is reduced in fetuses that have been challenged by poor placental function. Recently, however, the extent to which the control of liver function may be determined in fetal life has been emphasised by studies of fetal liver blood flow in relation to maternal diet and body composition (see also chapter 4). Thin women and those who consumed a less 'prudent' diet before pregnancy had fetuses in which the flow of blood to the fetal liver was increased at the expense of the blood normally shunted through the liver[7] to the fetal heart and brain. Studies in sheep fetuses in which the flow through the ductus venosus was artificially altered, producing in turn changes in liver blood flow, indicate that the effects on organ growth and function may be substantial, suggesting life-long changes in liver function.

## The heart and blood vessels

Despite the epidemiological studies suggesting that PARs alter the risks of cardio-vascular disease, there has been relatively little work on the induction of pathological effects on the heart and blood vessels. Animal studies have revealed that

---

[7] In the fetus there is a unique vessel called the ductus venosus, which shunts a substantial fraction of the blood coming from the placenta past the liver and straight to the heart. At birth this closes off when the umbilical cord is tied.

the function of the endothelial cells that line the blood vessels is impaired in the offspring of mothers fed an unbalanced diet. Such changes in function would be expected to produce elevated blood pressure, for some of the important stimuli that cause blood vessels to relax are mediated through these endothelial cells. Similar disruptions in endothelial cell function have been shown in children, and related to low birth weight. The size of the effects is similar to that produced by smoking in adult life, which disturbs endothelial cell function and is associated with high blood pressure. There are also changes in the function of the muscular layer in the wall of small arteries (smooth muscle), that regulate the calibre of the blood vessels and hence controls blood pressure. Structural changes in the blood vessels will also be expected to accompany such induced effects, making the effect on blood pressure worse and irreversible. Changes have indeed been seen in the amount of elastin, which is a protein that plays a role in making the vessels able to stretch in response to pressure changes. Elastin is secreted by the smooth muscle cells in the arterial wall, and this process is essentially complete early in life. Hence the 'stretchiness' of the arteries is less in the offspring of nutrient-deprived mothers. The combination of reduced elasticity, altered smooth muscle responsiveness and endothelial dysfunction is characteristic of aging and cardiovascular disease in humans.

Effects on the endothelium are also important in the onset of atheromatous plaque formation. In Western populations it is now clear that such atheroma, which used to be thought of as a disease of middle age, is now very much a feature of the young. Autopsies on the thousands of young, fit American GIs who were killed in action in Vietnam, many of whom were in their early twenties, revealed an astonishingly high level of atheromatous lesions in their arteries. Most recently, autopsies have even shown fatty streaks in the arteries of fetuses, an effect exacerbated by high levels of maternal cholesterol in pregnancy. Hence it is clear that vascular disease starts very early in the life of human populations in the developed world, demonstrating just how early the effects of inappropriate PARs can be manifest if the postnatal environment is rich. Studies in low birth weight guinea pigs similarly demonstrate altered cholesterol metabolism and increased plaque formation.

Metabolically active organs such as the heart and kidney are likely to be affected by PARs more than less energy-consuming organs. The heart of course develops to serve the circulating transport needs of the body, so if the fetal body-growth trajectory is down-regulated, we would expect the heart also to be affected. The heart is one of the few organs in the body in which the number of cells is essentially set before birth in the human. The heart muscle cells (cardiomyocytes) mature in late gestation and then do not divide. After birth any change in heart size, for example in response to the strain placed upon it by hypertension, results from increased growth of the muscle cells, not from an increase in their number. The effects of PARs on the heart are poorly studied but our experimental animal studies (MAH) are now beginning to show enlargement of the left side of the heart in adult offspring under-nourished in utero.

The endothelial cells lining blood vessels were referred to above. They also line the chambers of the heart, and of course the heart has an extensive blood supply of its own – the coronary vasculature. Endothelial cell function is important not only in the growth of the coronary blood vessels, as it is in other parts of the circulation, but it also links to both the growth and maturation of the cardiomyocytes and the specialised conducting tissue of the heart, which ensures the orderly and synchronous contraction of the separate parts of the myocardium. So it is possible that PARs may have drastic consequences for a range of components of cardiac function in later life. In the final analysis, cardiac function must be determined by the balance between the energy needs of the heart, which increase enormously in exercise or stress, and the supply of nutrients and oxygen in the coronary circulation. The latter is termed coronary reserve, and it is interesting that this appears to be altered in early life in fetuses exposed to anaemia (which lowers the oxygen-carrying capacity of the blood in utero). Whether nutritional and endocrine cues can induce similar influences on coronary reserve is not known.

## The kidney

In the adult animal or human, about one quarter of the blood pumped by the heart goes to the kidneys, which are metabolically highly active. As kidney size is related to body size, we therefore expect that PARs will affect this organ. The active unit of the kidney is the nephron, which conducts all the filtering and excretion of waste products from the blood stream and is also responsible for the control of water and solute (e.g. salt) excretion. It plays a vital role in the regulation of the body's fluid balance. In addition, because fluid balance is related to blood volume, and this in turn to cardiac output, the kidney plays a key role in cardiovascular and blood pressure regulation. It has been known for many years that a reduction in kidney function is associated with the development of high blood pressure. Nephrons are essentially all produced before birth in the human, and in rats they are produced by 10 days after birth. Growth-retarded human infants and nutritionally deprived fetal rats and pigs have reduced renal mass and an irreversibly reduced nephron number.

More detailed studies have used the fetal sheep as an experimental animal. The role of the kidney, and in particular of the renin–angiotensin system, has been confirmed in these. Renin is a hormone made by the kidney that activates a second hormone called angiotensin, which is a potent regulator of blood pressure by constricting blood vessels. One of the receptor types for angiotensin is increased in the fetus when placental function has been reduced. Further studies have explored the way in which fetal exposure to elevated levels of glucocorticoid can affect the kidney. It has been shown that exposure of the fetus to such steroids for only a few days at the critical time during renal development in early fetal life has drastic effects on kidney development and the blood pressure of the offspring as adults many years later. No such effect was seen if the cue was applied later in pregnancy. This evidence not only confirms the role of glucocorticoids in the induction of fetal development, especially the kidney, but it reinforces the concept that critical periods exist for such induction effects to be manifest.

Several groups around the world have therefore examined the effects of prenatal challenges on nephron number, usually measured by glomerular number. There is reasonable agreement that it is reduced by such challenges in animals. A recent study[8] in humans confirmed a hypothesis, originally proposed by Barry Brenner, that the number of nephrons in adult men who had hypertension was less than those who did not: the striking point about the study was the size of the effect, as the hypertensive men had only about 50 per cent of the glomeruli of the normotensive men.

We can begin to assemble a concept of a pathway to disease from such data, particularly with respect to the gradual development of high blood pressure in adulthood. If the number of nephrons in the kidneys is set before birth, it can be a target for a PAR, because the kidney is metabolically highly active. Thus the prediction that postnatal nutrition will be poor will lead to reduced kidney growth and nephron number, because a smaller body after birth needs a smaller kidney. The offspring will be able to cope initially with this reduced number of nephrons postnatally, partly because the body has still much growth to undertake so renal function is not at the maximum level required in life. In addition, the control of the kidney will allow those nephrons present to work harder, hyper-filtering the blood to achieve homeostasis. This will suffice to get the individual to reproductive age – a requirement of a PAR. But as the processes of ageing proceed, with arterial wall stiffening and endothelial dysfunction, the hyper-filtering nephrons will become less and less effective. Eventually they will lose control over blood volume, and this will place an additional strain on the heart. Hormones of the renin–angiotensin system will rise in the blood in an attempt to increase renal removal of sodium and, by increasing blood pressure, to drive more blood through the kidneys. This will lead to further remodelling of vascular structure and to further renal damage. The vicious circle of effects leading to pathologically high blood pressure and heart failure has begun.

---

[8] The number of glomeruli in the kidneys of men who died in car accidents was counted, and those with high versus normal blood pressure were compared.

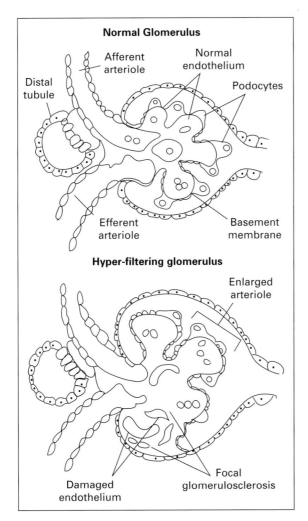

Fig. 6.2     The normal kidney glomerulus filters blood plasma to make a fluid that will form the basis for urine, after reabsorbtion and secretion of solutes. The driving force for the filtration is arterial pressure in the afferent arteriole. Normally this process is set, partly by the number of nephrons, to be appropriate for body size and metabolic demand. If nephron number has been reduced, e.g. as part of a predictive adaptive response, then those nephrons present have to work harder to achieve homeostasis. The continued hyper-filtration over time produces glomerular injury. This may cause blood pressure to rise; it may also damage the body's fluid control mechanisms. The result is hypertension and cardiovascular disease. The effect will develop slowly over life, accelerating in middle age. This concept (Brenner's hypothesis) is a good example of how an early structural change produces disease much later in life. Redrawn from Ingelfinger J. R. *New England Journal of Medicine* (2003), **348**: 99–100.

## Blood pressure control

The adult body has an intricate set of checks and balances that regulate its function either through hormonal or neural mechanisms. Many of these are reflex in nature and not under conscious control. We think of such reflexes as operating to control our skeletal muscles as in balancing to walk along a narrow path or ride a bicycle, or in defending the body from insult, e.g. the blink reflex or withdrawing a limb from a painful stimulus such as heat. But in addition to these interactions with our external environment, we possess many reflexes that regulate our internal environment. Examples are those involved in the control of blood pressure, cardiac and renal function and the integration of these components, which must be closely linked if we are to remain healthy. When we think about this, it seems rather odd that conditions such as high blood pressure arise. If the systems are so finely tuned, why does a persistent rise in blood pressure occur? We saw how this might occur owing to reduced nephron number above. But why isn't it compensated for by the other components of reflex control? One of the most important systems that controls blood pressure involves the baroreceptors. These are little sensory organs that are located in the walls of the major arteries in the chest and neck. If blood pressure rises, the arterial wall will be distended and this will stretch the receptors. As they are connected by fine nerves to the neurons in the brain that control the function of the cardiovascular system, the stimulus of increased pressure is communicated to the brain. Compensatory mechanisms are then brought into play – the forcefulness of the contractions of the heart is reduced, heart rate slows, the small arteries in the body relax. All these nervously induced changes will dampen down the increase in blood pressure. This of course will reduce the stretch of the arteries in which the baroreceptors lie, and so reduce their stimulatory effect on the brain. So the system will operate to control the blood pressure about a set-point, and the baroreceptors can be viewed rather like the thermostat that detects the temperature in the room and signals to the heating system whether more or less heat is required.

These various processes appear to be disturbed in animals with PARs but in slightly unexpected ways. It turns out that the function of the baroreceptors is normal in animals in which phenotypic changes have been induced; hence their ability to detect changes in arterial pressure and to signal this to the brain, while sometimes less, is not substantially altered. What *has* changed is the pressure set-point about which they operate. These receptors appear to have evolved to protect the animal against sudden changes in pressure, e.g. in life-threatening situations such as haemorrhage. They have not evolved to protect against hypertension – a disease of post-reproduction age. So what we find in animals is that the baroreceptors have reset, to retain their function of detecting changes in pressure, but with a higher set-point. This of course allows blood pressure to rise still further. In addition the neural output from the nerves that increase cardiac output and raise blood pressure[9] is higher than expected. At a time when the output from the neurones that control these nerves should be low, in an attempt to rein blood pressure in, it seems to be artificially high. Studies in several countries have shown that measures of this neural output, e.g. heart rate itself, are higher in people with low birth weight. Moreover, the response of such individuals to additional stress is greater, exacerbating the problem still further.

## Neural control systems

In view of the fact that it is the higher functions of the human brain that distinguish us so markedly from other species, it is perhaps surprising that mechanistic effects of PARs acting via the higher centres of the brain have not been much investigated. We have already reviewed experimental data suggesting that both appetite and willingness to exercise can be induced. There have been suggestions from the animal experiments that some aspects of behaviour – social grooming, exploratory and reproductive behaviour for example – can be determined by prenatal challenges. Effects on food preference and appetite in animals are discussed below. These ideas have been very little extrapolated to humans. Epidemiologists have also found associations between birth weight and the rate of cognitive decline in the elderly. Such observations will have far-reaching consequences if they are substantiated, and we await further research in this area. However at present we cannot say whether such effects are directly via patho-physiological effects on the brain, or whether they represent further examples of mechanisms involved in inappropriate PARs.

The extent to which intergenerational influences on behaviour are a result of PARs or are learned behaviours in the human is not known. This is an area meriting much more research. Recall the work of Michael Meaney described in chapter 5. It suggests that, at least in the rat, maternal–infant interactions at birth have lifelong effects on behaviour owing to alteration in the methylation of genes in the brain.

## Hormonal control systems

Several hormonal mechanisms play a part in PARs. They can operate via the mother's endocrine glands, and we have seen how changes in the level of the stress hormone cortisol in her blood can affect the developing placenta and fetus. In late gestation the fetal endocrine glands are maturing, and so the adaptations that form such an integral part of PARs may involve alterations in their development. Most of the attention in research has centred on the pituitary gland, as this is the 'master'

---

[9] The sympathetic nervous system.

endocrine gland, which controls many of the other hormonal systems. The effects of induction on the hypothalamo–pituitary–endocrine gland axes are subtle and graded, but they nonetheless have lifelong effects on the offspring. This is because the system involves a series of control mechanisms to regulate the secretion of hormones that determine reproductive function, growth and responses to stress, to name only some.

Periconceptional undernutrition in sheep alters the maturation of the HPA axis later in gestation and thus the rate of fetal development – recall that cortisol is a critical hormone in regulating maturation of some organs such as the fetal lung before birth. Other experiments involving fetal sheep, rats and guinea pigs show that exposing the fetus to either a nutritional stress or to steroids leads to permanent changes in the set-points of the HPA axis that, after birth, become manifest as increased levels of cortisol in the blood stream in response to stress. These changes appear primarily to reflect alterations in glucocorticoid receptors as described above. Chronic increases in glucocorticoids will tend to increase blood pressure and insulin resistance and promote fat deposition, as well as altering stress responses. This is not a healthy biochemical phenotype.

We saw in chapter 3 how the environment of the snowshoe hare induced the responses of its offspring: when the population numbers were low and the individual risk of predation was high, the offspring were more alert. Their levels of alertness are determined by HPA axis responsiveness, so we can see how the mechanism works. High maternal anxiety and hence elevated HPA-axis activity induces an increase in the responsiveness of the offspring's HPA axis and hence promotes alertness in them. If the environmental challenge lessens, because the risk of predation is reduced by rising population numbers or better food supplies, the pregnant hares are under less stress and their offspring will have reduced HPA-axis responses.

## Postnatal amplification

In chapter 4 we reviewed the evidence, both in humans and in rats, that there is an interaction between the fetal experience and the childhood growth pattern. Those that grow fastest after birth, particularly in the prepubertal years and particularly if they develop relative obesity[10] are at greatest risk of later disease. This may simply be an amplification phenomenon. In other words, if the organism is born small with a set of adaptations to stay small and the environment is such that catch-up growth and plentiful food is available, then the effects will be magnified by having a physiology designed for a small body operating in a large body.

---

[10]  Relative is the key word – it need not be gross obesity, merely a relative increase in fat compared to absolute height. The child may not look obese although the more obese the greater the risk.

The studies from Finland, to which we referred in chapter 4, suggest that after the period of slow growth in infancy the men who suffered coronary heart disease and diabetes later had shown accelerated growth in childhood. The children destined to develop diabetes gained weight somewhat earlier than those with heart disease. The importance of such 'catch-up' growth is debated by the paediatricians working in this area. It may simply be an indicator that earlier growth had been slowed and that the body is trying literally to catch up when food becomes available. If this is the case, then the earlier undernutrition is really the important thing. But the situation becomes more alarming if the children are followed further. They don't just catch up with their peers – many overtake them substantially. They are more likely to become obese and, given the discussion in the previous chapter, the reader will not be surprised by this observation.

The importance of the situation is brought home by data from young people in New Delhi. Those who went on to develop Type 2 diabetes had a very different pattern of growth from those who did not. Children tend to lose fat in their early childhood years and then to gain it again in the period running up to puberty, and this has been termed 'adiposity rebound'. In the New Delhi study the speed of this adiposity rebound was much faster in the children who would become Type 2 diabetics. This could be seen from the *rate* of increase in their body mass index (BMI) in mid childhood, even though their actual body weights did not differ from the young people who would remain healthy. Like the Finns destined to develop coronary heart disease or diabetes, the Indians destined to suffer from Type 2 diabetes went on to become relatively obese in childhood, magnifying this effect through adolescence. The scale of the problem is horrifying because in that group about 20 per cent of the subjects had overt diabetes by the age of 30.

We have already described that in the rat the origins of obesity, including dietary preference, a disinclination to exercise and increased appetite may be induced before birth as part of a PAR. If this is true in the human then it will be very difficult to rectify problems such as those in New Delhi just by postnatal interventions. But there is a deeper implication. Could it be that the relationship between catch-up growth (at least in weight) and fetal experience is not just interactive but is actually causally linked? The evidence we have presented, showing that obesity in part has a childhood origin, suggests that this may be the case; there are some snippets of data that hormonal axes that control growth might also contain some inducible elements. This area merits further research.

Other processes, including poor nutrition and infection, act directly on postnatal growth. These are likely to be particularly associated with poor living conditions and overcrowding, and it is easy to see how in large families in poor areas the younger children might lose out in the struggle for food. They may also be exposed to repeated infections, e.g. respiratory infections and diarrhoea, which will hamper their nutrition. There are data, to date very minimal, that support the idea that sensitivity to infection and the ability to mount an immune response may also be affected by the prenatal experience – this is an area that should be a research priority. But even in the developed world, many children are exposed to poverty and poor housing conditions. Population-based studies have shown that the effects of such poor conditions in childhood persist into adult life, regardless of the social class attained by the adult. We will return to the public health implications of PARs in chapter 9.

## Conclusion

As we have already shown, PARs induce some degree of structural change, whether in the walls of blood vessels or the enzymes in the liver or in the methylation of a gene. It is 'cheaper' to conduct these changes while the organism is growing, than to institute them later. The organism's ability to adapt becomes less as it grows and develops, as more and more structures and control mechanisms are laid down and the critical periods during which they could be modified have passed. Postnatal events may amplify or attenuate the effects on organs and systems of fetal induction, and the resulting consequences will depend on whether the adaptive responses are appropriate or inappropriate for the environment.

One of the most well-established epidemiological findings is the link between low birth weight and hypertension in later life, and we discussed the conflicting views over the actual size of the effect in chapter 4. Perhaps it is useful in concluding this chapter on mechanisms to return to that example. There are many reasons why high blood pressure develops. In part it is due to structural changes, with fewer small blood vessels developing in some tissues, leading to elevated peripheral resistance; in part it occurs because the kidney has a reduced nephron number; in part it occurs because of altered activity in the renin–angiotensin system; in part because of insulin resistance; in part because of altered endothelial function; and in part because of altered neural and reflex control. All these mechanisms are involved, but to varying extents in different individuals and when different challenges induce PARs. Insulin resistance and obesity further amplify the problem. This range of mechanisms leading to hypertension demonstrates the way in which there must be multiple paths to a single phenotypic attribute, in this case high blood pressure.

When we think of the ways in which the different phenotypic aspects of the body interact – cardiovascular and renal control, diet and feeding behaviour, neural function and growth etc. – it is not surprising that unequivocal correlations between stimulus and response do not always emerge even in the most tightly controlled study. Far from detracting from the concept that the appropriateness of a PAR plays a part in individual susceptibility to disease, this multiplicity of mechanisms underlines the strength of the PARs model. We would suggest that these diverse mechanisms, and the ease of their evocation, is strong evidence of the general evolutionary importance of these PARs. That is why they have been protected through evolutionary time. The critical issue may be that humans no longer live within the environment in which they evolved. A biological response that should generally produce an appropriate prediction now produces an inappropriate prediction. This is exacerbated by the mechanisms that have evolved in humans to push development towards the survival phenotype. Why this has occurred is the subject of the next chapter.

# 7

# Predictive adaptive responses – critical processes in evolution

## Our theory of predictive adaptive responses

We have introduced the term predictive adaptive responses by implication rather than by definition. It is now useful to define them more formally. We propose PARs as biological processes with the following characteristics:

1. They are induced by environmental factors acting in early life, most often in pre-embryonic, embryonic or fetal life, not as an immediate physiological adaptation, but as a predictive response in expectation of some future environment.
2. They are manifest in permanent change in the physiology or structure of the organism.
3. There are multiple pathways to the induction of these responses, involving different environmental cues acting at different times in development.
4. PARs are not restricted in direction, and occur across the full range of fetal environments.
5. The induction of PARs will confer a survival advantage in the predicted reproductive environment (that is appropriate prediction) and this will be manifest as increased fitness.[1]
6. The PAR thus defines an environmental range in which the organism can optimally thrive until and through the reproductive phase of its postnatal life.
7. However, these PARs may well lead to disease or disadvantage when the predicted reproductive or post-reproductive environmental boundaries are exceeded (that is inappropriate prediction).

The first three criteria in this list have been well described in the previous chapters and will not be discussed further. The remainder of these criteria will be covered in this chapter, and we also speculate on two further potential characteristics.

---

[1] *Fitness* refers to the life-time reproductive performance of an individual – that is a measure of the numbers of surviving children (or as we shall see, more strictly, grandchildren). It combines considerations such as fecundity, age at puberty, number of children born and number of children reaching reproductive age themselves. The traits that are selected, and amplified, by natural selection are those that improve the 'fitness' of a species.

8. PARs are likely to be neo-Darwinian adaptations[2] permitting a species to survive short-term environmental challenges while preserving maximum genotypic variation for later environmental challenges and evolutionary fitness.

9. It is likely that through a variety of processes, there will be transgenerational exhibition of PARs.

In the last three chapters our focus has been drawn to one subset of this phenomenon – namely inappropriate prediction and in particular the situation that occurs when the fetus anticipates a deprived environment and enters one that is better than predicted. Indeed we propose that the mechanisms of maternal constraint always shift the set-point of the normally growing human fetus to a position where it predicts some degree of postnatal nutrient limitation. Later we will discuss why we think that this had an evolutionary advantage. While this scenario has been our focus, the totality of the phenomenon – both appropriate and inappropriate prediction – is important to understand from a theoretical perspective.

Predictive responses are broadly based phenomena in the animal kingdom. They have been very easy to demonstrate experimentally in a variety of species including sheep, pigs, rats, mice and guinea pigs. We have also described some examples of similar phenomena in the natural habitat. The meadow vole's coat is a particularly striking example of a PAR with no immediate adaptive value. This universality implies that PARs have a survival value and that evolution has protected their persistence. If this is the case then it follows that, generally, PARs must confer an advantage, primarily when linked to a matched postnatal environment. We have termed this form of adaptive response, appropriate prediction. Through evolutionary history, it is indeed likely that a match between the fetal and postnatal environment has been the norm and this leads us to propose that the mechanisms of PARs, which themselves must be coded within the genome, are tightly conserved through evolution. This however, does not imply a single underlying mechanism. Indeed, it is obvious that, with multiple pathways to induce PARs, there must be multiple mechanisms underpinning them and that, if PARs have had survival advantage, the mechanisms underlying them will themselves have been selected.

In humans, inappropriate PARs can lead to disease. We argue that this is because the fetus has prepared itself for birth by developing its biological systems for independent life in the expectation that it is to be born into a relatively deprived or

---

[2] Why do we say *likely* to be an adaptation? Most people use adaptation to refer to any apparently useful response within a given environment, but evolutionary theorists use adaptation very precisely. In their language, adaptation means a response that has evolved through the processes of natural selection and has an advantage in terms of fitness. The phenomenon we are discussing is adaptive in that it is a response to a predicted environment and we suspect that it is a true adaptation. It would therefore be convenient to use the noun, adaptation, but the formal proof that it is an adaptation is lacking. If we are to be clear in our meaning to our scientific colleagues, despite its awkwardness we need to talk about predictive *adaptive* responses. These responses can either be an appropriate or inappropriate prediction depending on the match between the prenatal prediction and postnatal environment.

(more commonly) an enriched environment. The former arises because the signals given by the mother are interpreted as reflecting a poor extra-uterine environment. This may be an appropriate cue if the mother is living in a deprived or threatening environment and, as we shall see, has broader evolutionary appropriateness. But the signal, at least in modern humans, can be misleading if there has been maternal disease or placental dysfunction. If the child or adult faces a far better environment than was anticipated by the fetus, then there will be excessive catch-up growth and the development of obesity after birth. This postnatal amplification puts stress on the physiological phenotype set by the fetal PARs and this mismatch can lead to the development of disease in middle age. The converse can happen if the fetus is born into a poorer environment than predicted. This can also result from an environmental miscue – for example the fetus of a diabetic mother receives excessive glucose, suggesting a more energy-enriched environment than is actually the case after birth.

The biological basis of appropriate and inappropriate prediction is the same – this must be so because the fetus does not 'know' which category of prediction its 'choice' will become when it makes it – the fetus makes its choices based on its prediction of the future environment. In other words it takes a gamble based on information it receives from the mother across the placenta, which it interprets as reflecting the world into which it will be born. Depending on that interpretation, it commits itself to a set of biological changes that, because of the irreversible nature of developmental plasticity, it must live with for the rest of its life. If it got its prediction right then the choice is appropriate and generally adaptive; if it made a faulty prediction then the outcome is inappropriate and potentially maladaptive. Evolution will have operated to select the mechanisms underpinning a PAR on the basis that, in most situations for that population in that environment, the PAR will have conferred advantage. As we shall see, particularly in chapter 8, the evolution of life-style diseases in humans can be clearly understood from this perspective.

A continuum of predictive responses must exist, from the most appropriate at one extreme to the most inappropriate at the other, and the appropriateness may change at different phases in postnatal life – childhood, reproductive period and old age. Natural selection can essentially only reinforce processes operating during the first two periods.[3]

Predictive responses are not an 'all-or-nothing' process and of course the postnatal environment experienced can vary widely. The nature of the response that occurs is linked to the probability of environmental challenge and is determined by when, how strong and how prolonged the intrauterine triggering cues are. We argue that if the fetus is more certain that the postnatal environment will be extreme it

---

[3] One exception would be grand-maternal effects discussed in chapter 6.

will make a greater deviation from the norm than if it senses only a subtle change. Because of this continuum, and because the processes underlying appropriate and inappropriate predictive changes are the same, when we are discussing the common biological processes we will continue to use the generic term, *predictive adaptive responses*.

Our thesis is that the repertoire of PARs creates a set of biological processes that are a key element in the survival of a species. We think that evolution has used the PAR to 'tune' the fetus, in the absence of other cues, to adopt a default position – that of the survival phenotype: that is, the fetus is induced so that in the absence of other information it will be equipped to be born into a relatively poor nutritional environment. Certainly the evolution of hominids occurred in an environment very different from that which we now inhabit, and thus the processes underlying PARs may have led to the evolution of processes that may have been more generally appropriate in past evolutionary time but now are more likely to be inappropriate. Indeed we suggest that this is an important element in the rising epidemic of heart disease and diabetes, in both the developed and developing world.

In considering this we need to distinguish physiological constraints acting in all pregnancies, which have created the default phenotype, from those pathophysiological constraints that utilise similar mechanisms to generate a more exaggerated effect. We propose that the phenomenon of maternal constraint is a core process that served the evolutionary purpose of tuning the phenotype to be on the safe side in its prediction. This default pathway is one in which survival to reproductive age in an uncertain world is more likely. Hence we term this phenotype the default or survival phenotype. Humans are unusual in that their lives now extend well beyond the normal reproductive years and therefore the disease-enhancing effects of this phenotype, which generally appear relatively late in life in the modern world, were not subject to negative selection pressures.

## The role of PARs in the responses to environmental change

The fundamental focus of this book is on how the human species responds to environmental change. As we have detailed in chapter 3, the nature of the potential response depends on the duration of the environmental stimulus/change and when in development it occurs. Very short-term change involves homeostatic processes. A more prolonged environmental change, such as a seasonal change in food supply, may similarly be dealt with by selected physiological processes. For example in ruminants there are day-length dependent changes in growth hormone secretion that determine whether energy is diverted to fat storage or not. Similar processes underpin seasonal reproduction and daylight dependent changes in sex hormone secretion. Here the underlying physiological systems responding to environmental change have been selected because the environmental change, while transient, is reliably predictable and there is a clear fitness advantage in having mechanisms to respond to that change. Permanent environmental change obviously leads, through the processes of natural selection, to permanent change in the phenotype through genotypic change.

In contrast to these effects, irregular transient environmental change needs a different strategy, particularly if it occurs in early development. The fetus must choose a trajectory that adjusts its physiology to make it most likely to reproduce, and that is the basis of the PAR. There is enormous advantage in having a mechanism whereby, during early development, plastic changes are made that confer an advantage in a future environment. In energetic trade-off terms, a decision to make an irreversible plastic response in early development, while the fetus is still protected and nurtured by its mother, may confer great advantage on that animal in its period of reproductive life. Later trade-offs might be very costly. This is at the heart of our proposition of the role of evolved PARs.

There are many human examples of the costly nature of later biological trade-offs. Anorexia nervosa is a psychiatric disease leading to self-induced starvation. In females, it is inevitably associated with loss of menstruation and infertility. Clearly this is a homeorhetic response – energy supplies are limited – the body shuts down processes that are not essential to immediate survival, and obviously reproductive fitness is one. Similar processes occur when a population is exposed to famine. The exhaustion of energy supplies in high-performance female athletes that is associated with infertility is another example. Reproductive fitness cannot be preserved in such immediate responses but fortunately the biological changes underpinning them are reversible. In contrast, if the fetus can predict it will be in a nutrient-deficient environment as an adult, it can make a set of changes in its physiology so as to require less energy for maintenance and it will be able to reproduce – that is the advantage of early predictive responses and trade-offs.

There are important differences between a PAR and a homeostatic or classical adaptive response. In the case of homeostasis and classical adaptive response the survival benefit to the individual is immediate and at the time of the response. In the case of PARs, there need not be any immediate benefit but such benefit is manifest some time later. Obviously there is a gradation between classical adaptive responses and PARs: the response may have a small immediate benefit and a larger longer-term benefit or vice versa. Indeed it is probable that many mechanisms underlying PARs originally had some short-term benefit that led to their initial selection; subsequently this led to their magnification because, once present, added fitness led to the underpinning genes to be selected. However, natural selection could also act directly to select genes that only have predictive advantage.

## Environment

There are many environmental factors that might be considered as cues for the fetus to induce a predictive response. By far the most important is the nutritional environment and, in general, this is what we have focused on when talking of the prenatal environment. Nutrition is so central because the availability of food and its subsequent utilisation primarily determines growth and development. In all species, seeking food is a dominant activity. But there is a close and obvious interaction between food consumption and energy expenditure. The sum of these two factors creates a useful integrated view of the environment. We can term this the 'energy environment' – a high-energy environment is one in which there is high food availability and low energy consumption to obtain it. Conversely a low-energy environment is one in which the availability of food is low and the energy consumed in getting it is high. We can reasonably assume that the hunter–gatherer lived in a very low-energy environment. Agriculture enhanced the energy environment, with further changes following industrialisation. We think that a massive and rapid increase is now occurring in the energy environment owing to the development of enriched foods and sedentary lifestyles.

Another key environmental stimulus is 'stress'. Stress or anxiety are clearly critical survival factors when an individual is exposed to a high risk of predation. To be highly anxious and have powerful stress responses are logical reactions in a risky environment. Thus it is not surprising that stress cues and nutritional cues are interrelated and lead to similar PARs. There is no reason why multiple PARs triggered by different environmental stimuli cannot operate in the same organism.

In general when we use the term environment without qualification we will therefore be referring to the energy environment. This does not mean that these are the only possible predictive cues or that the responses we ascribe to nutritional and/or stress cues are the only possible predictive responses: however they will be the point of focus because of their relevance to human disease. The example given in chapter 1 of the development of sweat glands illustrates a PAR to another cue (temperature) and with a distinct phenotypic response. Similarly changes in how the body regulates salt and fluid balance are seen in the offspring of rats whose mothers were subjected to altered fluid loading.

## Evolution and selection

Darwin originally proposed that natural variation provided evolutionary selection on the basis of characteristics that suited a species for survival and reproduction in a particular environmental niche. These characteristics clearly had to be operating while the animal was still reproductively competent because in general selection pressures do not act to preserve characteristics that are favourable only after the individual has passed this age. We saw in chapter 2 that the variations in characteristics, which occur over an evolutionary timescale, are genomic – that is mutations, deletions or polymorphisms of the genes. So while it is phenotypic traits that determine whether an individual either survives or dies, and reproduces or does not, the effects in terms of the impact on the frequency of an allele in the gene pool can only be affected to the extent to which the phenotypic trait is coded genomically.

The issue of the level at which selection operates still leads to considerable debate – is it at the level of the organism, at the level of the species group, or at the gene itself? Dawkins has argued cogently for selection at the level of the gene and he sees the organism as the vehicle in which the replicator (the gene) is carried. Others see selection acting at the level of the whole organism – that is, one specific phenotypic trait may confer an advantage and to the extent to which it is reflected in the genotype, selection operates. Others still have argued that selection operates by group. These different perspectives are beyond the scope of this book.[4]

Evolution has two critical dimensions – diversity and time. Through the first, genetic variation produces a range of genotypes in the population, which are then expressed as phenotypes. Through the second dimension – time – the phenotypic traits are selected on the basis of fitness. This involves both natural and sexual selection. The two components of evolution operate sequentially: after the time needed for selection, another set of variations will be generated by mutation in the gene pool of the selected population, which will lead in time to another process of selection, and so on. Unless there is genetically determined phenotypic diversity underpinned by allelic variation there can be nothing on which selection can act. And selection can only act on genetically determined characteristics produced by genetic variation within the gene pool of a species, and this can essentially only be generated by mutation and recombination (see chapter 2). It is these processes that, along with the phenomenon of genetic drift, generate the stochastic elements (elements that have a random distribution that cannot be predicted precisely) underlying the evolutionary process.

Theoretically the wider the range of genotypes within a population, the greater the potential for evolutionary change. However in general the shift in phenotype associated with selection proceeds by miniscule steps: no one phenotypic trait can shift very far from other components because functional form and viability must be maintained. This creates constraints on the degree of change that can occur.

---

[4] But note that the simple genetic concept that a single gene leads to a single phenotypic trait has now been replaced by a much more sophisticated understanding of how one gene may have multiple non-parallel phenotypic effects (*pleiotopy*) and how multiple genes interact with each other (*epistasis*) and so can to some degree be coselected. Pleiotopy offers another possible mechanism for how PARs with no obvious prenatal advantage may have initially been selected.

Thus phenotypic change generally occurs slowly in the absence of a catastrophic event. When a single trait that has little impact on other traits is being selected, such as beak length in the finch, more rapid change is possible. But usually species survival depends on multiple associated traits and therefore change is restricted and showed by epistasis. For example in dog breeding multiple traits are usually selected in parallel. Even with strong inherited (genetically based) characteristics, it takes a dog breeder many generations before a new breed with distinct characteristics can be defined. Further, many traits are determined by the interaction of multiple genes. In mice it is not uncommon for experimentalists to select animals for or against a given characteristic (e.g. growth rate) – but it will take a minimum of perhaps 5, and probably 30 or more, generations to achieve divergence even on a single trait if multiple genes are involved in determining the phenotype.[5]

So evolution is a relatively slow process. It does not easily lend itself to enabling a species to survive a major and acute environmental transition. Imagine a field-mouse colony living on a hillside on a small volcanic island and feeding on wild wheat growing in a paddock below. An environmental catastrophe occurs – the volcano erupts and covers the field with ash. The nearest food supply, instead of being 20 metres away is now 2000 metres away on the other side of the island. Probably very few field mice would have the stamina to get to that food supply, and most would die. To survive as a species, both young males and females would have to get enough food over a long enough time period to survive and grow to reproductive competence. If a sub-population survived over several generations because they had genes that gave them more metabolic stamina to get to the food source, a new breed of field mice might emerge with greater stamina, and that is what can and does happen after such a dramatic, but relatively permanent, change in environment. But the above scenario is a high-risk strategy if the environment is unstable, shifting backwards and forwards within one or a few generations. Extinction could readily occur.

Evolution is a process that assumes a reasonably stable environment or one that is shifting in a constant direction.[6] However, PARs offer a highly effective strategy for survival, especially if the environment is only transiently changed. Evolution could not be effective (except in retaining highly plastic and adaptable genotypes like the finch's beak) if there were major shifts in the environment in one direction for say one or two generations, then there was shift back to the first environment again. Some other processes are needed to get the species through such short-term

---

[5] It has for example been suggested that over 100 genes are involved in determining just lower jaw shape.

[6] In the context of this discussion it is important to note that the capacity to mount plastic responses and induce phenotypic variation is itself a selected trait. Thus there are species that are 'generalists', which can adapt to a broad range of environments: the human is one. Other species are 'specialists', which exist in unique ecological niches, e.g. the polar bear.

environmental transitions. If the transitions are very short this is the process of homeostasis – for example increasing blood flow to our periphery when we are hot (cf. the rabbit's ears). But if the environmental change spans a lifetime, or at least a pregnancy, or perhaps one or two generations, some different strategy is needed. That strategy uses PARs.

Darwinian mechanisms operate on the assumption of a permanent environmental change. In contrast, PARs offer a more flexible solution, because in many cases the environmental change is transient. Such predictive responses fine-tune the phenotype in the offspring in a population. They bring the phenotype of those offspring close to an approximation of what is most likely to survive in the anticipated environment, without permanent change in the degree of genetic variation and in gene frequency, in the anticipation that the environmental change will be only transient. If the environmental change turns out to be permanent then there is time for natural selection to operate, in which case the genomic determinants of the favoured phenotype become selected, and over time the frequency of the relevant genomic alleles in the population changes.[7] Thus we see selection and PARs as interrelated responses ensuring species survival, although in different contexts – we shall return to this later.

There is a further Darwinian advantage conferred by the presence of PARs. Predictive adaptive responses allow a given genotype species access to a broader range of heterogeneous environments and to reproduce successfully. Thus a given genotype can survive in a broader range of ecological niches without loss of fitness.

## Developmental plasticity

The concept of developmental plasticity has led to an understanding that a single genotype can develop into a range of phenotypes – this range for a particular phenotypic trait is sometimes called the reaction norm or norm of reaction. For example, many identical twins with the same genotype have different phenotypes owing to environmental factors acting before and after birth; thus they can be different in height, weight, personality and so forth. The theoretical extreme of possible differences between the identical twins creates a norm of reaction for that genotype. The reaction norm for wing shape or colour or metabolic regulation in locusts includes very different phenotypes and it is clear that the dominant phenotype of a locust population is determined by the environment (see chapter 3). This is the key point – within the full theoretical range of phenotypes possible, the environmental history and the current environment will jointly determine the

---

[7] This phenomenon by which transient phenotypic advantage (fitness) is shifted over time into genetic change is known by several terms including *genetic assimilation* or *accommodation*.

distribution of phenotypes actually observed. This may well be less than the full range of possible phenotypes for the species.

The study of the finches on the Galapagos Islands illustrates this well. Clearly the genetic capacity to have shallow or deep beaks is present in the finch population.[8] But depending on the recent environmental history, the distribution of beak sizes we observe includes more shallow or more deep beaks. Thus the distribution and range of phenotypes present in a population may be less than the theoretical reaction norm.

Plasticity is a critical concept that we have already introduced. Through it, form can change either as a result of developmental process (developmental plasticity) or in response to an environmental change (environmental plasticity). Some plastic responses are reversible – for example when we exercise routinely we increase our muscle bulk by increasing the size of skeletal muscle fibres; when we get lazy, the muscles again become reduced in size. But most developmental plastic responses are irreversible. Once a tadpole has metamorphosed into a frog it cannot return to being a tadpole; once a human loses a limb it cannot regrow because it does not have that reversible plasticity (although the leg of an axolotl can!). Predictive adaptive responses are irreversible by definition – if they were reversible they would have no long-term significance, in that the body would be constantly adapting to its environment: they would then be no different from homeostasis.[9]

It is an intriguing question as to why so many plastic responses during development are irreversible. Some, like tadpole morphogenesis, must be irreversible because of the complexity of the tissue growth and differentiation processes involved. For others, such as the narrow window in which testosterone can masculinise the neonatal rat brain, or the change in fetal liver metabolism associated with maternal/fetal undernutrition in the rat, it is less easy to understand why they must be irreversible. We have to assume that these critical windows are set because a pathway must be chosen at that time in order for the remainder of development to proceed in an orderly manner. For example the period at which the gonad must become male or female must be chosen irreversibly (and early) so that gonadal stem-cell development can be completed in the right milieu for the oocyte or spermatid, given that the pathways for each type of gamete development are different. Then again, why is it that nephron number must be established irreversibly in fetal life – surely there would be advantages in being able to increase nephron number throughout life? Similarly, why is it that once the phase of neurogenesis is completed in the perinatal period, and essentially no brain cells can develop or regrow

---

[8] We are discussing the *Fortis* species in particular.

[9] Note here that we are thinking only of responses at the level of the individual. Predictive adaptive responses can and do change from generation to generation, so on that time scale they are reversible.

in most parts of the human brain after birth?[10] Surely there would be an advantage in being able to grow more brain cells in later life. Predictive adaptive responses only occur because much developmental phenotypic plasticity is irreversible. Yet in some systems it would not seem particularly complex to maintain continued plasticity – for example capillary density in some tissues, liver cell function etc. The only answer we can posit (almost by default) is that there is a presumption of high cost of maintaining plasticity. Presumably a trade-off has been made – give up reversible plasticity because of its cost in favour of some other advantage, linked to fitness.[11]

The concepts of life-history theory and biological trade-offs was introduced in chapter 3. Trade-offs arise because of the finite energetic capacity of the organism. Lactational amenorrhea is a trade-off by which the mother protects her energy reserves and energy intake capacity for lactation, i.e. for the support of her current progeny, rather than for another pregnancy. Another example in human reproduction is the age at menarche. It is well described that girls who are born small and have a deprived childhood are more likely to enter precocious puberty. A longer period of childhood growth to attain a larger adult size has been traded-off to ensure the capacity to reproduce. This seems logical and appropriate if one considers that this trade-off arose during the evolution of mammals (a similar trade-off is seen in many other species) and that it was protected during the hunter–gatherer phase of hominid evolution. Ageing has been proposed to occur as a trade-off between energy investment in cell repair versus reproduction. The processes of growth, cell replication and differentiation, and even programmed cell death, are all highly energy-dependent. We must assume that irreversible plasticity is itself a trade-off because of the costs associated with plasticity. During evolution higher priority has been given to maintaining functions that promote fitness rather than allowing continued plasticity in the components of the survival phenotype. Predictive adaptive responses reduce the need for energetically costly trade-offs and persistent plastic capacity and this underpins their advantage through evolutionary time.

## Transgenerational change

Predictive responses need not only operate over a single generation – that is solely as a set of mechanisms to convey environmental information from one generation to their offspring. For short-lived species such as small mammals, it may

---

[10] Neurogenesis is the process of growing brain cells from precursors. It essentially occurs between the 10th week of pregnancy and birth and there is no neurogenesis after birth, except for a very small amount in the area of the brain known as the hippocampus. In contrast, in some birds neurogenesis occurs throughout life.

[11] However, the issue of the high cost of plasticity remains an assumption and is poorly tested experimentally.

be particularly advantageous for the information to be transmitted beyond one generation. There is strong comparative data showing that some traits can be transmitted to a second, and perhaps further, generations. In a sense they create a transient form of non-genomic inheritance, and while they are well recognised in plant and comparative biology we are only now beginning to consider their role in human biology. They are not, as some people have thought, an echo of the discredited theory of Lamarck.[12] Instead these non-genomic transgenerational effects depend on developmental plasticity and a number of clearly defined functional and structural changes, some involving epigenetic change of DNA.

In the red deer, which have been studied in detail on the Isle of Rhum in Scotland, a period of starvation is reflected in lower birth weight not only in the offspring but also in the grand-offspring. We have already told the story of the Dutch Hunger Winter of 1944/5 and exactly the same thing happened there: the grandchildren born to mothers who were fetuses in the famine were born with reduced birth weight – interestingly this was most obvious in those exposed to famine in the first third of pregnancy. The mechanisms are speculative but remember that the egg that will form the second generation is formed within the female fetus in the first few weeks of gestation – that is the grandchild's egg can be informed by its grandmother's intra-uterine environment. An even more direct explanation is provided by studies suggesting that the uterus is smaller in women with lower birth weight and this would contribute to greater maternal constraint.

Another possibility is in epigenetic change to the genome. We discussed these possibilities in chapter 6. It turns out from studies in mice that such changes (e.g. in DNA methylation) not only determine the phenotype of the offspring but can sometimes be passed to the second generation. Until recently it was thought that imprinting was completely reversed at the time of gamete formation but we now know that the reversal can be incomplete and that the changes in DNA methylation can be copied into the germ cells (gametes – the sperm or the egg) of the offspring. From there they will be passed on in turn to the next generation. Such processes of transgenerational passage of changes in genomic DNA methylation can occur in both the female and male lineage, as the transmission is only via the gametes and this can equally apply to sperm and ova. We have told the story of how records in Scandinavia link the nutrition of the paternal grandparent to the risk of diabetes in the grandson. Interestingly, the effect seemed to be confined to nutrition during the grandfather's pre-pubertal growth phase, a time when the progenitor cells for making his sperm have formed, and presumably copying into them some changes in the methylation of his genomic DNA that had been driven by his diet. Much more

---

[12] Lamarck believed that acquired characteristics could be directly transmitted to the offspring of the next generation. If that were the case all Jewish boys would be born without foreskins!

research on this fascinating area of epigenetics[13] is needed – we are only beginning to see the size of the iceberg!

Other forms of transgenerational effect can occur through maternal behaviour. In chapter 5 we described the effects of grooming behaviour of the rat dam on her pups. It turns out that pups from mothers that groom their pups a lot groom their own pups a lot. Such effects cannot be purely genetic in origin but are associated with epigenetic changes in the brain. So in this case the intergenerational transmission of altered behaviour is epigenetic rather than simply cultural.

Intriguingly, the genomic determinants of the phenotypes initially favoured by these maternal effects, or learnt in response to environmental influences, can be subject over time to genetic selection. Thus they will be incorporated into changes in gene frequency giving stabilisation of the trait in genomic inheritance. These processes have been termed genetic assimilation, the 'Baldwin effect' or genetic accommodation.[14] Once a trait confers some advantage, and provided there is enough selection time and the change in the environment is fixed in direction, then selection can act on the genes underpinning that trait even though the initial source of the phenotypic variation selected was environmental. A key point however is that in many cases the initial short-term response to environmental change is not genomic. Another is that if the environmental change is only transient, then the genetic determinants cannot be magnified in the gene pool by selection – this is why PARs have been protected through evolutionary time, to deal with transient change.

## The survival, or default, phenotype

The 'developmental origins' story started with the identification of a certain human phenotype – people who were born smaller than optimal (which we now interpret as evidence of either physiological and/or pathophysiological maternal constraint) had elevated blood pressure and insulin resistance, tended to get relatively fat in childhood and to have reduced muscle mass and, in middle age, had a greater risk of developing heart disease and Type 2 diabetes. This is the 'metabolic syndrome' or Syndrome X phenotype.

It seems desirable, from our previous discussion, that all mammals should have evolved the capacity for the mother to inform the conceptus of its current environment and for the fetus to make predictive responses based on that information in order to have a phenotype most appropriate to its future environment. Such

---

[13] Epigenetics is the process(es) by which environmental factors change the chemical structure and thus the function of DNA – DNA methylation is the most well known of such epigenetic processes.

[14] There are subtle differences in what is meant by each of these terms to their authors, but these are beyond the scope of this book.

changes must be post-genetic because the genomic repertoire is set at fertilisation, yet the conceptus must have evolved some ability to detect its environment and to make the appropriate plastic responses.[15] Depending on when the environmental cues are sensed or occur, the fetus must make the best choices available to it. These choices become more limited the later in development the environmental change occurs or is sensed. In terms of species survival, the pathway to protect is that which will produce a phenotype surviving to reproduce during a transient environmental change that may last only one or two generations. As explained earlier, we call this phenotype the survival or default phenotype.

We have formulated this concept because we are impressed with how easy it is to generate features of this phenotype experimentally in a wide range of species and with a range of nutritional or hormonal cues from the mother. Phenotypes with considerable similarity appear to be generated by environmental cues operating both around conception and in gestation. As the biology of development is so different between the early and later stages of development, we have to infer that it is the phenotype that is common, not the process of getting there. There must be multiple pathways to the end-point, implying that multiple and redundant processes are encoded in the genome, which has been selected through evolution to preserve the survival phenotype.

In humans, rats, guinea pigs, sheep and mice, the phenotype produced by a maternal deprivation/stress cue seems to be strikingly similar.[16] It includes a degree of insulin resistance, a preference to lay down fat (in humans, omental fat), reduced skeletal muscle mass, reduced bone mineralisation, reduced capillary density in a number of tissues, altered endothelial function, reduced nephron number and reduced negative feedback in the hypothalamic–adrenal axis, leading to a tendency for greater stress responses. This is a phenotypic constellation that makes sense for maximising the chances of survival to reproduce in a deprived postnatal environment – it is a trade-off that ensures less resources will be committed to postnatal growth. Instead the resources will be diverted elsewhere in this constrained environment, ensuring reproductive fitness. A critical feature of this argument is that the prenatal selection is for an environmental range, not for precise and narrow conditions. Recall that a genotype can be expressed as a range of phenotypes (the reaction norm) given appropriate developmental stimuli. The reaction norm represents the total range of possible phenotypes – in practice a narrower range of phenotypes can tolerate a given environment. What is happening in a PAR is that the span of phenotypes that is expressed postnatally by a given

---

[15] This may even be at the one-cell stage where the sensor is a receptor for a nutrient or a maternally derived hormone.

[16] There are of course quantitative differences in the magnitude of its various components in different models, depending on the timing of the cue.

genotype is altered and, if hard times are predicted, generally the span will be narrowed.[17]

It is our hypothesis that the mechanisms for generating this phenotype evolved in small mammals and assisted their survival through transient environmental change. As the hominids developed, these processes remained critical at least until agriculture appeared and food supplies became more stable – we shall return to this discussion later. Indeed we suspect that through the evolution of the hominids, the survival phenotype was the optimal and dominant phenotype.

## Mechanisms underlying the default phenotype

But what mechanisms would ensure this default position? Obviously episodic events such as low maternal nutrient intake or high anxiety levels (which might accompany food shortage or risk of predation) might be the cue, but they might not have been sufficient to ensure that this phenotype would have persisted throughout evolutionary time. If a population had a multigenerational exposure to a very favourable ecological niche, then the genomic basis to allow survival in a poor environment would have been de-selected and then the species would have been at risk in a shift to a poorer environment. We propose that PARs reduce this risk and reduce the probability of such de-selection by reducing the pressure for a true adaptation. The advantage of maintaining the capacity to survive in the more likely environment of transient deprivation is ensured by the presence of maternal constraint, which is used to favour development of the default phenotype.

Maternal constraint operates in all pregnancies where, as we have explained before, it has the role of limiting fetal growth so that the fetal head can pass through the birth canal – otherwise neither mother nor baby could survive the birth process. But while maternal constraint operates in every pregnancy, the processes underlying it are magnified in several situations – adolescent pregnancy (where nutrients are still being diverted to maternal growth), the first pregnancy (where the uterine arteries are less distensible), multiple pregnancy (where there is competition for nutrients between the fetuses) and in small mothers (who are presumed to have a reduced capacity to increase uterine blood flow and for uterine growth). Maternal constraint is physiological and must be distinguished from pathophysiological influences on fetal growth caused by maternal or placental disease or maternal undernutrition. Maternal constraint has also been suggested to be a process by which the mother limits resource allocation to any one fetus, thus retaining reserves for further pregnancies. But we theorise that a further key role of maternal constraint has been to favour the default phenotype.

---

[17] From what we have said we can see that keeping a broad range of possible phenotypes is likely to be more energetically expensive than having a narrow one because it necessitates a broader range of energetically expensive homeostatic and adaptive responses.

Most small mammals are polytocous (i.e. have multiple fetuses), which in itself is a form of maternal constraint in that nutrient supply to each fetus is limited. But as larger mammals evolved – normally carrying only a single fetus – maternal constraint became important not only in preventing fetal overgrowth but in ensuring that, relative to its genetic drive to grow, the fetus was always receiving some degree of signal that nutrient supply was limited. This would ensure that the default phenotype developed through the predictive adaptive pathway, because maternal signals are biased towards signalling restricted nutrient availability. Assuming hominids evolved under uncertain nutritional conditions, (as primitive hunter–gatherers) for which there is considerable indirect evidence, thus survival of the species depended on being prepared in such a way.

Thus fetal growth is regulated very differently from postnatal growth. Postnatal growth is under growth hormone control and humans grow to an adult height that is largely genetically determined. In contrast fetal growth is constrained, being determined by the state of maternal metabolism and the limited capacity of the placenta to transfer nutrients to the fetus. The genetic determinants of birth size are far weaker than for adult size. This provides a mechanism whereby the fetus is constantly instructed that nutrient supplies are limited. It is not clear that the fetus has any strategy to increase its nutrient supplies. As a result in all pregnancies, but particularly when maternal constraint is greater or when pathophysiological situations are superimposed, PARs will prime the fetus to develop in expectation of some degree of postnatal nutrient limitation – that is towards the default phenotype. Only in (evolutionarily) rare situations such as maternal diabetes is this constraint overridden. This approach was critical to our evolutionary survival as a species.

But our fate changed when the nature of human nutrition and physical burdens changed. The phenotype ensured through the default pathway was no longer the better-suited phenotype. Thus PARs based on maternal constraint, which had been more often than not appropriate over evolutionary time, became more likely to be inappropriate. Throughout the bulk of hominid and human history this did not matter, in that the span of phenotypes humans could adopt, based on inherent genetic variation, was still within the range of energy environments that were compatible with health. But for the reasons we will discuss, human evolution has slowed down or largely stopped, while our energy environment has continued to change.

We propose that for the first time in hominid history, the energy environment may be such that the default phenotype will more often than not be inappropriate. An evolutionary echo exists because the survival phenotype was the appropriate phenotype until the period of agricultural development. Maternal constraint led to the prediction being one of a relatively deprived or uncertain energy environment, but postnatal environments are now generally very enriched. We are the victims of our bias to a default phenotype that is no longer appropriate.

We suspect that this has occurred because one mechanism, that of constraining fetal growth, has been used to subserve several objectives: regulating fetal size to prevent the risk of excessive fetal growth, regulating fetal size to prevent excessive nutritional investment by the mother in any one offspring, and being used as the environmental cue to ensure a survival phenotype through predictive adaptation. So in the modern human, the default phenotype has echoes in all pregnancies as a result of maternal constraint. Not surprisingly in view of the shift in the energy environment, these constraining factors are now associated after birth with a greater risk of inappropriate prediction and thus obesity, insulin resistance etc. But modern pregnancy is also confounded by maternal and placental disease, which in prehistoric times would have been associated with death of the fetus and/or mother. These pathological constraints serve as a cue for further degrees of inappropriate prediction.

It is useful to reiterate that a PAR is not appropriate or inappropriate at the time it is triggered. This classification can only be made retrospectively. The set of PARs that leads to the survival phenotype being the norm for humans evolved because, in general, it conferred a survival advantage (i.e. was appropriate) in the usual postnatal environment. Maternal constraint is part of the process used to achieve this set-point. Maternal size is likely to reflect the overall average environment the fetus will have been born into, and hence this is a direct way of reflecting longer-term environmental information to the fetus. In modern humans, the survival phenotype provides the mechanistic basis for health in some postnatal environments but also induces the latent potential for the survival mechanisms to be exaggerated in other environments. It is that second interaction that becomes manifest later in life as disease.

It is easy to fall into the trap of thinking about environments and responses in a dichotomous way – rich or poor, resistant or sensitive etc. Life is not like that. There is a continuum of energy environments and there is a continuum of physiological responses – for example degrees of insulin resistance, of change in nephron number etc. Predictive adaptive responses were retained because optimal reproductive success in the next generation depended on getting a close match between the predicted environment and physiological settings. The point about maternal constraint is not that it is the primary cause of PARs, merely that it shifts the default position in favour of the lower risk position for the species in expectation of some degree of nutritional limitation. But these responses would have been potentially valuable in situations of large and transient environmental shifts (drought, famine, flood etc.). We suspect protection against these episodes was a primary reason for the evolutionary retention of these responses.

## The evolution of predictive responses

We have been arguing that these predictive mechanisms are widely occurring biological phenomena that confer considerable survival advantage. We do not see evolutionary change and PARs as mutually exclusive, but rather as processes that confer different advantages on the species over vastly different time scales – from within one generation to millions of years. Therefore the multiple pathways and processes involved in predictive responses must themselves have evolved at some point. One wonders when, and at present can only speculate. They are easy to demonstrate in a wide variety of mammals and there are precursor responses that show similarities in plants and even in single-cell organisms. Thus while much of the focus of this book is on nutritional induction because of its importance to human disease, comparative studies demonstrate many other forms of environmental influences that have irreversible plastic consequences.

Perhaps this discussion is best linked to a consideration of the range of developmental plastic strategies that various classes of the animal kingdom appear to have evolved to ensure continuance of their species. The example of helmet formation in *Daphnia* is well known. These single-celled organisms can adapt, through a process of irreversible phenotypic plasticity, to a different shape in the presence of a high risk of predation. The helmet shape has a survival advantage in the presence of such predation. Subsequent generations return to the default non-helmet phenotype if there is a low risk of predation.

Egg-laying species such as reptiles have a limited ability to communicate with their offspring during their embryonic development, because this is taking place outside the mother's body. Moreover, in animals such as crocodiles and turtles, the parents cannot incubate the eggs because they are cold-blooded animals. So they must bury them in warm sand to protect the developmental process of the embryo. In addition, reptiles do not use chromosomes to determine gender – rather they use environmental stimuli. This is an extreme form of irreversible developmental plasticity because the temperature of the sand in which the eggs are buried influences whether the offspring will develop into males or females. It is not clear whether the selection of laying site is used by these species as a survival strategy but it is possible. Certainly in other species including some birds and mammals changing the ratio of male to female offspring is one way to survive transient environmental change.[18]

---

[18]  There are well-described examples of environmentally determined gender ratios in species such as the red deer. In general under poor conditions, more females are born, as the survival of the species is dependent on the number of fetuses that reproduce in later life, which is female-dependent. As conditions improve more males are born. There is far more contentious debate as to whether such environmental influences may occur in humans but there is at least one recent report in a deprived African population to support this idea. The mechanisms underpinning mammalian environmental sex determination are rather speculative but can be considered as an extreme form of predictive adaptive response in that a maternal environmentally

Birds have a greater range of ways in which the behaviour of the developing offspring can be influenced. For example where there are nutritional rushes,[19] some birds can manipulate the hatching of their clutch to capitalise on the environment by altering the incubation time. Late-laid eggs can be accelerated to hatch at the same time as those laid earlier. In a sense this is a maternal signal to the offspring in relation to anticipated environment. This is clearly vital to protect the young from predators and to ensure that the parents are not faced with the conflicting challenges of incubating unhatched eggs and finding food for hatched young.

Similarly some species of mongoose will ensure coordinated delivery of their pups – this is because they have a tendency to cannibalise each other's pups: to promote survival it is better for all pups to be born at the same time, because this reduces the risk for each pup of being eaten. Rats and mice (and the hares we discussed earlier) clearly base their survival strategy on the production of large numbers of progeny. The survival rate may however not be high. Predictive adaptive responses can thus confer a real advantage in such animals, as they promote the chance of survival to reproductive maturity. The presence of PARs in such animals has been well demonstrated. Because development is rapid in these species, e.g. gestation is only 21 days in the rat and a similar time is needed before the newborn pups are weaned, any adaptive responses initiated by a fetus are likely to be appropriate to the current environment and promote fitness.

But perhaps it is in the large mammals that PARs become the critical element in species survival – a concept we will explain later in this chapter. When the number of offspring produced is low, it is vital that each and every one is equipped with the most advantageous phenotype for survival. In most situations this means ensuring that the survival phenotype is the default and PARs become far more important. Their characteristics ensure that the default phenotype can persist to the second generation – hence why evolutionary biologists define fitness in terms of that generation. We would argue that once environmental stresses pass, the species must return to its equilibrium phenotype, which is genetically determined by much slower evolutionary processes.

## A model of predictive adaptive responses

Variation in phenotype, including indicators such as birth size, depends on the interaction between the environment and the organism's genotype. Indeed, as explained earlier, the genotype essentially informs a range of phenotypes that can be expressed under different circumstances – i.e. the reaction norm. Variation is provided by the

---

determined signal has induced an irreversible plastic response that confers a survival advantage in the future environment.

[19] A sudden increase in food availability, e.g. when berries ripen.

small genomic differences[20] that make each individual in a population unique. We have argued that it is the interactions in early development that have particularly profound effects not only on the mature phenotype but also on how the mature organism in turn interacts with its environment (this is actually tautologous because this mature environmental interaction is, itself, a phenotypic trait).

We have seen that some aspects of body function are plastic – that is they are altered by environmental conditions. Some of these changes are irreversible, for example the impact of male hormones on the development of the genitalia[21] or when a teratogen (for example thalidomide) acts to create development disruption. Some may be reversible but have immediate survival value – for example the conservation of fetal nutrients by reducing blood supply transiently to some organs to protect supply to the brain, heart and placenta. What we are talking about here however is a third type of plasticity – one in which the immediate advantage of an irreversible change in structure or function is not necessarily obvious. The advantage is conferred in the anticipated or predicted future environment. In fact some of these fetal responses also make sense as part of an immediate adaptive response (e.g. reduced muscle mass) but for some (e.g. altered fat mass) any immediate advantage is not obvious, and it can only be conferred in the postnatal phenotype that ensues.

We propose that PARs provide the strategy for a species to adjust transiently[22] to an environmental change that itself may be transient. Many environmental impacts last for more than one generation but do not last long enough for natural selection to apply. Without some short-term adjustment strategy, the gene pool would be put at risk. Just as Dawkins has stated, the driving force in evolution is the need to ensure that genes can survive to the next generation. Under threatening conditions, the individual must do all it can to survive to reproduce, irrespective of other consequences. Predictive adaptive responses provide just such a mechanism.

Mind experiments are a useful way in which to develop a general model from a particular set of data. Consider a cycle of famine, spanning one or two generations of early hominids. The pregnant female[23] carrying a single fetus signals to her fetus

---

[20] The use of the phrase 'small differences' may surprise some readers but while each human has many polymorphic differences from his or her peers that create the individual genotype, as a species we have very high homology in DNA sequences from individual to individual. This does not mean that these small genotypic differences are not important. Indeed as we know in some cases, only one base-pair change in DNA creates a disease like cystic fibrosis.

[21] An informative example is a syndrome called the adrenogenital syndrome. Because of a genetically determined enzyme defect, the adrenal gland makes insufficient amounts of cortisol and instead makes excess amounts of the male hormones (androgens). An affected female fetus becomes masculinised and, depending on the severity of the enzyme defect, may develop a full phallus and fused scrotalised labia (with no testes of course as the fetus has ovaries and a normal uterus and cervix that can only be corrected surgically). In contrast, in the affected male fetus, the effect is a somewhat enlarged phallus.

[22] That is transiently for the species but of course permanently for the affected individual.

[23] We will resist the temptation to call her Lucy or Eve!

that food supply is limited. The fetus adjusts its development to ensure it consumes minimal energy in utero and as a result also has reduced energy consumption after birth but can survive to reproduce. So it may be born smaller, have a slower postnatal growth rate, it will have insulin resistance to conserve energy, it will have fewer blood vessels in its tissues so that there is less delivery of nutrients to them, and the highest energy-consuming tissues such as muscle are smaller. While postnatal growth is slower, it can survive through puberty and can reproduce. This process can be repeated for several generations if necessary. But if the famine conditions are relieved, and the original better nutritional conditions are restored rapidly, within a generation or so the hominid will return to its original phenotype, which had been selected by evolution over a much longer time frame to be optimal for its ecological niche. There is no need for reliance on the mutated extreme outlying genotypes being selected to allow some members of the species to survive. Further, much of the original genetic variation in the population is preserved, which allows selection to continue to act if members of the species migrate to a new niche or if the environmental change turns out to be permanent.

Based on information provided by its mother, the fetus determines a phenotype that it predicts will optimise its chances of reproductive success postnatally. In turn this determines a range of postnatal environments in which the organism can live healthily after birth. If the environment falls within that range, then an appropriate prediction has occurred. If however the postnatal environment is outside this range (in either direction) then an inappropriate prediction has occurred. Disease occurs when the environmental conditions exceed the capacity of the phenotype to cope (i.e. the organism can no longer mount effective homeostatic responses) with a given set of environmental conditions. The safer position in general is to assume some risk of an adverse environment and this positioning is assisted by the presence of maternal constraint.

These ideas are shown diagrammatically in Figure 7.1. This figure shows the basic principle of PARs as defined by the interaction between the predicted and the actual postnatal environment in determining the risk of disease.

The horizontal axis shows the range of the postnatal environment as predicted from the environment to which the fetus is exposed. The vertical axis represents the range of energy environments *actually* experienced during reproductive adult life. Note that optimal fetal nutrition is close to the maximal because of the limitations that exist to such fetal nutrition. Hence the fetus is less able to predict a rich than a poor postnatal energy environment. The curves show the upper and lower limits of the combination of fetal prediction and postnatal environment for achieving health, especially that in post-reproductive life. If the postnatal environment is too poor or too rich in relation to that predicted, then the risk of disease will increase as indicated by the arrows. The dot shows an individual who should be in

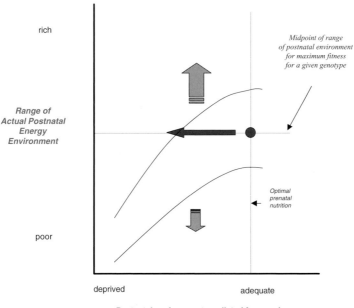

rich

*Midpoint of range
of postnatal environment
for maximum fitness
for a given genotype*

*Range of
Actual Postnatal
Energy
Environment*

*Optimal
prenatal
nutrition*

poor

deprived

adequate

*Postnatal environment predicted from early
environment*

Fig. 7.1     The interaction between the prenatal and postnatal environment as determined by PARs.

the safe zone. However, if maternal constraint operates more in this individual pregnancy than the average (e.g. owing to it being a first pregnancy, the mother being a teenager or being smaller) then the predicted postnatal environment shifts to the left as shown, and thus the acceptable upper limit of the postnatal energy environment associated with health shifts downwards. The situation is worse still in the presence of disease such as pre-eclampsia or placental dysfunction, and this will shift the individual's prediction further to the left, increasing the risk of disease from a postnatal environment that is richer than predicted.

Inappropriate prediction can involve one of two pathways leading to disease. The first is when the postnatal environment is predicted to be rich because the prenatal environment is good, yet the prediction is not accurate and the environment is poorer than predicted. Then disease risk is enhanced even in a moderate postnatal energy environment. This is the region below the lower curve in Figure 7.1. The extent to which this occurs is not known – but the infant of the diabetic mother does have a relatively high incidence of disease and it will have been well nourished in utero due to her high blood glucose levels. Such infants appear to have a less than optimal life course but more studies are needed.[24] In addition, we know

---

[24] We shall return to the infants of diabetic mothers later because there is an alternative pathway by which these infants can develop childhood obesity.

that animals fed a high-fat diet during pregnancy, which might indicate to their fetuses an enriched prenatal environment, have progeny that develop a number of pathological characteristics such as high blood pressure and endothelial dysfunction if reared on a normal diet.

The more common scenario is when the fetus with constrained fetal growth, owing to the combination of maternal constraint and/or maternal/placental pathophysiology, predicts a poor postnatal environment. The likelihood is that the environment will be adequate or even rich, and so the risk of disease is increased. This is the region above the upper curve in Figure 7.1. This makes a dramatic point: the postnatal environment does not have to be particularly enriched to be inappropriate for the offspring of a relatively deprived intrauterine environment to be put at risk of later disease.

Because of its importance we have focused on prenatal nutritional and postnatal energy environments. But similar curves are possible for other features of the environment. For example we could create curves for neonatal environmental temperature and the density of active sweat glands in adults. The Japanese soldier born in the cold climate, and collapsing in the heat in the tropics, would have been positioned in the upper left hand quadrant of such a graph.

The model we have described works well provided that the environment oscillates around the horizontal dotted line as the historical mean postnatal environment for the hominid. If that starts to shift rapidly, say because of much greater provision of cheap, high-energy food, then the risk of disease caused by inappropriate prediction becomes much increased. This is what we believe is happening to humans now. The set-points for the developed and developing world may differ, but the principles are the same. Because the babies of the developing world live in poorer environments in utero (on average) they are more likely to show disease because of inappropriate prediction than those from developed societies in a given postnatal energy environment.

The evolutionary process of natural selection will not be able to keep up with this problem if the postnatal energy environment changes rapidly, as has happened over the last generation. In any case, because the major diseases that result from inappropriate PARs occur predominantly in later life, natural selection operates weakly if at all. Our model would predict that the way of reducing disease risk would be for fetuses to grow bigger, that is to live in a supra-optimal prenatal environment. But fetal growth is always constrained and the opportunities to enhance it are extremely limited. There is no secular trend to an increase in birth weight in developed societies. Therefore the primary solution must be to manipulate the postnatal environment. Because it is not the *absolute* level of the postnatal energy environment that determines the risk of disease but the degree of match (or mismatch) between the predicted and the actual postnatal environment, and because the postnatal energy environment continues to be enriched in all developed and some developing societies, then the risk of disease related to inappropriate PARs is bound to increase worldwide.

## The implications of predictive adaptive responses for evolutionary theory

We now need to explore the relationships between this general model of PARs and current evolutionary thought. Darwinian (or strictly, neo-Darwinian as we must couch it in terms of the genes of which Darwin had no knowledge) models require that genetic variation be maintained as the substrate on which selection can act. This makes sense over evolutionary time to ensure that a species can evolve to survive in a variety of evolutionary landscapes. We propose that the presence of PARs has been an important component in preserving genetic variation through transient environmental change, and thus assisting the survival of species that demonstrate it.

Evolutionary success is generally determined by the persistence of a range of genomically influenced possible phenotypes. The greater the potential phenotypic variation, the more likely a set of specific genomic alleles determining that phenotype can survive a given environmental pressure. As implied from chapter 2, there are a wide variety of possible patterns of fetal development possible from a given genotype and these will be reflected in varying birth phenotypes. Thus the phenotype at birth is a consequence of genetic variation plus the various phenotypic changes made either in response to immediate needs for fetal survival and/or PARs. Similarly the mature phenotype is the consequence of genetic variation, phenotypic change made during development and the added impact of the postnatal environment. It is important to remember that it is the phenotype of an individual that determines its ability to survive and reproduce, not the genotype.

The dilemma for the individual maternal/fetal pair is that at the point when key choices are made, they cannot tell whether an environmental change is going to be transient or permanent. Evolutionary selection and PARs are two strategies that operate together to create a relatively fail-safe system to allow species to survive in either circumstance, albeit on different time scales.

The logic of our argument is set out diagrammatically in Figure 7.2. Imagine a population of animals – for example the snowshoe hares that we considered in chapter 3. Within that population there will be a range of genotypes (shown by the shaded dots) that may have evolved over millennia. They might be polymorphisms with a range of frequencies in the population, but the details do not matter. They code a range of theoretical adult phenotypes shown by the upper set of horizontal bars of the same shade – that is the reaction norm. The reaction norm is for a specific phenotypic characteristic, e.g. HPA responsiveness, ear-length, coat thickness etc. Each bar can be imagined to represent the maximal range of different phenotypes

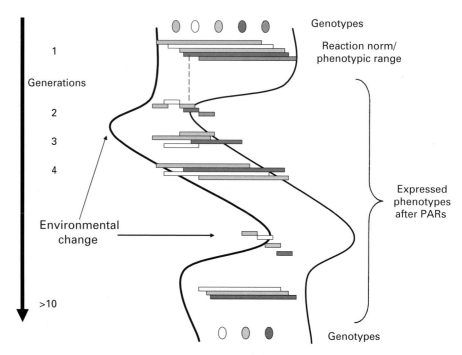

Fig. 7.2      The advantage of PARs in preserving genotypic variation in a population (shown by ovals of different shades) during rapid environmental changes occurring over the time frame of a generation. The curved lines represent the environmental range at each generation and the horizontal bars the phenotype corresponding to each genotype. See text for further details.

that identical twins (i.e. individuals with identical genotype) might have. Individuals within this genotypically homogenous population will be able to survive, as long as the capabilities of their homeostatic and other characteristics associated with the phenotype are not exceeded by an environmental challenge. When the population is in a stable state with respect to its environmental niche, the extent of the reaction norms bounded by the line and the varying environmental conditions, e.g. with seasons, coincide. But in practice, in any environment not all possible phenotypes arising from a genotype can survive and the expressed phenotypic range may be less than the reaction norm – these are shown in the lower sets of horizontal bars as indicated.

Now imagine that the environment changes quite drastically so that its boundaries shift between one generation and the next. By putting in the vertical broken line we can see that all of the chequered phenotype offspring in generation 2 will lie outside this range, and they may easily perish, and so will the majority of the black and striped phenotypes. The corresponding genotypes will be lost from the gene pool. The species is in trouble: these genotypes will be poorly equipped to deal

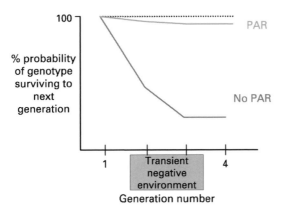

Fig. 7.3    PARs increase the probability of a particular genotype surviving a transient environmental change.

with the environment they will face and they are unlikely to survive to reproduce. Worse still, if we look down the diagram we can see that the environment shifts back again to beyond its original range – as it may well do if it were associated with a cyclical change such as *El Niño*. Under such circumstances we can see that any phenotypes that had survived the first shift will find themselves outside the range after the second. The species may actually become extinct in a few generations.

But now consider the effects of PARs. If the environmental change had occurred during the pregnancy of the first generation, then there will have been the chance for PARs to shift the development of generation 2 towards the traits that will convey a survival phenotype. The horizontal bars are now shifted, and also shortened. More individuals will be bunched up with phenotypic traits that convey a fitness advantage. The process is not perfect: even with the operation of PARs, the chequered phenotype will not have been able to shift far enough, and individuals with this phenotype may all die, as will a proportion of the black and striped phenotype. But the attrition rate will be far less than without this strategy. When the environment shifts back in the opposite direction, the stippled and some of the white phenotype (and hence their genotype) will be lost, but we can see that by the time the environment stabilises again at least three (white, striped and black) of the original five genotypes have been preserved.

Another way of looking at this is to calculate the probability of a genotype surviving through a transient environmental change in the presence or absence of PARs, as in Figure 7.3. One can see that without PARs the chances of a given genotype surviving two generations of transient environmental change falls dramatically. In the presence of PARs there is a far greater chance of this genotype surviving.

Earlier, we demonstrated that PARs had two advantages. First they allowed a fetus to optimise its development for survival in an uncertain world through ensuring the default position was towards a survival phenotype; second, they allowed a fetus to make the appropriate trade-offs early, to maximise its chances of survival in an environment predicted by information from its mother. The scenarios we have just described demonstrate a third value of PARs. They ensure that a greater pool of genotypes can survive a transient environmental change. This in turn protects the range of reaction norms for the species and makes it able to survive a broader range of environments both spatially (i.e. ecologically) and temporally. As the adverse effects of getting the prediction wrong generally occur after reproduction has ceased (at least in humans), the selection advantage in preserving the mechanisms of PARs would ensure that genotypes are maintained, to be acted on by natural selection, rather than lost. Thus PARs confer a range of strategies to ensure species survival. They allow a species to maximise diversity yet to achieve maximal survival of the range of genotypes to the next generation.

One implication of this theory should now be obvious. It relates to the speed of the biological response and so, by inference, to the speed of adaptive change. Most evolutionary biologists hold that only the slow process of natural selection can mediate the process of adaptation, whereby those genetic variants most suited to the environment have an advantage, and therefore survive to breed, ensuring that their genetic stock is passed on to future generations. The process inevitably takes many generations for the change to arrive at a point where a new species becomes apparent. A mechanism must exist to allow a species to survive the inevitable environmental changes that occur during this multigenerational process of selection. Predictive adaptive responses provide such a mechanism by providing a transient, but potentially intergenerational, strategy to allow species survival.

Predictive adaptive responses are rapid and reversible, and cyclic or episodic environmental change is common. Let us return once more to the population of snowshoe hares. Suppose that their environment changes just as we considered before, suddenly limiting the supply of food. Any such environmental change represents a threat to the population and only the best-adapted will survive. The problem is that if the hare population had to depend on the Darwinian processes alone to achieve adaptation to the changed environment, it would run enormous risks. The chance of some phenotypic variants actually being significantly better-adapted to the environment, as a result of a random mutation in the genotype, is very small. Mutations are actually rare events and any useful trait (faster running speed, better twilight vision) will involve an extensive fraction of the organs and systems in the body and hence the coordinated expression of thousands of genes. Clearly the chance of a significantly enhanced genotype being present in the population at the right time to cope with an unexpected transient environmental change is vanishingly small in a single generation. But it gets more problematic. Let us suppose that a relatively modest genetic change *has* in fact conferred an advantage in one member of the species: this cannot happen in more than one individual, because the genetic mutation is random. Even if that genetic variation were to be passed on 100 per cent faithfully to the next generation (which is far from certain), and even if the hare (male or female, it makes little difference) were the most reproductively fertile ever, it would still clearly take many generations and many seasons of breeding cycles for the useful variation to become prevalent in the population. It is all too slow: the threatening environmental change could easily have totally destroyed the population by then. It is also far too risky: if an eagle were to pick off the hare with the useful mutation, the story would be over.

There is therefore enormous advantage in a mechanism by which phenotypic change can occur very fast, actually within one generation. What this really means is that the change occurs in a large number of offspring so that, far from the Darwinian need for a long process of breeding to introduce a helpful phenotypic change, the change becomes manifest in large numbers of the population simultaneously. This is precisely what PARs achieves, as illustrated in Figure 7.2. Not only is it fast, producing a change in phenotype from one generation to the next, but it can act potentially on every member of the species in the next generation. During the breeding season for the hares, we might therefore see a sudden change in the phenotype almost overnight!

Genetic variation is non-directional and is based on random mutation. The direction that evolution takes arises from the accident of a mutation conferring an advantage (or a disadvantage) in any ecological niche. In contrast, PARs are driven entirely in a directional manner. The induced 'choices' that the embryo or fetus makes are in the direction of an appropriate adaptation to the environment into which it believes it will be born. The 'thrifty phenotype' is precisely that: a mother who detects a reduced nutritional level in her environment can programme her offspring's metabolic regulatory mechanisms to be nutritionally economical, and of course the process can operate in literally thousands of mothers simultaneously. We propose that in a more general sense this phenomenon offers an explanation of how mammalian species have survived many transient changes in environment. Thus the thrifty phenotype model must be seen as but one manifestation of PARs.

To summarise, we propose that PARs provide a fast, sensitive means by which the phenotype can be modified, using processes of environmental detection by the mother and passing the information to the offspring in the next generation. This produces a change in phenotype that is directional and can affect a large number of the offspring, and hence confers a definite survival advantage. The predictive adaptive processes, which modulate the genotype to phenotype transition, work on a different time scale from the processes of generation of variation by mutation, which is fundamental to natural selection. Working in concert, the two processes confer biodiversity for long-term evolutionary change (Darwinian selection) and rapid adaptation to the environment for short-term survival (PARs).

# 8

# Evolutionary echoes and the human camel

Humans are animals: but we are animals that evolved with a number of distinct characteristics. It is now believed that *Homo sapiens* appeared as a distinct species about 150 000 years ago – that is since our definitive speciation there have been perhaps less than 7 000 generations. All the diversity of human phenotypes has appeared in only that time[1] and, importantly, through that evolutionary time the human species has adapted to a wide range of environments. Humans can manipulate their own environment in a variety of ways and to an extent not available to other species – for example to make and wear clothing or make fire to regulate the thermal environment. With the development of agriculture less than 10 000 years ago humans developed the ability to manipulate their food supplies. There have also been dramatic changes in the nature of our food intake. Humans have developed a number of ways to reduce internal energy expenditure[2] from wheels to computers – this reduction in daily energy expenditure has been particularly accelerated in recent decades. With the development of religious beliefs and sets of cultural values, humans have developed a commitment to care for those in their species with a limited capacity to survive. Thus it has been suggested that, in humans, Darwinian evolution is no longer active or has been slowed dramatically because both environmental conditions and the processes of natural selection have been greatly attenuated by our human behaviour. As we will discuss, the implication of this is that, because the human environment has continued to become increasingly energy rich (that is less energy is needed to survive and access to high-energy food has become constant compared to when we evolved), the repertoire of adaptive responses that we developed by natural selection prior to the slowing down of our evolution may no longer allow humans to thrive optimally in the nutrient/energy environments in which we now live.

---

[1] And in reality in perhaps a third of that time, as there was a bottleneck when our ancestors migrated out of Africa about 65 000 years ago.

[2] But at the expense of course of enormous environmental energy consumption.

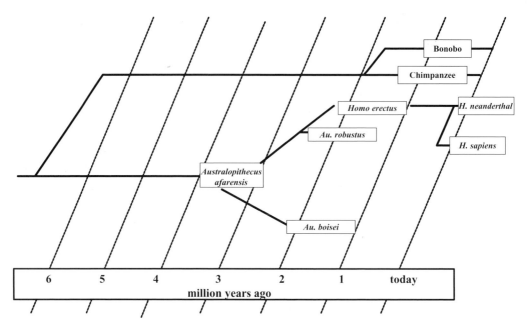

Fig. 8.1    Very simplified family tree (cladogram) of hominid evolution: About 6 million years ago there was a split in the ape family with one branch leading to the other great apes and one branch leading to the evolution of the first ape-like species to be dominantly bipedal (an *Australopithicus* species) which in turn led to the evolution of the *Homo* family about 2 million years ago. *Homo sapiens* only evolved as a distinct species about 200 000 years ago. While *Homo erectus* had spread through Euro–Asia as well as Africa over a million years ago, *Homo sapiens* did not leave Africa until about 65 000 years ago.

In evolutionary terms humans are relatively unusual in another way: whereas most species continue to reproduce throughout life (in the absence of disease), the phenomenon of reproductive failure well before death is essentially unique to the human female.[3] Therefore, natural selection has not acted significantly to reduce the probability of disease in humans where that disease appears in later life.

Putting these phenomena together, it is not surprising that modern humans often now live in environments that can induce disease in middle age. In itself this is not a novel conclusion. However what is novel is the increasing realisation that evolutionary echoes of other processes acting in early life interact with the current environment to increase the risk of such disease. These echoes are retained in the set of PARs, which have been essential processes over evolution to ensure the normal survival of mammalian species through transient environmental change. As humans have experienced recent and massive environmental change in the absence

---

[3] Chimpanzees retain fertility until old age, whereas rhesus monkeys have symptoms of reproductive failure in later life; human females lose reproductive competence in middle age.

of evolutionary progression, these responses now lead to a particular set of diseases being manifest.

This type of discussion and thought process has been surprisingly uncommon in human medicine. This is because there is a large cultural gap between clinicians interested in human disease on one hand and evolutionary biologists and ecologists on the other hand. Each has been reluctant to enter the field represented by the other. By and large, modern evolutionary biology has not focused on issues related to human development, except in the controversial field of socio-biology. While the understanding of phenotypic and developmental plasticity has greatly increased in the last two decades, the implications to human biology are little considered. Equally, human biology has hardly considered important concepts in comparative biology in its rather zealous focus on purely genetic explanations for non-communicable disease. This book (we hope) in part fills the space between these two worlds. In turn, the study of the developmental origins of disease has led us to develop concepts that are applicable in comparative biology across many species, but that have been overlooked because of the intellectual gulf between different spheres of biological understanding.

## The post-evolutionary human and PARs

The general model of PARs is easy to understand when considering wild populations of animals or laboratory rats. Is it more complex when extended to human biology? We have proposed that PARs have evolved to promote the chance of survival of a new generation through its reproductive period. But in our species a long period elapses between fertilisation of the egg and reproductive 'success' for the individual who grows from that egg. An increasing number of young women do not consider having children in Western societies until their 30s or later. The longer the interval between fertilisation and reproduction, the greater the risk of environmental mismatch. As modern humans (as opposed to prehistory hominids) we have far greater control over our environment and our biology, including our reproductive biology, than any other species. Viewing our species from the biological point of view, we can see that the PAR becomes an 'evolutionary echo' that may have become inappropriate in the twentieth and twenty-first centuries. It evolved as mammals evolved, and it persisted because it had advantage in the pre-agricultural era. But over the last 10 000 years its utility may have been displaced at a cost.

Let us explore this further by using the nutritional paradigm. Except in extraordinary conditions such as in the Dutch Hunger Winter, or in individual cases of anorexia nervosa, pregnant women are highly unlikely to be grossly undernourished in the developed world, although there is much evidence for milder forms of nutritional imbalance.[4] Generally a fetus will be grossly undernourished only when there is maternal or placental disease. However, fetal growth and development are exquisitely sensitive to very subtle changes in environment (see chapter 2) and these can change the trajectory of fetal development. That is why relationships between indices of maternal nutrition can be correlated with outcomes even in apparently healthy western populations (see chapters 4 and 6).

The genes and biological processes driving PARs exist in the human as they do in other species – indeed as we detailed earlier they would have been critical to the evolution of hominids. Thus the fetus exposed to an intrauterine environment that it perceives as less than optimal responds as we have described in chapters 3 and 4. It develops differently – there will be hormone resistance, fewer blood vessels will develop in some tissues, the growth trajectory will be reset. It is therefore born smaller (smaller than its genotypic potential but not necessarily smaller than the population average) and with a different biology. But if the cause of the predictive choice has been placental disease, then the fetus has misread the situation. In fact food is in good supply, so after birth it grows too fast, it gets obese and the physiological changes that were induced by induction of the 'survival phenotype' become pathological. The insulin resistance together with a large fat mass and high food intake manifests as Type 2 diabetes, the cardiovascular changes as endothelial dysfunction and hypertension, the metabolic changes as hyperlipidaemia and atheroma. These all combine to increase the risk of death from cardiovascular disease. The PARs phenomenon, which evolution ensured, is now pathological – its predictions are inappropriate. And to make matters worse, human growth has one further feature – human neonates are the fattest of any species at birth. This puts unusual demands on their nutrient requirements in late pregnancy and makes the fetus in late gestation very sensitive to nutrient limitation signals of environmental origin.[5]

The health significance of this evolutionary mismatch did not matter when life spans were shorter[6] and, in any event, the range of nutritional intakes and the reduction in energy expenditure has shifted most dramatically in the last one to four generations – depending on whether we examine a developing or developed society. In general the constraining mechanisms on fetal growth operating even in normal pregnancies trigger PARs appropriate for a limited postnatal environment (see Figure 7.1) but our postnatal environments are now very different. This mismatch makes the risk of an inappropriate prediction a common if not universal

---

[4] Recent data suggest over 30 per cent pregnant women may have suboptimal nutrition early in pregnancy.

[5] The reasons for human babies being fat may well relate to the high energy demands of the human brain and the need to have a buffer fuel supply to support it through its most critical periods of functional development and dangerous periods of weaning and infantile infection.

[6] In early Roman times the average life span was less than 30 years. In the UK as late as 1850 the average expectation of life for 'gentlemen' was only 45 years, and much less for 'tradesmen'.

phenomenon in modern *Homo sapiens*. The implications for the ecology of human disease are obvious.

For most of the last 150 000 years since *Homo sapiens* evolved,[7] food supplies have generally been limiting and necessary energy expenditure substantial. The hunter–gatherer state was our evolutionary normal state and the diet of palaeolithic humans was very different from the diets we now eat. While there is some debate as to the diets of our ancestral forebears and of the relevance of modern hunter–gatherer diets to the past, it is generally considered that the diets were higher in protein, (but protein intake was more episodic) and the carbohydrate intake was very low. Fat was primarily obtained from meat and nuts, and in some societies at least was only episodically available (as wild meat can have seasonal changes in fat content). The need to store energy when available was reflected in at least some hunter–gatherer societies in gorging behaviour – for example by North American Indians who gorged on buffalo in summer when the meat was fattest. Dramatic seasonal weight change has been observed in the Kalahari San people and other modern hunter–gatherer societies.

As well as a change in food supply, agriculture and modernisation have a second set of implications: reduced energy expenditure. Metabolic equilibrium depends on the balance between energy consumed in growth, exercise and body maintenance versus the intake of energy as food. Clearly as well as the major shifts in food supply over the last 10 000 years, the same is true on the demand side with less energy being expended in exercise – the hunter–gatherer had no easy life! This will magnify the effect of enhanced food supplies and thus the relative imbalance between PARs and postnatal existence in our recent past.

Much of the Third World still lives in relative nutritional deprivation, although with a dietary mix very different from that of our Palaeolithic ancestors. The mean weight of women in Southern India at the start of pregnancy is only 45 kg – about 60 per cent of that in the Western world. The fetuses of these pregnancies adopt a developmental trajectory such that they will thrive (reproductively) in a relatively limited postnatal energy environment. Until recently this type of PAR was highly appropriate, as that indeed was the environment these fetuses would be born into. It enabled them to survive to reproductive competence while staying small and thin and surviving on scarce food supplies. But in the last generation in India there has been a very rapid increase in food availability. The fetus makes the same predictive choice (the maternal signals are effectively similar because of the dominant role of maternal constraint) but instead of having made an appropriate PAR it has made an inappropriate PAR – hence the exploding incidence of diabetes and hypertension.

---

[7] The fossil record is still incomplete – *Homo sapiens* appeared somewhere between 300 000 and 100 000 years ago – not long in evolutionary terms.

This is the same phenomenon as we have seen in developed societies, the major difference being that the magnitude of the fetal constraint is such that the level of the inappropriate postnatal nutritional range is set much lower than in the developed world. In the West we have bigger better-fed mothers and less constraint, but still the processes of constraining fetal growth operate and fetuses make adaptive choices about a range of postnatal environments that are all too frequently exceeded.

One caveat is needed here: we have focused much of our discussion on the metabolic syndrome and its associated components. However, as we discussed in chapter 5, there may well be other components of importance, not the least being those associated with fluid balance and neural and behavioural function. Our lack of broader focus on these reflects a paucity of data. The animal data would suggest that stress responses, anxiety levels, willingness to explore, exercise tolerance and eating behaviour can all be modified by the processes of PARs. We can understand each of these responses as part of an extended survival phenotype. An animal programmed to trade-off growth for reproduction may be living in an environment at high risk of predation. Hence it will be more anxious, and the alterations in exercise and eating behaviour assist in meeting the environmental challenge. It is tempting to speculate that inappropriate prediction plays a role in the incidence of anxiety and other disorders in the modern world but we must point out that the necessary data are not available; much more research is needed.

## Are PARs a universal phenomenon in humans?

The original observations that led to the concepts of 'programming' and the 'fetal origins of adult disease' and that we now see as examples of inappropriate prediction, were made in studies of Caucasian populations born in the early and mid twentieth century in England. But they were rapidly confirmed in populations as diverse as those of Finland, Sweden, Holland, Australia and the USA. The story might have ended there, if the predictive adaptive concept was restricted to a problem of the so-called lifestyle diseases only within these Western societies. However, the association between low birth weight and high blood pressure, coronary heart disease and Type 2 diabetes was found similarly to occur in China, India, Jamaica and in South America. It is now clear that it is a universal phenomenon in humans – wherever it has been sought it has been found.

Populations around the globe differ enormously in terms of lifestyle, diet and even in birth weight itself. Thus in Southern India, the average birth weight is about 1 kg less than in most Western countries. Yet the graded inverse association between birth weight and the risk of cardiovascular disease exists in both that population and in the West. As we have already described (chapter 5), the consequences of inappropriate prediction relate to altered risks of the metabolic syndrome, obesity and its disease components, and extend to other diseases. But inappropriate prediction need not necessarily be manifest as disease – in population studies most of the population do not have overt diabetes or clinically relevant high blood pressure. What they *do* have are subtle but identifiable pathophysiological precursors and risk factors for the disease – for example graded changes in plasma lipid levels, in bone density, in insulin sensitivity and so on. Disease will be more likely to become manifest as the person gets older or if he or she has other causal factors (e.g. a particular genotype that independently confers an additional risk of insulin resistance). Disease will also be more likely if the amplification by postnatal factors takes the individual out of a physiological zone in which he or she can cope, because the particular genotype of that individual is, in effect, sensitising. For example inappropriate prediction will have set the individual on a path to have a degree of insulin resistance, but Type 2 diabetes mellitus will be more likely to develop if the individual has particularly bad eating behaviour, or has a polymorphism in the PPARγ gene, which in itself interferes with insulin action. Disease is often a result of double 'hits', and our proposition is that one of these 'hits' is the early life environment.

A most important factor in this regard is ageing. One would predict that, if evolution protected the development of PARs, it would not do so at a cost to reproductive fitness. Indeed the whole point in evolutionary and reproductive terms is to make predictive adaptations that will allow an animal in a risky environment to survive and reproduce, even if there are longer-term consequences. It is well established that natural selection works primarily in early life and in the reproductive phase, and there is little evidence for it operating once reproduction is over.[8] Humans are virtually unique in that females in particular live well past reproductive age.[9] Thus it is easy to see that natural selection may have selected for processes that have some advantage in the reproductive period, but are not selected against later in life when they are manifest as disease.

Ageing itself is a complex process that is beyond the scope of this book. Simplistically it can be viewed in terms of the cost of maintaining our cells in good order. Within each cell there are many such processes, for example to repair damaged DNA, but they all consume energy. Other cells may have finite capacity to divide. Over time in many tissues the capacity for repair and maintenance falls and more cells die.[10] For example the reduced nephron number of the challenged fetus

---

[8] This is a bit of a simplification; the exception may be in some species such as man and elephants where there is some evidence that there are grandparent-effects that play a role in species survival – for example the matriarchal elephant leading the herd to a water hole in a severe drought. New evidence for 'grandmother effects' in promoting survival of their grandchildren is now emerging for humans.

[9] This is primarily true of females whereas males have declining but active sperm formation throughout life.

[10] Skin is a good example – with age it becomes thinner as there is difficulty maintaining cell replication to replace shed skin cells. The ability to maintain the proteins such as the keratins, which waterproof skin,

may not matter until middle age when the accumulated effects of other changes in cardiovascular function, in part as a result of lifestyle and age-related nephron loss, mean that the kidney can no longer conduct its role to maintain normal blood pressure; pathological hypertension needing treatment appears and itself leads to an increased risk of heart disease and stroke.

## The significance of the 'continuum'

Central to our hypothesis is that the fetus can alter its development in response to its immediate environment for two separate reasons: instant survival (i.e. fetal homeostasis and homeorhesis), and for ultimate postnatal fitness (i.e. PARs). We have pointed out that this choice is not a once-only choice made at one point in development, but rather that the embryo/fetus is constantly responding to environmental information and adjusting its physiology for these two separate purposes accordingly. We have focused primarily on nutrient-related signals because they are the most obvious and probably the most important in terms of species survival. Because altered nutrition may often affect absolute fetal weight, there is a dangerous tendency to fall into the trap of thinking that it is birth weight itself that is mechanistically involved in phenotypic induction. Of course it is not. It is just a surrogate that reflects some information about some indices of fetal nutrition. Birth size could not for example reflect a deficiency in one critical nutrient – iodine deficiency may cause gross functional abnormality of brain development (cretinism) but not alter birth weight. It is indeed likely that much programming is triggered by changes in the environment that specifically do not affect birth weight – for example changes in nutrient mix rather than absolute amounts of food can trigger PARs. Predictive adaptive responses are not usually all-or-nothing switches in trajectory – they are adjustments in physiology and structure to match a developing organism to its predicted postnatal environment.

The risk of heart disease is not just increased in babies who were very growth-retarded at birth,[11] nor diminished only in those who were exceptionally large at birth. We have emphasised that nothing could be further from the truth: being very small or very large at birth is associated with different, additional health risks reflecting the pathologies that create extremes in fetal development and may well involve developmental disruptions. Predictive responses are manifest in babies born

also declines. Wound repair is slower. Skin cancers become more common as the impact of accumulated ultraviolet and other insults becomes apparent.

[11] Again we caution the reader of the following paragraphs not to fall into the trap of assuming birth weight as anything more than a poor surrogate for summing up the fetal experience. But because there are relationships between birth weight and measures of inappropriate prediction, we can draw from a study of these relationships the important conclusion that PARs operate across the full spectrum of fetal environments, and not just at the extremes.

within the *normal range* of birth size phenotypes for their population. The baby born weighing 3.5 kg has a different risk profile to the baby born weighing 3.2 kg: yet both are of 'normal' birth size. Similar observations have been made in animal studies using sheep, guinea pigs and rats. For example in guinea pigs we know that smaller pups at birth are more likely as adults to develop higher blood pressures and reduced insulin sensitivity. These occur within the normal range of guinea pig birth sizes, arising from the varying degrees of the maternal constraint that is operative in all pregnancies. Maternal constraint will vary in degree according to maternal size, whether it is the first pregnancy and whether it is a multiple birth. We have already suggested that, for humans and other species with small litter sizes, maternal constraint is the key mechanism in ensuring a tendency for induction of the survival phenotype to be the default strategy.

But why are there relationships between birth size and PARs across this full spectrum of human fetal development? There would appear to be two, not mutually exclusive, explanations for this. First, as we saw in chapter 2, fetuses rarely grow to their full genetic potential – their growth is held in check to some extent by the processes of maternal constraint to ensure that the fetal head does not get too large and obstruct delivery. It is of course not possible to do the experiments in humans that were done by Walton and Hammond in 1938 when they crossed horses of very different size. However the relatively rare incidence of pelvic disproportion, in which the fetus cannot be delivered vaginally in monotocous species including the human, suggests that maternal constraint operates in most situations. Further evidence in humans is provided by the relationship between birth size and the size of the *recipient* (but not the *donor*) mother in pregnancies that originated in ovum donations. This shows that constraint is not a genetic phenomenon. All other things being equal, a fetus who has large parents may reach 4 kg; but if he or she only reaches 3.8 kg at term, then that fetus has experienced a 5 per cent constraint for weight. This would reflect a less than optimal fetal environment and that may have triggered an adaptive response, but most would still consider the baby to be a big baby. Thus across the full range of birth weights we would expect that the smaller the size at birth, the greater the degree of constraint that has operated in utero – and the greater the PARs-mediated as deviation in physiological settings from the population mean.

The second reason also comes from our understanding of fetal growth. As we have seen in chapter 2, short periods of undernutrition of the fetus affect its growth but it will show catch-up growth and return to its original growth trajectory. If the period of nutritional restriction is longer, then the fetus may have to reset its growth trajectory permanently. What is clear is that from at least a third of the way through pregnancy, the fetus is able to sense its nutritional milieu and change its growth rate accordingly. Then it is constantly setting and resetting this growth trajectory.

If the maternal environment creates repetitive triggers either because of repeated stresses and disease or because the placenta is inadequate – then the fetus must adjust continuously. This too will lead to the fetus constantly decelerating and accelerating its growth in trying to determine the appropriate trajectory for its perception of the postnatal environment – and this will create a continuum of birth weights, where the smallest has been exposed to greatest cumulative insult and the largest to least insult. The smaller fetuses are thus more likely to have developed a more overt survival phenotype through the processes of PARs than the larger fetuses. This phenomenon is at the heart of understanding the evolutionary and biological significance of PARs.

## The human camel

There is a final implication and one on which we shall focus in the remainder of the book – the exploding epidemic of obesity that we believe partly has its origins early in life. The camel's hump is made of fat. It is designed as an organ that is highly labile. This means that the fat in the hump mobilises readily to provide energy when the camel treks across the desert, and stores fat readily when it has access to food. The camel evolved for survival in an environment where the expectation of episodic food supply was the norm. The camel's hump is on the back because it serves a second purpose – that of protecting the camel from the desert sun (because fat is a poor thermal conductor – which is why whales and seals have so much blubber)[12] and also permits its limbs to be thin for maximal heat loss.

However, other species that have episodic access to food also have labile fat stores. Humans evolved these too – but it is located somewhere else – within the omentum. Omental fat is stored in the membranes attaching the intestines to the abdominal wall. It is very labile and has different biochemical properties to fat under the skin. Its location gives it unique potential to regulate insulin sensitivity in the liver because when fat is mobilised free fatty acids are formed. Blood from the omentum flows to the liver, and fatty acids act on the liver to change the properties of its cell membranes to make them more insulin resistant.[13] This happens every night to help us maintain our blood sugar levels during the overnight fast (relative to many species we have a long overnight fast) – then during the day we eat, and under the action of insulin we use nutrients for our energy needs and store excess energy as fat and glycogen. Several related mechanisms operate when we go to sleep. We release growth hormone from our pituitary gland, which stimulates fat breakdown and

---

[12] This may be another reason why the hairless human neonate is so fat compared to neonates of other species.

[13] The use of some drugs to treat insulin resistance has its origin in this piece of biology. Some of these drugs reduce fatty acid mobilisation from the omentum.

the release of glucose from glycogen. The fat breakdown causes insulin resistance in the liver, which also allows glucose to be released from glycogen. Fasting lowers our insulin levels, which has an additional effect.

The fat under our skin is called subcutaneous fat and appears less labile than omental fat. This difference in lability is owing to some differences between chemical signals made in omental and subcutaneous fat. In some indigenous African populations, a further fat store is found on the thighs and buttocks. This condition is called steatopygia. It has been suggested that this distinct fat store is due to mutation in the genes regulating the properties of fat stores. It acts as a further storage depot for high-energy fuels but it does not have the mobility of omental fat.

Omental fat probably evolved in ancestral early hominids to allow them to sustain energy supplies over longer periods – hunter–gatherers typically went several days without eating then gorged when high-fat food was available. The omental site is more appropriate to an upright posture than is the positioning of the camel's hump! It is reported that hunter–gatherers in some populations (e.g. Australian aborigines) have relatively high waist–hip ratios suggesting a propensity to omental fat deposition. Even placing the major shift in nutrient supply and energy demands in the recent decades alongside this evolutionary echo, it would not necessarily have adverse consequences if postnatal diet and exercise were appropriate. Further, the processes of satiety might limit food intake appropriately and omental fat would not become pathologically enlarged. But add in the context of PARs, the universally constrained nature of fetal growth, and the dramatic change in our energy environment, and a different picture emerges. We know from animal experiments that the default phenotype includes degrees of altered appetite, fat preference and leptin resistance. Leptin is a hormone made by fat that normally inhibits appetite, and leptin resistance provides a mechanism for the increased food intake. There are also data showing abnormalities in other hormones controlling appetite. We know that these animals exercise less and have reduced muscle mass. All this predisposes them to obesity. If this applies in humans, it suggests a new hypothesis – namely that the rising epidemic of truncal (omental) obesity has its origin in the mismatch between the predicted and actual postnatal environment – i.e. it is a consequence of PARs.

New evidence for this idea is rapidly appearing. We know that children born slightly smaller owing to greater maternal constraint are relatively obese by five years of age although they tended to be thinner at birth. We also know that children born small are more likely to get obese later, and that this also applies to children of mothers who had poor weight gain in mid-pregnancy. Children of mothers who smoke are more likely to be obese – smoking is a major cause of pathophysiological restraint of fetal growth through a number of mechanisms. Perhaps most surprising of all is recent data from India. Babies born in South India may have a birth weight of only 2.6 kg. This is largely because of the extreme maternal constraint operating, owing to small maternal stature and poor nutritional status. Despite these babies being some of the smallest in the world, they do not have reduced body fat at birth – while all other body proportions are reduced compared to babies of the same gestational age in the UK, the amount of central fat is actually the same, thus their relative proportion of body fat is greater. This is compelling data. It suggests that in humans the problem of obesity may be induced in utero. Being born small or constrained, and then exposed to a *relative* increase in nutrition over the plane predicted in utero, sets up a likelihood of relative obesity[14] appearing in childhood with increased risk of progression to disease later in life.

In general the observations in humans born small or in adults with the metabolic syndrome have remarkable similarities to those made in experimental animals. What we do not yet know is whether the other pathophysiological observations made in animals, and which might contribute to the obesity, also occur in humans. Animals that have been prenatally undernourished have reduced muscle mass, high food intakes, a preference for fatty food, alterations in their appetite regulatory centres in the brain and tend to be less active. There is some evidence that humans have reduced muscle mass as a consequence of an adverse intrauterine environment but, as yet, studies of appetite, exercise and food preference are lacking. It will be intriguing to see if these do contribute to the human condition – we suspect they will, because of the great problems there are in inducing weight loss and exercise in subjects with features of the metabolic syndrome. If this is the case, then public health measures to combat obesity in adults may be of limited value. The very individuals most at risk may have been hardwired in utero not to want to exercise and to prefer high fat intakes. A longer-term preventative strategy may require intervention prior to birth!

Thus we propose that childhood obesity it not just a feature of a television set and French fries – it is the inevitable consequence of PARs. We are a species that evolved as a hunter–gatherer – we developed a potential for a camel's hump in our abdomen as a fat-fuel reserve. We evolved in the expectation of rather poor nutrient environments and high-energy expenditures. Predictive adaptive responses, and the consequent default/survival phenotype were the norm, and the presence of maternal constraint assisted in ensuring this position. Thus primitive man survived and became modern man. Now we live much longer and have very high nutrient supplies. But the echoes of these survival mechanisms persist –we find it easy to put on omental fat, some of us find it difficult to exercise and to restrain our food intake, and truncal obesity develops. This in itself magnifies the problems of insulin resistance and cardiovascular changes, such that disease develops in later life.

---

[14] The key measure is relative fatness for height, not absolute weight.

Is it necessary to invoke PARs as part of the story? We believe so because the weight of evidence shows that antenatal factors are involved, and there are metabolic changes and altered fat mass at birth or in childhood, well before obvious obesity has developed. The childhood patterns of fat gain may well be determined prenatally and there is ample evidence that childhood and adolescent weight gain predict disease in adulthood. No doubt excess food intake at any age can lead to gross obesity – this is implied at the upper extremes for the well-nourished fetus in Figure 7.2. However when there is an inappropriate prediction, there is a greater disease risk in a lower-energy environment than would be the case if PARs did not occur. Thus while bad environments after birth always increase disease risk, the presence of a deficient fetal environment greatly increases the risk of disease. The implications of how and when to intervene in this pathway are complex and are the subject of the next chapter.

There are marked ethnic differences in the risks of insulin resistance in different populations. For example, in general Europeans have relatively lower risks compared to Australian aborigines, or Asian Indians. One suggestion is that Europeans have been exposed to higher carbohydrate diets (which come with agriculture) for longer than the other ethnic groups and have selected against insulin resistance. This idea cannot be excluded – at the very beginning of agriculture the capacity for selection would have been greater than it is now, but the adverse effects of insulin resistance are largely post-reproductive. The alternative explanation (which is not mutually exclusive) is that the difference is explained by PARs. In the developed societies, the fetal environment is better than in developing societies – mothers are taller, less likely to be adolescent, have less infection (and its associated stress), and less likely to be undernourished. As a result the fetuses of these mothers predict a higher postnatal nutritional level than those from developing societies. Thus the absolute postnatal nutritional level at which disease risk increases substantially (see Figure 7.2) in India is much lower than in developed societies; more fetuses will as adults cross the boundary to diabetes, particularly as high-carbohydrate foods have become more common in developing countries.

## The alternative fetal pathway to obesity and diabetes

Before we leave this topic, we must note that there is an alternative pathway to postnatal obesity and disease: it occurs when the *fetus* lays down too much fat. One of the important adaptations to pregnancy is for the mother to become relatively insulin resistant so that she uses fat for her own energy needs and provides glucose to the placenta and fetus. This relative insulin resistance is induced by placental lactogen, a hormone made by the placenta. In normal situations this appropriately balances the nutritional needs of mother and fetus. But if the mother has a diabetic tendency the situation is different. Infants of diabetic or prediabetic[15] mothers are relatively obese. This occurs because insulin drives fat synthesis. The mother will have higher blood glucose levels, and more glucose than normal crosses the placenta. This stimulates the fetal pancreas to make insulin, which drives the excess energy available into fat deposition. Such children therefore have more fat laid down at birth. In the energy-rich environment of the modern world these children continue to get more obese and may be at particular risk as increased fat mass is associated with greater insulin resistance. When this is considered in the light of the boundaries of postnatal nutrition associated with health (Figure 7.2) such individuals are at greater risk of crossing the lower nutritional boundary than those from non-diabetic pregnancies. In turn these children – when they become adults – are at risk of developing gestational diabetes if they are female, and so the cycle extends to the next generation. Breaking this cycle may require attention as to how we can restrict the increase in neonatal fat mass being amplified throughout childhood.

There is an intriguing complexity to the story that is now unfolding in India but is also relevant to the developed world. Women who were in adverse intrauterine environments and live postnatally in nutritionally relatively better environments are more likely to have gestational diabetes or to be prediabetic even though their body size is still small because of the effects of PARs acting in the mother.[16] On one hand, growth of the fetus is severely constrained by maternal size but, on the other, fetuses are receiving excessive glucose because of the maternal prediabetic state. The result is relatively low birth weight children who have relative adiposity. They have the same risks as larger-size infants born to diabetic mothers in Western populations. The zone of security, in terms of the ranges of birth weight associated with a low risk of disease, may be much reduced in Indian babies. This is shown diagrammatically in Figure 8.2.

## Populations in transition

The intriguing issue that then arises concerns the pathway for transition of populations between these two curves. What is the set of conditions that allows one population to move from a particularly high-risk profile to a lower-risk profile? We can see that a historically deprived population such as India is more likely to face disease because of PARs at a relatively low postnatal energy environment

[15] The prediabetic woman has a slightly higher glucose level through pregnancy and this is sufficient to affect the fetus and cause a larger, fatter baby.
[16] The relative insulin resistance induced in utero by PARs is exposed and magnified by the insulin resistance-inducing effects of placental lactogen when the female offspring in turn becomes pregnant.

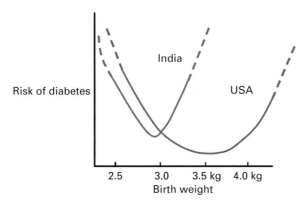

Fig. 8.2    The risk of insulin resistance in adulthood related to birth weight in India compared to the USA. The U-shaped curve shows that risk increases at both low and high birth weight. The low limb we attribute to inappropriate PARs, at least until the dotted portion for very low birth weight when other processes may also operate. The data on the upper limb is less substantial. Again, part of the risk may be caused by inappropriate PARs, amplified by gestational diabetes (including that associated with low *maternal* birth weight).

(Figure 7.1) and also problems secondarily to an enriched fetal environment at a relatively low maternal intake (Figure 8.2).

In such a population the postnatal environment has shifted rapidly and dramatically, even within a single generation. However with respect to PARs, the fetal environment can only shift more slowly. The first developmental signals to which the fetus is exposed occurred within the grandmother's uterus when the egg destined to become the mother first developed,[17] and that exposure will have echoes into the grandchild. The uterus develops during the embryonic period and so the fetus lives in a uterus whose development was determined a generation earlier. But perhaps the most dominant influence on the fetal environment is maternal size, metabolism and body composition. Maternal size and metabolism are strongly influenced by the mother's early life experience as a fetus as is her metabolism as a result of PARs. Her body composition is influenced both by current and by past (i.e. as a result of PARs) experience. Thus the fetus develops in an environment where many of the important influences concern maternal history rather than the current environment. And thus in a rapidly changing environment the risk of mismatch between fetal and postnatal environments is greater, with its consequences for PARs-related disease.

Similar considerations apply to the overnourished fetus – the high current food intake of a mother who is adapted for a rationed food intake and strong maternal constraint because of small body size, will lead to greater risk of fetal hyperglycaemia.

---

[17] Eggs start development in the first few weeks of female gestation, developing as the primitive ovary forms.

This, in turn, will lead to increased fetal fat mass and increased long-term risk even at a relatively small fetal size. This too is a manifestation of inappropriate PARs where constrained maternal growth in utero programmes the future mother towards relative insulin resistance, which is exposed by pregnancy.

As we will discuss in the next chapter, it is the speed of the nutritional transition that therefore determines the population disease risk. A slow transition over many generations will be associated with a gradual reduction in the degree of maternal constraint, as the uterine environment improves with both maternal health and size in successive generations. In turn this will allow (see Figure 7.1) a richer postnatal energy environment to be tolerated without disease.[18]

## Putting it all together

Human obesity and its complications are best understood within a conceptual framework that takes into account both prenatal life and the role of PARs.

We have suggested that humans evolved in a nutritional and energy environment that was very different from that which we enjoy today. Thus the regulation of fetal growth evolved in such a way that the constrained environment of the fetus was largely matched to the postnatal environment. The mean fetal phenotype would have been programmed by the maternal environment to a default phenotype that was highly appropriate for the hunter–gatherer. This phenotype includes the propensity to grow our abdominal hump i.e. omental fat. PARs were protected through evolution because, as was discussed in chapter 7, they allow a genetic lineage to survive a transient environmental change, and during Palaeolithic evolution they would have been valuable in maintaining the survival phenotype. Given the short life spans of Palaeolithic humans, there would be no pressures to select against PARs. Hence, under these conditions, most predictions would have been roughly appropriate for the postnatal environment.

But humans now live in a very different environment from that in which we evolved and the speed of environmental change has been particularly dramatic in the last few generations, both in developing and developed societies. The regulation of fetal growth has not changed – it is still physiologically and pathophysiologically constrained. Under these circumstances, PARs operate to produce an adult best-equipped to live in relatively nutritionally poor conditions and with the physiological characteristics of the survival phenotype. But this is no longer an appropriate prediction. Hence we see a rising incidence of childhood obesity, with its longer-term consequences. The characteristics of inappropriate prediction are such that, in the developing world, the upper boundary of the healthy postnatal environment

---

[18] Including the risk of maternal hyperglycaemia and thus diabetic-prone fetuses.

is at a lower energy/nutritional level than in developed countries. This is because fetal growth is more restricted and constrained in developing countries. However, our nutritional intakes in either setting now frequently exceed the boundaries set by the combination of our genotype and PARs: an epidemic of cardiovascular disease and Type 2 diabetes results.

There is a second path that leads to the obesity in infancy and that becomes magnified through life, that of the fetus exposed to excessive glucose levels caused by maternal prediabetes or gestational diabetes. In developed countries this is only seen at very large birth weights, but in countries such as India where maternal size is still small but nutrition is changing, this increased adiposity can be seen even at relatively low birth weights. This becomes a form of inappropriate prediction but processes additional to PARs also operate.

# 9

# Improving human health

## Disease, evolution and ageing

Since the evolution of *Homo sapiens*, some 150 000 years ago humans have made enormous strides in the battle for survival through the use of shelter, clothing, fire and weaponry and, since civilisations developed, through the development of social structures, religion, medication and healthcare. These strategies, which started to appear with the discovery of tool making, the control of fire and the development of culture, meant that humans have been able to sustain a very broad variety of phenotypes (and hence genotypes) across a range of environments. It is sometimes said that the control humans have over their environment means that we have stopped or, at least slowed, our evolution.

In evolving, humans traded-off reproductive performance for longevity. Contrast humans to rodents. Rodents invest their resources in getting large numbers of individuals to reproductive age as quickly in the life cycle as possible, but invest very little in promoting survival beyond that period. Humans have evolved the opposite strategy – later attainment of reproductive competence, a smaller investment in the number of offspring, and a considerable investment in preservation of members of the species beyond the reproductive period. Such older members assist with the child care associated with our slower development and ensure the passage of complex cultural traditions to these offspring.

But evolution primarily selects for advantage up to and during the reproductive period of life.[1] We are left in middle and old age to cope with the inevitable diseases associated with lifelong exposure to pathogens, oxidants etc., and are equipped with adaptive responses that were selected for their ability to get us to reproductive age and no further.[2] Life continues to be a battle to defend and repair our bodies against

---

[1] There are arguments that there are some selection advantages for grandparental survival as alluded to in the previous paragraph but, if present, they are probably of minimal overall significance.
[2] For example, even if one of our ancestors had developed a beneficial mutation that protected against prostate cancer (which is very rare in younger men), it would not have been selected by evolution unless it had other advantages. Thus the gene would not have entered our gene pool with high frequency.

the ravages of the environment. There is little or no selection for defences against problems that beset us in old age if these problems do not also compromise us when we are younger. Predictive adaptive responses operate against this background. The mechanisms underpinning PARs were selected in the evolving hominid because they provide survival advantage in an uncertain world up to and through our reproductive age, assuming there is a match between the predicted and actual environment. As we discussed in chapter 8 this would have been the case in our Palaeolithic and Neolithic ancestors. Disease arises when our predictions turn out to be wrong and, not surprisingly, most of this disadvantage appears in middle and old age.

## The prenatal origin of inappropriate PARs

As we have discussed, all fetuses are cognisant of their environment and thus PARs are a normal part of fetal development. Inappropriate predictions can arise at any level of prenatal environment if the prediction and the postnatal environment are mismatched. As shown in Figure 7.1, even if the prenatal environment is optimal there will be a defined postnatal-energy environmental range compatible with good health as an adult, and outside this range there will be increased risk of disease. The most common pathway to PARs-related disease in the modern world is that from a constrained pattern of fetal growth to an over-rich postnatal environment, and we will focus on this. However, the principles extend across the full range of prenatal environments from most deprived to excessive[3], and from our focus on available energy to other environmental components (e.g. thermal environment). It is thus obvious that to reduce the burden of disease later in life there are two interdependent approaches – first to improve the fetal environment and second, to address the postnatal management of the programmed infant.

In earlier chapters we pointed out the two major ways in which the prenatal environment is affected – first, a set of physiological constraints operative as part of 'normal' pregnancy and termed maternal constraint; second a set of pathophysiological restraints caused by maternal or placental disease. Maternal constraint can be of varying impact depending on maternal size, maternal age, parity etc. and thus has a variable effect in determining the fetal growth trajectory. But whatever the degree of constraint, PARs position all infants to have some survival phenotype characteristics and thus to be at greater risk of lifestyle disease at any postnatal

---

[3]  The concept of an 'excessive' fetal environment is difficult. In monotocous species like the human, maternal constraint essentially always restricts the level of fetal growth. However the fetus can still receive signals that it interprets as suggesting a rich postnatal environment – maternal diabetes may do this is if glucose is the signalling molecule. On the other hand, if the fetus is seeking signals about protein supply as an indication of the postnatal environment, the diabetic state might even be interpreted as deficient. One can interpret the available data either way.

nutritional level than would be the hypothetical case if maternal constraint were not operating.

In wild animals the consequences of inappropriate PARs are not often obvious because such animals are likely to die before they become elderly. Situations such as the population cycles of snowshoe hares, however, demonstrate that PARs do occur in the natural environment. In contrast, inappropriate PARs are common in humans because we preserve through the combination of mothering, protection and medicine, the offspring of mothers with diseases such as pre-eclampsia or malfunctioning of the placenta. The presence of such disease results in inappropriate information about the external environment being transmitted from the mother/placenta to the embryo and fetus. There is an enormous amount of medical evidence that the offspring of such pregnancies have an increased risk of a range of diseases.

## The postnatal origins of inappropriate PARs: the role of environmental transition

As well as prenatal causes of the inappropriate prediction, there are postnatal causes: the most important occurs because human beings often change their environments. The fetus can grow in an environment appropriate to that which the mother is signalling to it, but the postnatal environment is then changed by human intervention – changing living standards, migration etc. There is inevitably a lag in time and thus the potential exists for an environmental shift between what the conceptus predicts will exist in adult life and the actual environment it is born into, and if the environment starts to change rapidly this can be a significant factor. The speed of the nutritional transition is such that in some societies it is not uncommon for the diet of the mother in her reproductive phase and that of her offspring as they reach adulthood to be very different – inappropriate PARs occur as a result. We believe that this change is a major contributor to the patterns of human disease in different societies. Essentially the fetus grew exposed to one nutritional situation but the nutritional environment it now faces as an adult is very different: the homeostatic set-points it chose in utero may be very wrong.

Let us consider this issue of nutritional transition further, taking the example of France. France was the first country to adopt a major nutritional intervention programme to protect the health of mothers and children in the nineteenth century. This was not entirely altruistic – the French authorities were worried about the fitness of their future soldiers in the recurrent Franco–Prussian wars and recognised the need to protect the production line of strong young men! Thus France is a country where nutritional standards have been high over several generations, although the fad for American-style fast foods may now be causing disequilibrium.

At the other extreme we have populations such as those in urban India and China where a very fast transition from a low- to a high-fat diet is underway. Here we find millions of children born to mothers of small stature and poor muscle development, and these children are exposed after birth to much higher levels of nutrition than those they were exposed to in utero. This is a problem on a global scale, and it has occurred over only one generation, faster than any previous change in human lifestyle. Recent data from the International Obesity Taskforce show that for the first time more people in the world suffer from the effects of over-nourishment than of starvation! In some of the countries particularly affected such as China, the problem is made worse by the legislation introduced to limit population numbers. When family size is limited, sometimes to one child, more children are born with greater maternal constraint (i.e. to first pregnancies) and these children are over-nourished because of the high parental investment in them. We envisage that the public health consequences of this will be enormous.

The focus of this discussion is on transition and change – we have used the Indian example to illustrate how a population as a whole may experience environmental change within a generation. But humans have another major way of changing their environment suddenly – migration. The last 300 years have seen some enormous human migrations. Many have been associated with movement from one nutritional environment to another – often a much-improved environment. For example more Samoans now live in New Zealand than in Samoa. In Polynesia their diet was unrefined with a high content of fish, taro[4] and coconut. In New Zealand their diet is very different with a very high intake of fat, meat and refined foods.

The Falasha Jews come from the highlands of Ethiopia. They lived in poor rural areas and believed themselves to be descendants of the biblical King Solomon and the Queen of Sheba. Following the terrible civil wars in Ethiopia in the late-twentieth century, many Falasha Jews were transported virtually overnight to Israel. There were many adjustments these people had to make.[5] They were moved from a remote rural environment into a modern and technologically advanced state.[6] But the transition that may have had the biggest impact of all was the change in nutritional environment. They had lived in Ethiopia under very deprived, subsistence conditions; in Israel they were exposed to a modern diet with essentially no

---

[4] A potato-like tuber.
[5] There were rabbinical debates over their status as Jews because they had no knowledge of the Talmud, that component of Jewish law written after they separated from the rest of Judaism – Talmudic law is the basis of modern religious Jewish practice.
[6] Unfortunately they were not moving from a war-torn country to a peaceful one!

limitations of carbohydrate or fat availability. It will therefore not be a surprise that the Falasha Jews, like the Samoans and the Indians described above, now face an epidemic of Type 2 diabetes. In each of these cases the fetus grew in a nutritional environment that was relatively deprived compared to that which the child later experienced. In the Indian case this was caused by maternal constraint, in the Falasha by maternal famine, and in the Samoans the baseline nutrition was adequate but there was a substantial change in the nutritional intake on moving to New Zealand. The fetuses of these different populations all made what we can now see, with the wisdom of hindsight, to be inappropriate PARs, although they lie on different parts of the spectrum that we showed in Figure 7.1.

What speed of nutritional transition is possible for a population while minimising the risk of inappropriate PARs? We would suggest the rate limiting step lies in utero. But the in utero environment of the current fetal generation has been in no small part determined by the environment of the mother when she herself was a fetus. That is, the current fetus is influenced by its grandmaternal environment.[7] The egg that a mother provides at ovulation for fertilisation first develops when the mother was herself an embryo[8]. Similarly the uterus develops during fetal life and there is evidence that the uterus of mothers who had experienced intrauterine growth retardation is smaller and thus will be more constraining. And as we have seen, one's metabolic status as an adult is partially determined in utero and thus the mother's metabolic status in pregnancy will have in turn been influenced by her fetal experiences.

The rate of environmental change therefore becomes critical. If the change is very fast, then the risk of inappropriate PARs will be very high and the consequences for later disease will be large. If the rate of transition is very slow then the degree of mismatch between the fetal and postnatal environment will be small, and the risk of inappropriate PARs will be less. Could this explain the declining incidence of heart disease in the Western world? There have been many other factors suggested (including maybe the intake of red wine!) but our contention is that early-life factors cannot be ignored. Predictive adaptive responses can be inappropriate either because the fetus has predicted wrongly, or because the postnatal environment has changed. Therefore we would in fact argue that the rise in high-fat and high-calorie nutrition in childhood has been so fast and so large that the current generation of fetuses will inevitably have made PARs inappropriate to the environment in which they will live. Further, the problem will continue in a somewhat different nature

---

[7] And the argument can continue back with diminishing effect to the great-grandmaternal and great-great-grandmaternal environments and so on.

[8] The ovary develops in the first half of gestation and during that time, all the eggs the ovary will ever have form and then lie in suspended development until puberty when in each cycle one egg is activated and fully develops.

into the next generation, because these children as adults are likely to be obese and to have increased insulin resistance because of inappropriate PARs. In turn women of this generation, when they become pregnant, will have a greater risk of gestational diabetes with its ongoing consequences for the following generation. Those believing largely in adult 'lifestyle' factors are reassured by the fall in incidence of coronary heart disease. We think that we might be sitting on a time bomb, and that the incidence of lifestyle disease may fall a little more, flatten out and then rise again.

## A chain reaction

There is no doubt that postnatal obesity on its own carries very significant health risks. Some medical researchers therefore argue that there is no need to invoke a prenatal element at all. We would counter with three points. First, the data in many populations consistently show that those who had the greater prenatal insults, as evidenced by small maternal size, are at greatest risk. Second, the experimental data show that it is possible to induce this phenotype purely with antenatal insults in animals. Thus both humans and rats undernourished in utero develop truncal obesity. This can be seen in gross situations like the Dutch Hunger Winter, more subtly in the relationship between maternal weight gain and truncal obesity in the offspring of British women, and in the laboratory. Third, in India it appears that there are two paths to Type 2 diabetes and both involve antenatal components – these paths start with either being overnourished or being undernourished in utero. The children who show a rapid adiposity rebound are more likely to get diabetes, and in both India and Finland the pattern and timing of the adiposity rebound is partly determined prenatally. The data from Finland show similar influences on the risks for coronary heart disease.

Then it has been suggested by some critics that the magnitude of the antenatal effect is so small that it cannot be important. This is because if we ask the question, 'How much of the variation in, say, adult blood pressure can be accounted for by variation in birth weight?' the answer will be, 'Not very much.'[9] It is much easier (and quicker) for epidemiologists to start at the end of life and to look retrospectively than it is for them to start at the beginning of life and do prospective studies. The latter gives us a very different answer – namely that the fetal experience plays a major role in defining our adult cardiovascular status. It determines the phenotype, which in turn determines the risk of disease in any given postnatal environment.

[9] It is a very different answer if the question that is posed is 'What is the evidence that metabolic diseases are more likely to occur if there is a past history suggesting a constrained or restricted fetal environment?'

Quite different data collection and statistical approaches are needed for the prospective and retrospective approaches, and they have quite different reliability. It is like looking at a triangle of snooker balls that has just been hit by the cue ball. We can start at the end and see balls scattered all over the table and have no idea how this happened. But if we look with a different perspective and start at the beginning we get a very clear view of what caused them to be moving. When the cue ball hits the first ball it in turn gives momentum to the next two, which in turn give momentum to the next three, which in turn give momentum to the fourth and then to the fifth row, until all the balls are moving. This is a very simple illustration of the concept of an amplifying cascade. Moving one ball just a small distance (at the apex of the triangle) in the end leads to the five balls in the last row moving. Although the time scale is very short, the first ball must move before the second row moves, and so on. The initial impetus imparted to the cue ball is transmitted over time so that five balls are moving long distances (if the cue ball is hit hard enough), even if the cue ball itself may not move very far if it is hit with a lot of backspin.

So it is with inappropriate PARs leading to disease. The initial effect on phenotype may be very small or subtle but it must happen. The PARs triggered in antenatal life are like the first snooker ball being hit – not much may be obvious but the infant is now primed to put on weight in the situation of a relatively high-calorific and, especially, a high-fat, diet. This leads to rapid weight gain during childhood, which magnifies the subtle degree of insulin resistance that had developed in utero. In turn the snooker ball effect becomes magnified into young adulthood with an even greater degree of obesity and insulin resistance until the final row of balls is reached, and Type 2 diabetes and other problems such as heart disease are manifest in the adult. Type 2 diabetes now affects some 25 per cent of Indians in South India, by the age of 40. This epidemic is greatest in the cities, because the postnatal diet there is less balanced and is fat- and carbohydrate-enriched compared to that of rural India. We have repeatedly stressed that these effects have become manifest in a generation: this of course is a fundamental aspect of the biological consequences of inappropriate PARs – they occur in the next immediate generation. We can now imagine the potential human consequences. Type 2 diabetes is associated with peripheral vascular disease and thus severe damage to the extremities. If we cannot rectify the problem, such Indian and Chinese cities may need armies of surgeons dedicated to vascular treatment alone. The humanitarian and financial costs will be enormous.

The alternative argument, which we have addressed in chapter 8, suggests that these patterns can be explained solely by genetic factors. There can be no doubt that as a result of genetic drift, migration through genetic bottlenecks,[10] and selection,

---

[10] A genetic bottleneck is a point in time where a new population was formed from a very small founder population, thus limiting the allelic variation in all successors.

different populations do have different allelic frequencies and some of these differences will influence the risk of disease. But we hope that by now the reader will see why it is not possible to explain PARs produced in laboratory rats by genetics, and why we feel confident in extending the theory to humans. This book has tried to show how the environment interacts with the genome at critical periods in development to induce a specific phenotype. It is the phenotype that in the end determines the risk of disease, otherwise identical twins or genetically homogeneous members of strains of laboratory rats would always have the same lifecourse of disease. This does not mean that there are no critical genetic elements. For example in chapter 4 we described one polymorphism that interacts with birth size to influence the risk of Type 2 diabetes in adults, and in chapter 6 we discussed the role of 'thrifty genes'. Both actually provide strong support for the validity of our model – that there are genomic and non-genomic (environmental) components, including epigenetic mechanisms, just as there are antenatal and postnatal components. The particular point we are making is that two environments matter – the environment of the present (e.g. current food intake, level of physical activity etc.) and the environment of the past (in utero).

There are several messages in this discussion: first, disease ecology is influenced by the rate of transition in a society or population, with slower transitions being beneficial as they create adequate time to make appropriate prenatal predictions. Second, nutrition is clearly an important factor but, as we will see, it is not simply a matter of the total volume of food – it is more about the balance and composition of the diet, and sadly our knowledge of what constitutes optimal nutrition in a given situation is very limited. Third, inappropriate PARs are a phenomenon that become magnified over many years from a subtle start, to be fully exhibited in adulthood, and may explain a considerable amount of the changing ecology of disease in both the developed and developing world.

## How important are inappropriate PARs to the pattern of human disease?

The most difficult issue is to determine how much of the current patterns of disease has a contribution from inappropriate predictive adaptive responses. At the Harvard School of Public Health a major project called the Global Burden of Disease has been undertaken to ascertain the likely patterns of disease in different societies over the next few decades. Diabetes, heart disease, depression and cancer remain in the top ten. In each of these it is realistic to imagine elements of inappropriate PARs at work.

As we noted in chapter 4, the most complete epidemiological analysis comes from Finland, where there has been careful population-based monitoring for over 60 years. Researchers have looked retrospectively at the records of those who develop heart disease or diabetes and compared their growth patterns with those who did not develop these diseases. They found that the growth patterns of these two groups of individuals are substantially different from the normal population, in terms of birth size and patterns of infant and childhood growth. The researchers have examined three components; height, weight and body-mass index. They have shown that those men who develop heart disease are born small, show poor infant growth then develop obesity prior to puberty at a faster rate than those who did not. Not dissimilar patterns are seen in those who develop Type 2 diabetes although there are differences in the details. These data demonstrate the chain reaction we have already described – there is a prenatal component that is magnified by an infancy component; this is then grossly amplified by a childhood component, and the result is an increased risk of disease.

The researchers have also tried a reverse analysis – they have estimated what would happen to the incidence of hypertension, heart disease and Type 2 diabetes if every neonate were born at least average in size, gained weight and height normally in the first year of life and did not develop obesity as a child. The results of the calculations are astounding and certainly need evaluation in other populations (if only the data were available). They found that the incidence of heart disease in adults would be reduced by 45 per cent, that of hypertension by 31 per cent and that of Type 2 diabetes by 62 per cent. If this extrapolation is valid and the calculation makes many assumptions, then these are much greater impacts on disease incidence than can be achieved by many other measures, such as prevention of smoking, reducing salt intake and minimising occupational stress.

Sorting out how much of this is prenatally – and how much is postnatally – determined is difficult – remember the snooker ball analogy. Moreover, the postnatal components, such as the role of postnatal growth and the adiposity rebound, may in turn be determined by the prenatal component – indeed that is what we suspect.

Such studies and interpretations are problematic because they have all the dangers of any retrospective study – looking at it from the end rather than from the beginning. And here lies the conundrum: there is no way to undertake these studies prospectively and achieve a rapid answer. If we were to study aspects of pregnancy and childhood growth to see how they relate to the incidence of disease, we would have to wait 50 to 70 years for the results. What would we do in the meantime – refrain from trying to prevent disease? Obviously if we introduce any interventions now they would confound the issue and ruin the interpretation of the study. But clearly not to intervene when we can is unethical.

One intermediate solution has been to seek surrogate markers of risk of future adult heart disease and diabetes, e.g. by measuring insulin resistance or vascular endothelial function in childhood, as these are known to be precursors to the development of the adult disease. Such studies show quite clearly that prenatal and childhood events associated with inappropriate PARs do lead to a much-increased risk of such precursors of adult disease. But the range of markers available at present is limited and their predictability is not necessarily good enough.

## Preventing diseases caused by inappropriate PARs

These various lines of enquiry, indirect as some must be, lead to only one conclusion – namely that improving prenatal wellbeing will make it easier to prevent inappropriate PARs and greatly reduce the burden of adult disease. Just as the most effective way to stop all the snooker balls moving is to stop the first ball moving, we suspect that the best way to stop the inappropriate predictive cascade is to intervene at the early steps.

In chapter 4 we described rats with inappropriate PARs caused by maternal undernutrition during pregnancy. These rats, especially if given a high-fat diet postnatally to exaggerate the inappropriateness of the prediction, exhibited changes in their appetite regulation and in their willingness to exercise. Currently the major public health measures being applied to reduce the risk of diabetes and heart disease are to encourage the middle-aged population to eat less and exercise more, as well as to stop smoking. These are laudable approaches and have had a significant impact on the incidence of heart disease and *must* be encouraged. But it is also well established that those most at risk of the metabolic syndrome and its component parts are relatively unresponsive to exercise and dietary programmes. That is, those who may benefit most from adult lifestyle change are most resistant. The rat experiments suggest that this may be no accident. The PAR cascade has led to postnatal phenotypes with obesity, hypertension and insulin resistance that have altered brain control of eating, and of the willingness to exercise, in an exaggeration of the survival phenotype. If extrapolation can be made from these experiments to the human, then it is obvious that the focus of an intervention restricted only to the adult population is doomed to failure.

So how can we intervene to reduce the incidence of disease caused by inappropriate PARs? Either we have to prevent the inappropriate PARs or we have to alter the postnatal environment so that the PARs are no longer inappropriate. As in other areas of medicine there are two broad approaches that we can adopt – either prevention or active intervention in the chain of cause-and-effect that leads to disease. Prevention depends on optimising the environment of the embryo, fetus and infant and trying to minimise the risks of environmental change postnatally. Intervention assumes that there may be ways of stopping the cascade even after it has started so as to reduce the impact of inappropriate PARs. Unfortunately in both areas we are limited by a serious lack of knowledge. We believe that addressing this knowledge gap needs urgent action.

## Primary prevention

The primary approach to reducing the problem must be to match the fetal environment to the postnatal environment. In general this means minimising the risks of false signals to the fetus through maternal or placental disease and optimising maternal and fetal health.

There are some very obvious strategies that will improve the probability of a healthy fetus. The most obvious concerns maternal age. Teenage mothers tend to have poorly growing fetuses. This is because the mother's uterus and pelvis may not be fully grown and the degree of maternal constraint is greater. It is also probable that the hormonal adjustments to pregnancy of the adolescent mother are somewhat different from the woman who has ceased to grow. Whereas in a mature woman the placental hormones act to direct nutrients from mother to the placenta and fetus, in the growing girl the drive to promote maternal growth persists and this limits the capacity of nutrients to be diverted from the mother to her fetus. Adolescent pregnancy is a world-wide problem but is particularly so in less-developed countries where childhood marriage and pregnancy soon after menarche are common. The strategies to break this cycle are complex and involve the empowerment of women, major cultural shifts and enhancing gender equality in matters such as education.

The problems must not be underestimated. It has been shown that a number of key factors can operate to limit the effectiveness of preventative educational strategies. First it is essential to decide whether a broad population-based approach will work, or whether it is better to focus on a target group. For example, should the perils of teenage pregnancy be taught as part of the core curriculum for young people in school, or will it be more effective if publicised on a national level – e.g. via television? The most effective strategy is not always obvious and may require a feasibility study in itself, something that is not always easy in a society that shows a high level of deprivation. Nor is it safe to assume that, just because we do not know the best strategy, we should use blanket and multiple educational approaches: more is not always better, and in fact parallel educational campaigns can sometimes occlude each other and lead to audience fatigue and poor uptake of the advice.

Advanced maternal age is also associated with poorer fetal growth, especially in first pregnancies. The reasons for this are less clear but may relate to a reduced capacity to make the cardiovascular and other adaptations necessary for optimal nutrient supply to the fetus. In developed countries, the increasing tendency of women to delay pregnancy until after they have established a career, gained some financial independence or experienced a series of relationships, presents us with a problem.

As women delay pregnancy longer, the risks of infertility grow. Likewise, the drastic fall in sperm count in Western males produces unwanted infertility even in many younger couples. Both trends have occurred at a time when assisted reproductive technologies have been broadly available. This has led to a great increase in multiple pregnancies and to the associated maternal constraint. The available data also raise the probability that the abnormal environment of the pre-embryo cultured in vitro may have long-term effects – it is too soon yet to know.

While the evidence is still preliminary, there are increasing clues that for both mother and father there are factors to consider *prior* to conception. We have already reviewed the evidence in chapter 6 that inappropriate PARs may have been triggered in this period. There may also be sperm effects as well as the egg effects that we have described in some detail. Exposure of the sperm during spermatogenesis to less than optimal conditions may influence the imprinting status of paternal genes after fertilisation and thus produce epigenetic effects. As we noted in chapter 5, data from Sweden reveal that the risk of Type 2 diabetes in men is determined in part by the diet of their grandfathers in the period before they reached puberty. So the challenge may extend to both parents.

We have already described animal experiments that suggest that nutrition around the time of conception has important inductive effects.[11] Only now are the necessarily very complex studies being started, in which data on nutritional status at the beginning of human pregnancy are collected and then related to the outcome of pregnancy.[12] This is information we badly need. Such data create a real challenge. It may not be sufficient to focus on nutrition once the woman knows she is pregnant – much may have already happened before then that will have lifelong consequences. If that is the case we then need strategies to address how to improve the nutritional status of women prior to conception – a difficult and culture-specific challenge.

It is apparent that nutritional factors are the most important environmental factors. We have seen that the nature of the impact of nutritional signals may differ at different times in pregnancy and that nutritional information is a major pathway of signalling to the fetus. It can reflect the actual status of the mother and her environment or it can be a false signal that arises from placental dysfunction or maternal metabolic disease (e.g. diabetes). What this suggests is that, maternal and placental disease apart, maternal nutrition may be by far the most important

---

[11] Sheep that are undernourished in the time around conception have abnormal placental and fetal development. Indeed these fetuses appear to grow normally for the first 80 per cent of pregnancy then slow their growth. Extrapolated to the human, if one had not known that the cause of the growth failure had occurred at the time of conception one would have assumed it to be a late-pregnancy problem. In the sheep study there was also a higher incidence of premature labour and there is a well-described relationship between being born small and being born premature. In Indian women with a reduced body mass at the start of pregnancy there is a tendency to have shorter gestational lengths by about 10 days compared to European women with high body weights at the start of pregnancy.

[12] The most comprehensive and detailed is the Southampton Women's Survey.

component of any preventative strategy to reduce the probability of inappropriate PARs.[13]

But we face a knowledge crisis. We actually know very little about what constitutes the optimal nutrition for a woman at different stages before and during pregnancy. We have already discussed what little we know and perhaps should summarise it again now. The studies we have reviewed show clearly that maternal nutrition is not just a question of adequate calories, unless the mother is under starvation conditions. Assuming that the total caloric intake is adequate, the balance of carbohydrate to protein and the source of that protein (dairy, meat or vegetable) have important influences on optimal fetal growth. Folate, an important vitamin regulating amino acid metabolism, has an essential interaction with the amount of protein ingested. High maternal protein intakes without folate will lead to fetal growth retardation. The major source of folate is green leafy vegetables. We also know that some critical micronutrients are important to the development of specific organs, e.g. iodine for the thyroid gland, calcium for bone. Based on animal experiments we predict, but do not know for sure, that many other micronutrients such as zinc, vitamin D and members of the vitamin B family are also important for optimal fetal development.

While we know that the most likely focus for a preventative strategy will be nutritional, we are also very cautious. There are many examples of well-meant preventative measures that, when implemented, did not reduce the size of the problem but in fact made it worse. For example babies were put to bed on their bellies for apparently logical reasons during the mid-twentieth century and yet this caused an increase, not the predicted decrease, in cot death. In a sense the public health emphasis on promoting big infants as healthy babies, and the consequent overfeeding of infants leading to obesity has contributed to the problem of inappropriate PARs. These of course are strategies that assume a level of choice in the degree of uptake by the population, and humans are by nature somewhat irrational and like to take risks. But they can also take advice too seriously and exacerbate problems by overdoing things. There are many health warnings about the dangers of excessive use of vitamin and mineral supplements, for example.

A good deal of attention to date has been on folate because it plays a range of metabolic roles (assisting in DNA synthesis, breakdown of toxic substances such as homocysteine and DNA methylation) and we have growing belief that such mechanisms play a major role in the origin of PARs. The Indian data and the Motherwell data both point to folate deficiency in pregnancy as a cause of inappropriate PARs. Folate supplementation at the beginning of pregnancy is known to reduce the risk of spina bifida. But what is the appropriate amount and timing of

---

[13] And the emerging information on the influences of maternal body composition and metabolism in initiating PARs are related to nutrition on a longer time scale.

folate administration? We do not know enough to be certain. Preliminary experiments show that the beneficial effects of folate supplementation in pregnancy on the offspring of undernourished rat dams are in fact converted into deleterious effects on the offspring if well-nourished dams are given excessive dietary folate supplementation during pregnancy. One reason for this might be that such normal offspring will become adapted to high folate levels before birth, make PARs accordingly and may develop pathology unless they are able to access such high folate levels postnatally.

So we are left with a gaping hole in our knowledge. We simply do not know the optimal or normal nutritional profile either for a pre-pregnant or a pregnant woman. If we have to focus on the periconceptional period, then for most of the world we must focus on optimising the nutritional status of adolescent females. For cultural and political reasons this is a real challenge in many societies, but particularly so in developing societies. Many studies have shown that the nutrition of girls in developing countries is worse than that of boys, that they grow less in consequence and that this is not necessarily rectified when they marry or commence childbearing. But even there we are uncertain whether the focus should just be on macronutrients (fat, carbohydrate, protein) or whether there needs to be a greater emphasis on micronutrients such as folate, zinc and vitamins. In other words, can micronutrient supplementation correct dietary macronutrient imbalance? It may even be that the optimal nutritional balance is different prior to, in early and in late pregnancy.

But some progress is being made. Knowledge about treating the fetus as a potential patient is growing.[14] Could fetal growth be enhanced or placental function improved in situations where it appears to be inadequate? There are data, particularly in the sheep, suggesting that experimental hormonal therapies can enhance placental function and thus might promote fetal growth. But we still do not know whether enhancing fetal growth in late pregnancy would reverse the impact of inappropriate PAR events earlier in pregnancy. This is a 64-billion-dollar question for which there are no data at present.

## Secondary prevention

The second preventative approach is to adjust the postnatal environment to match the phenotype induced in utero. Recall the Falasha story – the Falasha that stayed in Ethiopia had a low incidence of diabetes, but after moving to Israel the incidence increased dramatically. Clearly if the nutritional regime had stayed closer to that

---

[14] The first attempts to treat the fetus as a patient involved giving an intrauterine blood transfusion for rhesus isoimmunisation disease. This was introduced by Sir William Liley in 1963.

predicted in utero, the risk would have been lower. This is an extreme example and raises other ethical and philosophical issues – it is clearly unacceptable to maintain a Falasha child in Israel on near-famine rations just to stop him or her getting diabetes. But take the more common scenario. The nutritional energy burdens we allow our children to be exposed to are far higher than the nutritional status predicted by the fetus of any normal pregnancy and needed for optimal postnatal growth. Pregnancy is a constraining environment in which the amount of nutrients that reach the fetus is normally limited by placental function. So we can see that the consequences of inappropriate PARs operate in both the developed and developing world, just at different levels of postnatal nutrition – recall Figure 7.1. In the developed countries the philosophical issues of managing childhood nutrition to a more appropriate level are certainly challenging but the dilemmas are less.

We suspect the time is approaching when the birth-size phenotype and the pregnancy history (supported by markers of the level of PARs, e.g. the degree of epigenetic change on specific genomic regions, the amount of omental fat, blood hormonal levels etc.) may lead to individual-specific recommendations about the optimal growth curve for a given child. A neonate born weighing 3800 grams and 52 cm in length will have a different postnatal nutritional range from one weighing 3300 grams and 58 cm in length, even if both are born at the same gestational age. We need to use the available data, and collect more prospective data, to identify optimal growth curves for these two children – for example the latter may well require a lower postnatal nutritional level to be optimally healthy. These will give enormous but important challenges to public health and nutrition scientists and to pediatricians.

## Treating the inevitable

How should we approach intervention beyond the perinatal period? Obviously there is the 'ambulance at the bottom of the cliff' approach, in which we treat hypertension with antihypertensive drugs and diabetes with insulin-sensitising drugs or insulin itself. But after all that we have said above, couldn't we intervene earlier? The simple answer is that we just do not know. It would seem probable that if we can stop childhood obesity developing we would have an effective intervention in the cascade. Whether this justifies the use of agents that aggressively reduce fat mass in children is far from certain. In the meantime, where can we turn for support? We cannot count on the food industry for help, as many of the larger companies have little interest in stemming the enormous flow of junk-food consumption by youngsters worldwide. To be fair to these companies, many of them merely provide what their customers wish for, and it is sad that such fast foods (considered 30 years ago almost a luxury item) are now among the cheapest forms of nutrition, offering enormous appeal in low socio-economic societies and to parents who are pressed for time.

Nor, unfortunately, can the pharmaceutical companies be expected to lend their wealth and resources to the endeavour. Their market models and the requirements of regulating agencies mean that they just simply cannot afford to invest in pharmaceutical approaches that have only a long-term benefit. To be cynical, we would say that the very reverse might be true: the prospect of as much as 25 per cent of the vast populations of the developing world suffering from Type 2 diabetes by the age of 30, and needing to be maintained on glycaemic-control drugs for decades, spells profits on an unheard of scale. Moreover, the health effects of inappropriate PARs in the increasingly ageing populations of the developed world should fill the coffers too. We have to temper this cynicism once again by reminding ourselves that the pharmaceutical industry provides what is acceptable and usable. We cannot at present see the prospect of a unique drug that would prevent the consequences of inappropriate PARs, and even if such a drug were available, the ethical and practical issues of using it would have to be resolved. There have been too many examples of unforeseen side effects of new drugs, especially if they are used during human development.

These gaps in our knowledge are enormous. The challenges for different societies – those of the developed and those of the developing worlds – are very different. We have no doubt that if we knew how to address these challenges the burden of disease would fall dramatically.

# 10

# Fetal futures

We have seen how the theory of PARs helps us to understand the aetiology of some of the common chronic diseases of adulthood, especially components of the metabolic syndrome (Syndrome X), which include high blood pressure, Type 2 diabetes, a disordered blood-lipid profile and clotting-factor levels, obesity and increased risk of atheroma, coronary heart disease and stroke. Such diseases have a high prevalence in the developed world and are increasing at an alarming rate in populations in transition in the developing world. The humanitarian and financial burden they convey is enormous. The growing epidemic of obesity in young people further magnifies the problem.

But what of other common chronic diseases – breast and prostate cancer, asthma, Alzheimer's disease? Is it possible that the biological phenomenon of PARs could underlie the aetiology of such diseases? We can only speculate. For each of these conditions there is some evidence but as yet it is either preliminary or unconfirmed, so we felt that it would not be responsible to include it in our discussions at this stage.

Not everything that happens in early life and has lifelong consequences is a result of PARs. Teratogenesis is an irreversible developmental disruption which can have no predictive or adaptive value. In addition, some responses the fetus must make to survive (e.g. preterm delivery in the face of amniotic infection) must have inevitable costs after. The obesity of adults who had diabetic mothers may similarly just be a consequence of increased fat mass laid down in fetal life by virtue of the high insulin levels, or alternatively there may be a predictive element – we do not yet know, but an experimental approach to answer this question is possible.

It is important that those who think about PARs do so within the framework of the definition we laid down at the start of chapter 7.

## Predictive adaptive responses: the evolutionary perspective

Our primary goal has been to examine how the environment and genome interact at critical points in early development, thus determining biological destiny and, in particular, having consequences for subsequent postnatal gene–environmental interactions. Our theory is that the mechanisms underlying PARs have been preserved through evolution because they provide a species with a way of surviving short-term environmental challenges while still retaining maximal genotypic variation. Many environmental changes are transient, and because PARs can be reversed over a few generations, they permit phenotypic changes to follow these environmental changes. We saw in chapter 7 that while the Darwinian processes of natural and sexual selection provide a way of surviving an environmental challenge for some members of the species, these members will only be those with a genotypically determined phenotype that confers advantageous characteristics; other members whose genotypes produce less advantageous characteristics will be more likely to perish, and their genetic information will not be passed on to future generations. Thus this component of the genetic variation of the species will be lost and may never be recaptured unless a random mutation throws it up again at some future time. Darwinian evolution is not only usually very incremental, but also permanent. Darwinian responses to an environmental challenge that turns out to be transient are extremely costly as they produce (probably irreversible) loss of a component of the gene pool.

We have argued that PARs are a natural phenomenon whereby the developing conceptus makes some short-term choices to allow intrauterine survival, but that it also makes a series of choices that will establish biochemical and physiological phenotypes intended to assist survival to adulthood and to promote species survival through reproduction. By preserving the maximal amount of variation in the gene pool, PARs are likely to assist population survival by preserving genotypic variation. In one sense this aids the evolutionary process by sustaining genetic variation – the substrate for selection – and certainly this will allow a species to survive in a variety of ecological niches. In another sense it dilutes selection by preserving genotypic variation rather than concentrating gene frequencies. However, it is the capacity to sustain a population through transient change as well as maximising the individual's chances of reproductive success that confers the overall advantage of PARs.

In most situations in most species, the predictions made by the fetus will be correct and these mechanisms will be largely silent players. In humans, the evolutionary echo is seen in the phenomena, driven by maternal constraint, that created a default phenotype to protect against the historically most likely and risky scenario – a transient lack of food. Predictive adaptive responses become important when the environment changes because they allow the developing conceptus to makes choices that should turn out to be appropriate for the changed postnatal environment. But misinformation from the mother or a rapidly changing environment can lead to the in utero prediction of the postnatal environment being incorrect. In animals this usually means that the affected offspring dies, but in humans there are enormous longer-term consequences.

## The nature of the problem

Diseases are always easier to treat if we understand their causes. The problem with PAR-related disease is that we do not know the underlying mechanisms in sufficient detail. There are several reasons for this.

First, the phenomenon has only recently been described – the major impetus to its study arose from epidemiological observations made in the last 15 years or so. It has taken time for the scientific community to catch up, and of course during this period there have been debates about the validity of the epidemiological observations themselves.

Second, it has taken considerable time to generate animal models to demonstrate that PARs are a biological phenomenon in other mammalian species, especially laboratory animals such as rats, mice and guinea pigs, but also in large animals such as the sheep and pig. This has been necessary not only to confirm the validity of the concept, but also to show that it occurs in species with very different degrees of maturity at birth. It has also been necessary to rule out purely genetic explanations. Now established, such animal models should speed the investigation of the mechanisms underlying PARs and PAR-related disease.

But herein lies the third problem: the discipline of integrative biology, which is needed to investigate such mechanisms, has been chronically under-funded for decades and the expertise needed to make rapid progress in this area has been all but lost. As active researchers in this field, the authors know only too well how hard it has been to get funding for research in the area and, once funded, how difficult it is to recruit young scientists to it. Biomedical research has taken an increasingly reductionist approach, and this has been fuelled recently by the human genome project. While we do not deny the importance of such work, its fashionable style and the sheer resources it has commanded have drawn bright young scientists and funding away from the integrative biology that will now be needed to put the genes back into the environment in which they operate. Nowhere is this more true than in the field of developmental origins of disease.

The experiments necessary to advance our knowledge are complex and of very long duration. To prove experimentally aspects of the theoretical construct we have put forward will require very difficult and careful experimental design. Proving the relationship we model in Figure 7.1 will be difficult but is feasible. It is worth the effort in clarifying both our biological understanding and its application to disease prevention.

Defining the mechanisms requires good models and good clinical studies. But to plan intervention studies will require both expensive and lengthy experimental studies and clever epidemiological and clinical enquiry.

Last of all, to make real progress in this field requires a marriage of disciplines, from theoretical biology to health policy and economics. As we discussed in the preface, there has been a large gulf between the theoretical and evolutionary biologists on one hand and medical scientists on the other. Humans are animals and we need to get better at bridging this gap in approach.

## What we do know

Despite this somewhat gloomy prelude to the final chapter of this book, the fact is that the knowledge we have in this field is far from negligible. The phenomenon of so-called 'fetal origins of adult disease' is now widely accepted,[1] as a result of the plethora of experimental, epidemiological and clinical studies conducted around the world by many groups. Particularly as a result of animal studies, we now have some idea of the maternal processes that initiate PARs, primarily via the balance of nutrition but also through body composition and hormonal status For hormonal status a range of stimuli loosely grouped under the heading 'stress' – emotional, environmental and nutritional – may be included, and it is possible that changes in hormones such as the steroid cortisol in the maternal (and hence potentially the fetal) bloodstream are of key importance.

The explosion of knowledge about genes and cells, introduced in the first two chapters, has fuelled a rapid expansion of knowledge in developmental and perinatal biology. This has helped us to improve our knowledge of the very early life components of PARs more than those that operate in late gestation. It is clear that the induction of a PAR can occur in the periconceptional period, before implantation of the blastocyst. This suggests that induction involves changes in the expression of genes that control this early development, and we have now progressed to the point where we have some good candidates for such genes, especially those that can be imprinted, and that regulate the growth and development of the early embryo and the placenta. This in turn has led to investigation of epigenetic changes induced by environmental stimuli in such responses. Because DNA methylation depends on the provision of methyl groups from amino acids such as glycine and on cofactors such as folic acid and vitamin B12, the links between such early embryonic PAR processes and maternal nutritional balance can be drawn. But there is much yet to

---

[1]   These days usually referred to as developmental origins of health and disease (DOHaD), for which an international learned society now exists.

understand about the scope of these changes, of the environmental cues and the impact on cell growth and differentiation.

Then we will start to get an idea of the range of disorders that might be caused by inappropriate PARs. There are many gaps – understanding the effects on the nervous system, on the origins of obesity, and on immune function and the susceptibility to infection – would appear to be priorities. This cannot be done in isolation from understanding the window in which environmental cues might act and the nature of the cues involved. Even with something apparently as fundamental as nutrition, we still do not really know how to feed the mother optimally and what guidance to give about nutrition for children of different birth phenotypes in different populations. Research in this area must be given a high priority.

## PARs and the genome

In chapter 1 we pointed out that every phenotypic response depends on interaction between the genome and the environment. This is clearly the case with respect to the special set of interactions we have termed PARs.

What PARs do is to set up a two-stage interaction. An irreversible choice is first made in fetal life as a result of an environmentally cued prediction and that irreversibility is reflected, at least in part, in epigenetic change. That choice (e.g. in growth trajectory), once established, becomes the framework on which the postnatal interactions between the organism and its environment occurs. Depending on the choice made in early development, the consequences of that second interaction will be different. Because ultimately all such interactions involve changes in gene expression, one would expect there to be genetically determined differences in the nature of these responses, both in the primary and in the secondary interactions. We are starting to find out that this is indeed the case. Polymorphisms influence the relationship between the fetal environment and long-term consequences[2], and over time we expect to identify many more polymorphisms influencing both reactions.

Many clinicians and clinical researchers have fallen into the trap of thinking about familial disease either in terms of purely genetic considerations (on the model of a monogenic inherited disease such as cystic fibrosis) or in terms of clustered and common environmental factors (e.g. all members of a family being exposed to cigarette smoke). There is a third pathway which is well recognised in plant and comparative biology but has received little attention in human medicine – that of maternal effects or epigenetic inheritance. Studies arising from PARs research show

---

[2]  Good examples of this were given in chapter 4, where we showed how the risk of Type 2 diabetes associated with low birth weight was greater in individuals with a PPAR$\gamma$ polymorphism.

that this phenomenon is relevant to human disease. We described both animal studies of dietary-induced PARs and human population studies (e.g. the Dutch famine) that demonstrate its relevance. The extent to which familial clustering of diseases such as Type 2 diabetes mellitus is epigenetic and PARs-related rather than genetic therefore needs to be given much more attention.

## Preventing PAR-related disease

In chapter 9 we examined how this developing knowledge might be applied to reduce the burden of disease. We are reluctant to make sweeping statements that extend beyond the available data. First, with the exception of one estimate based on one population (Finland), there are no data available on which we can predict the size of the impact of successful intervention – we suspect it to be large. Second, as we have been careful to point out, societies by definition have very different genetic and environmental histories, and therefore the nature of any intervention and the magnitude of the resulting effect may be very population-specific.

From first principles we can identify two preventative approaches – primary prevention by optimising the fetal environment, and secondary prevention by adjusting the postnatal environment to make it closer to that which the fetus predicted. But we are immediately faced with difficulties. One is that we simply do not know the optimal nutrient delivery for an embryo/fetus at different points in development. Nor do we have good tools for identifying the level of nutrition a fetus is receiving. We certainly do not know how to intervene in populations to optimise nutrition prior to conception. We do not have markers of when a neonate has made a PAR and we have yet to understand the optimal range of childhood growth for a given birth phenotype. These are all good research questions and there is an understandable urge to leap ahead.

But at this stage we can but be cautious. It would appear to us that a balanced and micronutrient-adequate nutritional intake starting well before conception is essential for optimal fetal outcome. So is optimal maternal age, avoiding smoking, minimising the risk of disease and perhaps moderating maternal exercise. We still have insufficient data about placental disease and its management and even about gestational diabetes. And of course we must remember that some factors can never be avoided, e.g. primiparous pregnancy.

It would also seem to us that excessive catch-up growth and excessive weight gain in infancy and childhood must be avoided. Much more work is needed to understand optimal nutritional regimes for childhood growth and these must be individualised to the birth phenotype. The challenging possibility remains that childhood obesity constitutes such a risk factor that it merits therapeutic intervention with agents that will inhibit fat deposition – a research question that should not be ignored. We do not know whether epigenetic change can be specifically reversed, or indeed the consequences of doing so.

We have focused the discussion in this book largely on the metabolic syndrome and its components. At its conclusion we should note that we suspect a much broader set of PARs might be associated with altered disease risk. The study of the Japanese soldiers,[3] for example, illustrates PARs operating in a different physiological framework.

## The scientific agenda

As we hope will be clear from this book, the theory of PARs has considerable implications for science. This applies not only to developmental biology and fetal physiology, but also to epidemiology, clinical research and evolutionary biology. Progress in research will be much faster with greater collaboration between these fields, and happily such wide-ranging collaborations are now becoming more common in science. Achieving funding for them is of course vital. We have alluded to this earlier, but here would make two points. The first is that such research really does need to break the mould of current concepts about collaborations. It will have to be based on a true exchange of staff, ideas and expertise, not just on Laboratory A doing some experiments and collecting some samples which are of interest to those in Laboratory B, who proceed to analyse them and publish the results as a dissociated exercise. This gives no added value to the endeavour.

The second issue is that the work now needed involves conducting very long-term studies, whether in the following up of children born to mothers in whom pre-pregnancy characteristics have been measured in detail, or in establishing how experimental diets in pregnancy influence cardiovascular function and responses to stress in subsequent generations of experimental animals. There is a matrix of questions that need to be answered and there is a need to develop a coordinated approach to filling in this matrix. This requires a 'big science' approach as used in high - energy physics or in the human genome project, rather than ad hoc individual isolated research efforts where key questions are left unanswered. The research paradigm is changing and research agencies need to adjust their approach to fit it or the public health applications of potential collaborations will never be realised.

## A final commentary

Understanding PARs changes our view of prenatal development and health. Logic would suggest that a greater emphasis on the well-being of women of reproductive

[3] See chapter 1.

age, even before pregnancy, must be made in medical research, in healthcare delivery, in economic policy and in the political process. It is no longer possible to see the embryo or fetus as the larval stage of human development, not needing particular care or attention because it will be nourished, nurtured and defended from a hostile environment by its mother. Instead it is now apparent that by taking a developmental perspective, radical changes in priorities are demanded that will impact on many components of our lives.

We believe that this has implications both for individuals, be they parents or politicians, and for society. It has immediate implications for how potential parents make choices about their lifestyle, health care and rearing of their children. In society, it must influence scientific, medical, philosophical and economic thought. This in turn will have implications for decisions about priorities made by policymakers and politicians, whether with respect to fiscal allocations to medical research, healthcare delivery, education, or aid to the developing world.

We now know that even periconceptional events can have an impact that extends through and beyond fetal life and early childhood. While this has most easily been demonstrated in the animal experiments we have discussed, the careful observations on the offspring of those exposed to famine in the Dutch Hunger Winter demonstrated that the biology is equally applicable to the human. The implications of this to human healthcare and to preventative medicine are immense. It should be obvious that it is critical to focus on the health of the developing adolescent and to promote planned pregnancy within an optimal window of maternal age. Maternal care must start before pregnancy. In both developed and developing societies achieving this goal will challenge prevailing attitudes.

This discussion has implications for how people live and the choices they make. Many of these choices are those of the mother. The modern lifestyle creates attitudes and a self-centered focus that is not necessarily in accord with an optimal outcome for a pregnancy. The fad for thinness, the tendency to delay first pregnancy and advance maternal age in the Western world, the converse prevalence of adolescent pregnancy in many populations, the use of tobacco, of recreational drugs, are all relevant. These are all factors that impact on prenatal development. Most people, and particularly our youngsters, do not want to think too much about longer-term implications of their behaviour. We know that simply stating that the body composition and diet of young women may affect the health of their children in middle age is unlikely to provide much of an incentive for them to change their lifestyle. We have to find new ways of educating them, to make their current health status itself fashionable and to focus on the short-term benefits to them.

Just as those controlling medical research need to take greater account of the issues we have addressed, so too must those determining healthcare policy. In the developed countries, the demographic shift towards an ageing population carries with it an increasing redistribution of healthcare resources towards the middle aged and elderly and on public health measures focused on an adult lifestyle. It seems obvious that a greater investment in healthcare services for adolescent females, for those who wish to become or are pregnant, and in fetal and perinatal medicine must pay great dividends over time to society. Because the costs of incorrect healthcare investment decisions are so high, there is an even greater reason for further research to establish how important and how far-reaching the consequences of inappropriate PARs may be.

So economists have a challenge. The new paradigms of economic development place great weight on human capital. In the developed world the burden of diseases that are PAR-related is enormous. As has been suggested, we may find in time that the burden extends to include elements of mental health and social behaviour. Yet the burden of investment in healthcare has shifted from mother and child to other elements of society. Is this economic rationalism?

Ultimately all resource allocation decisions are the responsibility of politicians. They should reflect on the lives of their young female voters and indeed on the prenatal lives of future voters! It seems extraordinary to us that in some countries politicians will make stands over abortion, a matter that is clearly one of individual belief, yet they do not champion measures to promote the health of the young woman and her fetus.

A focus on female health before and during the reproductive phase would be a powerful tool for human capital development in the developing world. Only through female literacy and education and by empowering women is it likely that female children will receive optimal nutrition. This of course will have effects throughout society, including on males. A healthy female population is far more likely to contribute to economic growth, and the cycle of gender disadvantage leading to a catastrophic epidemic of diabetes and heart disease may then be broken. Again this perspective should inform aid agencies, developing governments and non-government organisations. It should also be taken up by the feminists of the newer international women's movements. Their predecessors who were closely identified in the first half of the twentieth century with campaigning for women's health and maternal welfare in pregnancy,[4] led to more recent revolutions in reproductive choice for women. It will be a great pity if contemporary feminism does not now focus on the issue of fetal development and its consequences.

[4]  See Margaret Llewelyn-Davies, *Maternity: Letters from Working Women (1915)*, (London: Virago, 1978); and Margery Spring-Rice, *Working-Class Wives: Their Health and Conditions* (Harmondsworth: Penguin, 1939).

Hippocrates (450 BC) was the first to write about the fetus. He was the original systematic fetal scientist. He dissected eggs at each stage of embryological development and recorded his findings. From his observations, he recognised that the health of the fetus and the subsequent child depended on the health of the mother. Two-and-a-half thousand years later, we understand significantly more but still have an enormous number of critical questions left to answer about the fetal matrix.

# Further reading

We recognise that this book will appeal to a range of readers. Thus we have provided a reading list that, while not referencing every statement, addresses those areas that may be of most interest to the reader. Those references marked with an asterisk are particularly recommended to the general reader. Because we return to the same topic over several chapters we have grouped the suggested reading by field rather than by chapter. We have given a particularly comprehensive list of reading on topics related to prenatal induction. Five reading lists are provided:

   i. Comparative and evolutionary biology.

  ii. The biology of the fetus, pregnancy and growth.

 iii. Genetics and developmental biology.

 iv. Clinical medicine.

  v. Developmental origins of health and disease.

Within each we have sub-categorised further to assist the reader.

## Comparative and evolutionary biology
### Comparative biology

Applebaum, S. W. and Heifetz, Y. Density-dependent physiological phase in insects. *Ann. Rev. Entomol.* **44** (1999), 317–41.

Blanckenhorn, W. U. Adaptive phenotypic plasticity in growth, development, and body size in the yellow dung fly. *Evolution* **52** (1998), 1394–407.

Boonstra, R., Hik, D., Singleton, G. R. and Tinnikov, A. The impact of predator-induced stress on the snowshoe hare cycle. *Ecological Monographs* **68** (1998), 371–94.

Bromham, L. and Harvey, P. H. Behavioural ecology: naked mole-rats on the move. *Curr. Biol.* **6** (1996), 1082–3.

Cant, M. A. Social control of reproduction in banded mongooses. *Anim. Behav.* **59** (2000), 147–58.

Cichón, M. Evolution of longevity through optimal resource allocation. *Proc. Royal Soc. Lond. B* **264** (1997), 1383–8.

Cresswell, W. and McCleery, R. How great tits maintain synchronization of their hatch date with food supply in response to long-term variability in temperature. *J. Anim. Ecol.* **72** (2003), 356–66.

Denver, R. J. Environmental stress as a developmental cue: corticotropin-releasing hormone is a proximate mediator of adaptive phenotypic plasticity in amphibian metamorphosis. *Horm. Behav.* **31** (1997), 169–79.

Ferguson, M. W. J. Temperature of egg incubation determines sex in *Alligator mississippiensis*. *Nature* **296** (1982), 850–3.

Forchhammer, M. C., Clutton-Brock, T. H., Lindström, J. and Albon, S. D. Climate and population density induce long-term cohort variation in a northern ungulate. *J. Anim. Ecol.* **70** (2001), 721–9.

Goldman, B. D., Goldman, S. L., Lanz, T., Magaurin, A. and Maurice, A. Factors influencing metabolic rate in naked mole rats*(Heterocephalus glaber)*. *Physiol. Behav.* **66** (1999), 447–59.

Janzen, F. J. and Morjan, C. L. Repeatability of microenvironment-specific nesting behaviour in a turtle with environmental sex determination. *Anim. Behav.* **62** (2001), 73–82.

Krebs, C. J., Boonstra, R., Boutin, S. and Sinclair, A. R. E. What drives the 10-year cycle of Snowshoe Hares? *BioScience* **51** (2001), 25–35.

*Lavers, C. *Why Elephants have Big Ears: Understanding Patterns of Life on Earth*. (Victor Gollanz, London, 2000).

Lee, T. M., Spears, N., Tuthill, C. R. and Zucker, I. Maternal melatonin treatment influences rates of neonatal development of meadow vole pups. *Biol. Reprod.* **40** (1989), 495–502.

Lee, T. M. and Zucker, I. Vole infant development is influenced perinatally by maternal photoperiodic history. *Am. J. Physiol.* **255** (1988), R831–8.

Metcalfe, N. B. and Monaghan, P. Growth versus lifespan: perspectives from evolutionary ecology. *Exp. Gerontol.* **38** (2003), 935–40.

Miller, R. A., Harper, J. M., Dysko, R. C., Durkee, S. J. and Austad, S. N. Longer life spans and delayed maturation in wild-derived mice. *Exp. Biol. Med.* **227** (2002), 500–8.

Newman, R. A. Adaptive plasticity in amphibian metamorphosis. *BioScience* **42** (1992), 671–8.

Packer, C., Tatar, M., and Collins, A. Reproduction cessation in female mammals. *Nature* **392** (1998), 807–10.

Shine, R. Why is sex determined by nest temperature in many reptiles? *Trends in Ecology and Evolution* **14** (1999), 186–9.

Stefan, C. I. and Krebs, C. J. Reproductive changes in a cyclic population of snowshoe hares. *Can. J. Zoology* **79** (2001), 2101–8.

Stenseth, N. C., Falck, W., Bjørnstad, O. N. and Krebs, C. J. Population regulation in snowshoe hare and Canadian lynx: Asymmetric food web configurations between hare and lynx. *Proc. Nat. Acad. Sci. (USA)* **94** (1997), 5147–52.

*Weiner, J., *The Beak of the Finch. A Story of Evolution in Our Time*. (New York, NY: Alfred A. Knopf, Inc., 1994).

West, P. M. and Packer, C. Sexual selection, temperature, and the lion's mane. *Science* **297** (2002), 1339–43.

Williams, C. K. and Moore, R. J. Phenotypic adaptation and natural selection in the wild rabbit. *Oryctolagus cuniculus*, in Australia. *J. Anim. Ecol.* **58** (1989), 495–507.

Winterhalder, B. P. Canadian fur bearer cycles and Cree-Ojibway hunting and trapping practices. *Am. Naturalist.* **116** (1980), 870–9.

*Evolutionary biology*

\*Darwin, C. *The Origin of Species by Means of Natural Selection*. (London: John Murray, 1869).

\*Darwin, C. *The Descent of Man* (with introduction by R. Dawkins), (London: Gibson Square Books 1871, 2003 edn.).

Dawkins, R. *The Extended Phenotype*, ed. R. Dawkins (Oxford: Oxford University Press, 1982).

\*Dawkins, R. *The Blind Watchmaker: Why the Evidence of Evolution Reveals a Universe Without Design*. (New York, NY: W. W. Norton & Company, 1986).

Futuyma, D. J. *Evolutionary Biology*, 3rd edn. (Boston, MA: Sinauer Associates, 1998).

Grant, B. R. and Grant, P. R. Evolution of Darwin's finches caused by a rare climatic event. *Proc. R. Soc. Lond. B* **251** (1993), 111–17.

Halder, G., Callaerts, P. and Gehring, W. J. New perspectives on eye evolution. *Curr. Opin. Genet. Dev.* **5** (1995), 602–9.

Kirkwood, T. B. L. Evolution of ageing. *Nature* **270** (1977), 301–4.

Kirkwood, T. B. L. and Austad, S. N. Why do we age? *Nature* **408** (2000), 233–8.

Land, M. F. The evolution of eyes. *Annu. Rev. Neurosci.* **15** (1992), 1–29.

\* Mayr, E. (2001). *What Evolution Is*, ed. E. Mayr (New York, NY: Basic Books).

McComb, K., Moss, C., Durant, S. M., Baker, L. and Sayialel, S. Matriarchs as repositories of social knowledge in African elephants. *Science* **292** (2001), 491–4.

Price, T. D., Qvarnström, A. and Irwin, D. E. The role of phenotypic plasticity in driving genetic evolution. *Proc. R. Soc. Lond. B.* **270** (2003), 1433–40.

Schlichting, C. D. and Pigliucci, M. *Phenotypic Evolution: A Reaction Norm Perspective*. (Boston, MA: Sinauer Associates, 1998).

Williams, G. C. Pleiotropy, natural selection, and the evolution of senescence. *Evolution* **11** (1957), 398–411.

Yokoyama, S. Molecular evolution of color vision in vertebrates. *Gene* **300** (2002), 69–78.

*Human evolution*

Cordain, L., Eaton, S. B., Miller, J. B., Mann, N. and Hill, K. The paradoxical nature of hunter–gatherer diets: meat-based, yet non-atherogenic. *Eur. J. Clin. Nutr.* **56** (2002), S42–52.

Cordain, L., Miller, J. B., Eaton, S. B. *et al.* Plant-animal subsistence ratios and macronutrient energy estimations in worldwide hunter–gatherer diets. *Am. J. Clin. Nutr.* **71** (2000), 682–92.

\*Diamond, J. *Guns, Germs and Steel: A Short History of Everybody for the Last 13,000 Years*. (London: Vintage, 1998).

Eaton, S. B. Paleolithic vs. modern diets : selected pathophysiological implications. *Eur. J. Nutr.* **39** (2000), 67–70.

Eaton, S. B. and Konner, M. Paleolithic nutrition. A consideration of its nature and current implications. *N. Engl. J. Med.* **312** (1985), 283–9.

Gagneux, P., Wills, C., Gerloff, U., *et al.* Mitochondrial sequences show diverse evolutionary histories of African hominoids. *Pediatr. Res.* **96** (1999), 5077–82.

Hawkes, K., O'Connell, J. F., Jones, N. G. B., Alvarez, H. and Charnov, E. L. Grandmothering, menopause, and the evolution of human life histories. *Proc. Nat. Acad. Sci. (USA)* **95** (1998), 1336–9.

Kuzawa, C. W. Adipose tissue in human infancy and childhood: an evolutionary perspective. *Yearbook of Physical Anthropology* **41** (1998), 177–209.

Mann, N. Dietary lean red meat and human evolution. *Eur. J. Nutr.* **39** (2000), 71–9.

Miller, J. C. B. and Colagiuri, S. The carnivore connection: dietary carbohydrate in the evolution of NIDDM. *Diabetologia* **37** (1994), 1280–6.

Promislow, D. E. L. Longevity and the barren aristocrat. *Nature* **396** (1998), 719–20.

* Ridley, M. *Nature Via Nurture: Genes, Experience, and What Makes Us Human.* (London: HarperCollins, 2003).

Shanley, D. P. and Kirkwood, T. B. L. Evolution of the human menopause. *Bioessays* **23** (2001), 282–7.

Sherman, P. W. The evolution of menopause. *Nature* **392** (1998), 759–61.

Speth, J. D. and Spielmann, K. A. Energy source, protein metabolism, and hunter–gatherer subsistence strategies. *J. Anthropol. Archaeol.* **2** (1983), 1–31.

Truswell, A. S. and Hansen, J. D. Medical research among the !Kung. In *Kalahari Hunter–Gatherers. Studies of the !Kung San and Their Neighbors*, ed. R. B. Lee and I. DeVore (Cambridge MA: Harvard University Press, 1976), pp. 168–95.

Walker, A. R. P., Walker, B. F., and Adam, F. Nutrition, diet, physical activity, smoking, and longevity: from primitive hunter–gatherer to present passive consumer – how far can we go? *Nutrition* **19** (2003), 169–73.

Wells, J. C. K. Natural selection and sex differences in morbidity and mortality in early life. *J. Theor. Biol.* **202** (2000), 65–76.

*Wells, S. *The Journey of Man: A Genetic Odyssey*, ed. S. Wells (Princeton, NJ: Princeton University Press, 2003).

Westendorp, R. G. J. and Kirkwood, T. B. L. Human longevity at the cost of reproductive success. *Nature* **396** (1998), 743–6.

## Biology of the fetus, pregnancy and growth
### Biology of pregnancy

Bauman, D. E. and Currie, W. B. Partitioning of nutrients during pregnancy and lactation: a review of mechanisms involving homeostasis and homeorhesis. *J. Dairy Sci.* **63** (1980), 1514–29.

Beaconsfield, P., Birdwood, G. and Beaconsfield, R. The placenta. *Sci. Am.* **243** (1980), 80–9.

Bell, R. and O'Neill, M. Exercise and pregnancy: a review. *Birth* **21** (1994), 85–95.

Burton, G. J., Hempstock, J. and Jauniaux, E. Nutrition of the human fetus during the first trimester – a review. *Placenta* **22** (2001), S70–6.

Duggleby, S. L. and Jackson, A. A. Relationship of maternal protein turnover and lean body mass during pregnancy and birth length. *Clin. Sci.* **101** (2001), 65–72.

Georgiades, P., Ferguson-Smith, A. C. and Burton, G. J. Comparative developmental anatomy of the murine and human definitive placentae. *Placenta* **23** (2002), 3–19.

Grieve, J. F. Prevention of gestational failure by high protein diet. *J. Reprod. Med.* **13** (1974), 170–4.

Haig, D. Genetic conflicts in human pregnancy. *Q. Rev. Biol.* **68** (1993), 495–532.

Harman, C. R. and Menticoglou, S. M. Fetal surveillance in diabetic pregnancy. *Curr. Opin. Obstet. Gynecol.* **9** (1997), 83–90.

Lacroix, M. C., Guibourdenche, J., Frendo, J. L., Muller, F. and Evain-Brion, D. Human placental growth hormone : a review. *Placenta* **23** (2002), S87–94.

Lotgering, F. K., Gilbert, R. D. and Longo, L. D. Exercise responses in pregnant sheep: oxygen consumption, uterine blood flow, and blood volume. *J. Appl. Physiol.* **55** (1983), 834–41.

Rondo, P. H., Ferreira, R. F., Nogueira, F. *et al.* Maternal psychological stress and distress as predictors of low birth weight, prematurity and intrauterine growth retardation. *Eur. J. Clin. Nutr.* **57** (2003), 266–72.

Sagawa, N., Yura, S., Itoh, H. *et al.* Role of leptin in pregnancy: a review. *Placenta* **23**, *Suppl. A. Trophoblast Res.* **16** (2002), S80.

## Fetal physiology and medicine

Brace, R. A, Hanson, M. A., and Rodeck, C. H., eds. *Fetus and Neonate: Physiology and Clinical Applications. Vol. 4, Kidney and Body Fluids.* (Cambridge: Cambridge University Press, 1988).

Gluckman, P. D. and Heymann, M. A. eds. *Pediatrics and Perinatology: The Scientific Basis*, 2nd edn. (London: Arnold, 1996).

Gunn, A. J. and Gluckman, D. The response of the fetal brain to asphyxia/ischaemia. In *Fetal Medicine: Basic Science and Clinical Practice, ed.* C. H. Rodeck and M. J. Whittle. (London: Churchill Livingstone, 1999), pp. 241–62.

Hanson, M. A., Spencer, J. A. D. and Rodeck, C. H., eds. *Fetus and Neonate: Physiology and Clinical Applications. Vol. 1, The Circulation.* (Cambridge: Cambridge University Press, 1993).

Hanson, M. A., Spencer, J. A. D. and Rodeck, C. H., eds. *Fetus and Neonate: Physiology and Clinical Applications. Vol. 2, Breathing.* (Cambridge: Cambridge University Press, 1994).

Hanson, M. A., Spencer, J. A. D. and Rodeck, C. H., eds. *Fetus and Neonate: Physiology and Clinical Applications. Vol. 3, Growth.* (Cambridge: Cambridge University Press, 1995).

Liggins, G. C. (1994). The role of cortisol in preparing the fetus for birth. *Reprod. Fertil. Dev.* **6**, 141–50.

*Nathanielsz, P. W., ed. *Life in the Womb.* (New York, NY: Promethean Press, 1999.)

Schwarz, R. H. and Jaffe, S., eds. *Drug and Chemical Risks to the Fetus and Newborn* (New York, NY : Alan R. Liss, Inc., 1980).

Walker, D. W., Hale, J. R. S., Fawcett, A. A. and Pratt, N. M. Cardiovascular responses to heat stress in late-gestation fetal sheep. *Exp. Physiol.* **80** (1995), 755–66.

## Fetal and postnatal growth

Allen, W. R., Wilsher, S., Turnbull, C. *et al.* Influence of maternal size on placental, fetal and postnatal growth in the horse. I. Development *in utero. Reproduction* **123** (2002), 445–53.

Bauer, M. K., Breier, B. H., Harding, J. E., Veldhuis, J. D. and Gluckman, P. D. The fetal somatotropic axis during long term maternal undernutrition in sheep: evidence for nutritional regulation in utero. *Endocrinology* **136** (1995), 1250–7.

Brooks, A. A., Johnson, M. R., Steer, P. J., Pawson, M. E. and Abdalla, H. I. Birth weight: nature or nuture? *Early. Hum. Dev.* **42** (1995), 29–35.

de Jonge, L. V. H., Waller, G. and Stettler, N. Ethnicity modifies seasonal variations in birth weight and weight gain of infants. *J. Nutr.* **133** (2003), 1415–18.

Fowden, A. L. The role of insulin in prenatal growth. *J. Dev. Physiol.* **12** (1989), 173–82.

Gluckman, P. D. The endocrine regulation of fetal growth in late gestation: the role of insulin-like growth factors. *J. Clin. Endocrinol. Metab.* **80** (1995), 1047–50.

Gluckman, P. D. Endocrine and nutritional regulation of prenatal growth. *Acta Paediatr.* Suppl. **423** (1997a), 153–7.

Gluckman, P. D. Endocrine mechanisms and consequences of intrauterine growth retardation. *Clin. Pediatr. Endocrinol.* **6** (1997b), 135–40.

Gluckman, P. D., Breier, B. H., Oliver, M., Harding, J. and Bassett, N. Fetal growth in late gestation: a constrained pattern of growth. *Acta Paediatr. Scand.* Suppl. **367** (1990), 105–10.

Gluckman, P. D. and Harding, J. E. The regulation of fetal growth. In *Human Growth: Basic and Clinical Aspects*, ed. M. Hernandez and J. Argente (Amsterdam: Excepta Medica, 1992), pp. 253–60.

Gluckman, P. D. and Harding, J. E. Nutritional and hormonal regulation of fetal growth-evolving concepts. *Acta Paediatr.* Suppl. **399** (1994), 60–3.

Gluckman, P. D. and Harding, J. E. The physiology and pathophysiology of intrauterine growth retardation. *Horm. Res.* **48** (1997), Suppl. 1, 11–16.

Gluckman, P. D. and Liggins, G. C. The regulation of fetal growth. In *Fetal Physiology and Medicine*, ed. R. W. Beard and P. W. Nathanielsz (New York and Basel: Marcel Dekker,1984), pp. 511–58.

Gluckman, P. D., Morel, P. C. H., Ambler, G. R. *et al.* Elevating maternal insulin-like growth factor-I in mice and rats alters the pattern of fetal growth by removing maternal constraint. *J. Endocrinol.* **134** (1992), R1–3.

Gluckman, P. D. and Pinal, C. Maternal–placental–fetal interactions in the endocrine regulation of fetal growth: role of somatotrophic axes. *Endocrine* **19** (2002), 81–9.

Ha, J. C., Ha, R. R., Almasy, L., and Dyke, B. (2002). Genetics and caging type affect birth weight in captive pigtailed macaques *(Macaca nemestrina)*. *Am. J. Primatol.* **56**, 207–13.

Hales, C. N. and Ozanne, S. E. The dangerous road of catch-up growth. *J. Physiol.* **547** (2003), *1*, 5–10.

Han, V. K. M. and Carter, A. M. Control of growth and development of the feto–placental unit. *Curr. Opin. Pharmacol.* **1** (2001), 632–40.

Harding, J. E. and Johnston, B. M. Nutrition and fetal growth. *Reprod. Fertil. Dev.* **7** (1995), 539–47.

Johnston, L. B., Clark, A. J. and Savage, M. O. Genetic factors contributing to birth weight. *Arch. Dis. Child. Fetal Neonatal Edn.* **86** (2002), F2–3.

Milner, R. D. G. and Gluckman, P. D. The regulation of intrauterine growth. In *Pediatrics and Perinatology: The Scientific Basis*, ed. P. D. Gluckman and M. A. Heymann (London: Edward Arnold, 1996), pp. 284–9.

Oliver, M. H., Harding, J. E., Breier, B. H., Evans, P. C., and Gluckman, D. Glucose but not a mixed amino acid infusion regulates plasma insulin-like growth factor-I concentrations in fetal sheep. *Pediatr. Res.* **34** (1993), 62–5.

Oliver, M. H., Harding, J. E., and Gluckman, P. D. Duration of maternal undernutrition in late gestation determines the reversibility of intrauterine growth restriction in sheep. *Prenat. Neonat. Med.* **6** (2001), 271–9.

Ostlund, E., Bang, P., Hagenas, L., and Fried, G. Insulin-like growth factor I in fetal serum obtained by cordocentesis is correlated with intrauterine growth retardation. *Hum. Reprod.* **12** (1997), 840–4.

Owens, J. A. Endocrine and substrate control of fetal growth: placental and maternal influences and insulin-like growth factors. *Reprod. Fertil. Dev.* **3** (1991), 501–17.

Pardi, G., Marconi, A. M. and Cetin, I. Placental–fetal interrelationships in IUGR fetuses – a review. *Placenta* **23** (2002), Suppl. A, S136–S41.

Parks, J. S. The ontogeny of growth hormone sensitivity. *Horm. Res.* **55** (2001), 27–31.

Rees, S., Bocking, A. D. and Harding, R. Structure of the fetal sheep brain in experimental growth retardation. *J. Dev. Physiol.* **10** (1998), 211–24.

Robson, E. B. The genetics of birth weight. In *Human Growth: Principles and Prenatal Growth*, ed. F. Faulkner and J. M. Tanner (New York: Plenum, 1978), pp. 285–97.

Smith, G. C. S., Stenhouse, E. J., Crossley, J. A. *et al.* Early-pregnancy origins of low birth weight. *Nature* **417** (2002), 916.

Spencer, N. and Logan, S. Social infuences on birth weight. *Arch. Dis. Child. Neonatal Ed.* **86** (2002), F6–7.

Stephenson, T. and Symonds, M. E. Maternal nutrition as a determinant of birth weight. *Arch. Dis. Child. Neonatal Edn.* **86** (2002), F4–6.

Tchirikov, M., Kertschanska, S., Sturenberg, H. J., and Schroder, H. J. Liver blood perfusion as a possible instrument for fetal growth regulation. *Placenta* **23** (2002), Suppl. A, S153–8.

Tchirikov, M., Rybakowski, C., Huneke, B. and Schroder, H. J. Blood flow through the ductus venosus in singleton and multifetal pregnancies and in fetuses with intrauterine growth retardation. *Am. J. Obstet. Gynecol.* **178** (1998), 943–9.

Themmen, A. P. N. and Verhoef-Post, M. LH receptor defects. *Semin. Reprod. Med.* **20** (2002), 199–204.

Wallace, J., Bourke, D., Da Silva, P. and Aitken, R. Nutrient partitioning during adolescent pregnancy. *Reproduction* **122** (2001), 347–57.

Wallace, J. M., Aitken, R. P. and Cheyne, M. A. Nutrient partitioning and fetal growth in rapidly growing adolescent ewes. *J. Reprod. Fert.* **107** (1996), 183–90.

Walton, A. and Hammond, J. The maternal effects on growth and conformation in Shire horse–Shetland pony crosses. *Proc. Royal Soc. Lond. – Series B: Biol. Sci.* **125** (1938), 311–35.

Wi, J. M. and Boersma, B. Catch-up growth: definition, mechanisms, and models. *J. Pediatr. Endocrinol. Metab.* **15** (2002), 1229–41.

### Nutrition in pregnancy

Black, R. E. Micronutrients in pregnancy. *Br. J. Nutr.* **85** (2001), Suppl. 2, S193–7.

Bhutta, Z. A., Jackson, A. and Lumbiganon, P., eds. Nutrition as a preventive strategy against adverse pregnancy outcomes. *The Journal of Nutrition* (2003), 1589S–767.

Centers for Disease Control. Recommendations for the use of folic acid to reduce the number of cases of spina bifida and other neural tube defects. *MMWR* **41** (1992) (RR14), 001.

Erickson, J. D. Folic acid and prevention of spina bifida and anencephaly: 10 years after the U.S. Public Health Service recommendation. *MMWR* **51** (2002) (RR13), 1–3.

Popkin, B. M. Nutrition in transition: the changing global nutrition challenge. *Asia Pac. J. Clin. Nutr.* **10** (2001), S13–18.

Smithells, R. W., Sheppard, S., Schorah, C. J. *et al.* Possible prevention of neural-tube defects by periconceptional vitamin supplementation. *Lancet* **1** (1980), 339–40.

Stewart, R. J. C., Preece, R. F. and Sheppard, H. G. Twelve generations of marginal protein deficiency. *Br. J. Nutr.* **33** (1975), 233–53.

Winick, M. and Noble, A. Cellular response in rats during malnutrition at various ages. *J. Nutr.* **89** (1966), 300–6.

## Genetics and developmental biology
### *Developmental biology and plasticity*

Baehrecke, E. H. How death shapes life during development. *Nature Rev. Mol. Cell Biol.* **3** (2002), 79–87.

Campbell, K. H., McWhir, J., Ritchie, W. A. and Wilmut, I. Sheep cloned by nuclear transfer from a cultured cell line. *Nature* **380** (1996), 64–6.

Duke, R. C., Ojcius, D. M. and Young, J. D. Cell suicide in health and disease. *Sci. Am.* **275** (1996), 80–7.

Finch, C. E. and Kirkwood, T. B. L. *Chance, Development, and Aging*, ed. C. E. Finch and T. B. L. Kirkwood. (New York, NY: Oxford University Press, 2000), pp. 1–278.

Greider, C. W. and Blackburn, E. H. Telomeres, telomerase and cancer. *Sci. Am.* **274** (1996), 92–7.

Kalter, H. Teratology in the 20th century. Environmental causes of congenital malformations in humans and how they were established. *Neurotoxicol. Teratol.* **25** (2003), 131–282.

Klip, H., Werloop, J., van Gool, J. D. *et al.* Hypospadias in sons of women exposed to diethylstilbestrol in utero: a cohort study. *Lancet* **359** (2002), 1102–07.

Schwartz, R. H. and Jaffe, S. J. *Drug and Chemical Risks to the Fetus and Newborn* (New York, NY: Alan Liss, 1980).

West-Eberhard, M. J. *Developmental Plasticity and Evolution.* (New York, NY: Oxford University Press, 2003).

### *Genetics and epigenetics*

Avner, P. and Head, E. X-chromosome inactivation: counting, choice and initiation. *Nat. Rev. Genet.* **2** (2001), 59–67.

Beutler, E. Glucose-6-phosphate dehydrogenase deficiency. *New Engl. J. Med.* **324** (1991), 169–74.

Blott, S., Kim, J.-J., Moisio, S. *et al.* Molecular dissection of a quantitative trait locus: a phenylalanine-to-tyrosine substitution in the transmembrane domain of the bovine growth hormone receptor is associated with a major effect on milk yield and composition. *Genetics* **163** (2003), 253–66.

Daniels, R., Zuccotti, M., Kinis, T., Serhal, P. and Monk, M. Xist expression in human oocytes and preimplantation embryos. *Am. J. Hum. Genet.* **61** (1997), 33–9.

Goto, T. and Monk, M. Regulation of X-chromosome inactivation in development in mice and humans. *Microbiol. Mol. Biol. Rev.* **62** (1998), 362–78.

Haig, D. and Graham, C. Genomic imprinting and the strange case of the insulin-like growth factor II receptor. *Cell* **64** (1991), 1045–6.

Hedborg, F., Holmgren, L., Sandstedt, B. and Ohlsson, R. The cell type-specific IGF2 expression during early human development correlates to the pattern of overgrowth and neoplasia in the Beckwith–Wiedemann syndrome. *Am. J. Pathol.* **145** (1994), 802–17.

*Henig, R. M. *A Monk and Two Peas: The Story of Gregor Mendel and the Discovery of Genetics.* (Weidenfeld & Nicolson/Houghton Mifflin, 2000).

Hollon, T. Human genes: how many? *The Scientist* **15** (2001), 1.

Jaenisch, R. and Bird, A. Epigenetic regulation of gene expression: how the genome integrates intrinsic and environmental signals. *Nature Genetics* **33** (2003), 245–54.

Miozzo, M. and Simoni, G. The role of imprinted genes in fetal growth. *Biol. Neonate* **81** (2002), 217–28.

Reik, W. and Maher, E. R. Imprinting in clusters: lessons from Beckwith–Wiedemann syndrome. *Trends in Genetics* **13** (1997), 330–4.

Sapienza, C. Parental imprinting of genes. *Sci. Am.* **263** (1990), 26–32.

The Huntington's Disease Collaborative Research Group. A novel gene containing a trinucleotide repeat that is expanded and unstable on Huntington's disease chromosomes. *Cell* **72** (1993), 817–18.

*Tudge, C. In *Mendel's Footnotes*, ed. C. Tudge (London: Vintage, 2002).

Waterland, R. A. and Garza, C. Potential mechanisms of metabolic imprinting that lead to chronic disease. *Am. J. Clin. Nutr.* **69** (1999), 179–97.

Waterland, R. A. and Jirtle, R. L. Transposable elements: targets for early nutritional effects on epigenetic gene regulation. *Mol. Cell Biol.* **23** (2003), 5293–300.

Wolff, G. L., Kodell, R. L., Moore, S. R. and Cooney, C. A. Maternal epigenetics and methyl supplements affect agouti gene expression in A$^{vy}$/a mice. *FASEB J.* **12** (1998), 949–57.

## Maternal and trans-generational effects

Agrawal, A. A., Laforsch, C. and Tollrian, R. Transgenerational induction of defences in animals and plants. *Nature* **401** (1999), 60–3.

Alekseev, V. and Lampert, W. Maternal control of resting-egg production in *Daphnia. Nature* **414** (2001), 899–901.

Bernardo, J. Maternal effects in animal ecology. *Am. Zoology* **36** (1996), 83–105.

Engh, A. L., Esch, K., Smale, L. and Holekamp, K. E. Mechanisms of maternal rank 'inheritance' in the spotted hyaena, *Crocuta crocuta. Anim. Behav.* **60** (2000), 323–32.

Herbst, A. L., Ulfelder, H. and Poskanzer, D. C. Adenocarcinoma of the vagina. Association of maternal stilbestrol therapy with tumor appearance in young women. *N. Engl. J. Med.* **284** (1971), 878–81.

Kruuk, L. E. B., Clutton-Brock, T. H., Slate, J., *et al.* Heritability of fitness in a wild mammal population. *Proc. Nat. Acad. Sci.* **97** (2000), 698–703.

Lacey, E. P. What is an adaptive environmentally induced parental effect? In *Maternal Effects as Adaptations*, ed. T. A. Mousseau and C. W. Fox. (Oxford: Oxford University Press, 1998), pp. 54–66.

Mousseau, T. A. and Fox, C. W., eds. *Maternal Effects as Adaptations.* (New York, NY: Oxford University Press, 1998.)

Pembrey, M. E. Time to take epigenetic inheritance seriously. *Eur. J. Human Genetics* **10** (2002), 669–71.

Rossiter, M. C. Incidence and consequences of inherited environmental effects. *Annu. Rev. Ecol. System* **27** (1996), 451–76.

## Clinical medicine

### *Cardiovascular disease*

Keller, G., Zimmer, G., Mall, G., Ritz, E. and Amann, K. Nephron number in patients with primary hypertension. *New Engl. J. Med.* **348** (2003), 101–8.

McNamara, J. J., Molot, M. A., Stremple, J. F. and Cutting, R. T. Coronary artery disease in combat casualties in Vietnam. *JAMA* **216** (1971), 1185–7.

Renaud, S. and de Lorgeril, M. Wine, alcohol, platelets, and the French paradox for coronary heart disease. *Lancet* **339** (1992), 1523–6.

### *Diabetes mellitus*

Diamond, J. The double puzzle of diabetes. *Nature* **423** (2003), 599–602.

Groop, L. Genetics of the metabolic syndrome. *Br. J. Nutr.* **83** (2000), s39–48.

Hill, D. J. and Duvillie, B. Pancreatic development and adult diabetes. *Pediatr. Res.* **48** (2000), 269–74.

McIntyre, E. A. and Walker, M. Genetics of type 2 diabetes and insulin resistance: knowledge from human studies. *Clin. Endocrinol.* **57** (2002), 303–11.

Neel, J. V. The "thrifty genotype" in 1998. *Nutr. Rev.* **57** (1999), s2–9.

Pizzuti, A., Frittitta, L., Argiolas, A. *et al.* A polymorphism (K121Q) of the human glycoprotein PC-1 gene coding region is strongly associated with insulin resistance. *Diabetes* **48** (1999), 1881–4.

Plagemann, A., Harder, T., Kohlhoff, R., Rohde, W. and Dörner, G. Glucose tolerance and insulin secretion in children of mothers with pregestational IDDM or gestational diabetes. *Diabetologia* **40** (1997a), 1094–100.

Plagemann, A., Harder, T., Kohlhoff, R., Rohde, W. and Dörner, G. Overweight and obesity in infants of mothers with long-term insulin-dependent diabetes or gestational diabetes. *Int. J. Obes. Relat. Metab. Disord.* **21** (1997b), 451–6.

Pugliese, A. and Miceli, D. The insulin gene in diabetes. *Diabetes. Metab. Res. Rev.* **18** (2002), 13–25.

Reaven, G. M. and Laws, A. *Insulin Resistance: The Metabolic Syndrome* X, ed. G. M. Reaven and A. Laws. (Humana Press, 1999).

Reece, E. A. and Coustan, D. R., eds. *Diabetes Mellitus in Pregnancy.* (Churchill Livingstone Inc., 1995.)

Sobngwi, E., Boudou, P., Mauvais-Jarvis, F., *et al.* Effect of a diabetic environment in utero on predisposition to type 2 diabetes. *Lancet* **361** (2003), 1861–5.

Stanhope, J. M. and Prior, I. A. The Tokelau island migrant study: prevalence and incidence of diabetes mellitus. *NZ Med. J.* **92** (1980), 417–21.

### Obesity

Björntorp, P. Thrifty genes and human obesity. Are we chasing ghosts? *Lancet* **358** (2001), 1006–8.

Bougnères, P. Genetics of obesity and type 2 diabetes. *Diabetes* **41** (2002), S295–303.

Bujalska, I. J., Kumar, S. and Stewart, P. M. Does central obesity reflect "Cushing's disease of the omentum"? *Lancet* **349** (1997), 1210–13.

Crescenzo, R., Samec, S., Antic, V. *et al.* A role for suppressed thermogenesis favoring catch-up fat in the pathophysiology of catch-up growth. *Diabetes* **52** (2003), 1090–7.

Cuthill, I. C., Maddocks, S. A., Weall, C. V. and Jones, E. K. M. Body mass regulation in response to changes in feeding predictability and overnight energy expenditure. *Behav. Ecol.* **11** (2000), 189–95.

Dulloo, A. G., Jacquet, J. and Montani, J. P. Pathways from weight fluctuations to metabolic diseases: focus on maladaptive thermogenesis during catch-up fat. *Int. J. Obesity and Related Metab. Disorders* **26** (2000), S46–57.

Friedman, J. M. The function of leptin in nutrition, weight, and physiology. *Nutr. Rev.* **60** (2002), S1–14.

Grinspoon, S., Gulick, T., Askari, H. *et al.* Serum leptin levels in women with anorexia nervosa. *J. Clin. Endocrinol. Metab.* **81** (1996), 3861–3.

Jones, C. O. and White, N. G. Adiposity in aboriginal people from Arnhem Land, Australia: variation in degree and distribution associated with age, sex and lifestyle. *Annals. Human. Biol.* **21** (1994), 207–27.

Lee, R. B. The allocation of nutritional stress. In *The !Kung San. Men, Women, and Work in a Foraging Society*, ed. R. B. Lee. (Cambridge: Cambridge University Press, 1979), pp. 281–305.

Lev-Ran, A. Human obesity: an evolutionary approach to understanding our bulging waistline. *Diabetes Metab. Res. Rev.* **17** (2001), 347–62.

Montague, C. T., Farooqi, I. S., Whitehead, J. P. *et al.* Congenital leptin deficiency is associated with severe early-onset obesity in humans. *Nature* **387** (1997), 903–8.

Montague, C. T. and O'Rahilly, S. Perspectives in diabetes. The perils of portliness. Causes and consequences of visceral adiposity. *Diabetes* **49** (2000), 883–8.

Pond, C. M. Paracrine interactions of mammalian adipose tissue. *J. Experimental Zoology* **295A** (2003), 99–110.

Schroeder, D. G., Martorell, R. and Flores, R. Infant and child growth and fatness and fat distribution in Guatemalan adults. *Am. J. Epidemiol.* **149** (1999), 177–85.

Wilmsen, E. N. Seasonal effects of dietary intake on Kalahari San. *Federation Proc.* **37** (1978), 65–72.

Zhang, Y., Proenca, R., Maffei, M. *et al.* Positional cloning of the mouse obese gene and its human homologue. *Nature* **372** (1994), 425–32.

Zierath, J. R., Livingston, J. N., Thorne, A. *et al.* Regional difference in insulin inhibition of non-esterified fatty acid release from human adipocytes: relation to insulin receptor phosphorylation and intracellular signalling through the insulin receptor substrate-1 pathway. *Diabetologia* **41** (1998), 1343–54.

## Osteoporosis

Cooper, C., Cawley, M., Bhalla, A. *et al.* Childhood growth, physical activity, and peak bone mass in women. J. Bone Mineral Res. **10** (1995), 940–7.

Cooper, C., Eriksson, J. G., Forsen, T. *et al.* Maternal height, childhood growth and risk of hip fracture in later life: a longitudinal study. *Osteoporos. Int.* **12** (2001), 623–9.

Cooper, C., Fall, C., Egger, P. *et al.* Growth in infancy and bone mass in later life. *Ann. Rheum. Dis.* **56** (1997), 17–21.

Cooper, C., Javaid, M. K., Taylor, P. *et al.* The fetal origins of osteoporotic fracture. *Calcif. Tiss. Int.* **70** (2002), 391–4.

Cooper, C., Walker-Bone, K., Arden, N. and Dennison, E. Novel insights into the pathogenesis of osteoporosis: the role of intrauterine programming. *Rheumatology* **39** (2000), 1312–15.

Geusens, P. P. M. M. and Boonen, S. Osteoporosis and the growth hormone-insulin-like growth factor axis. *Horm. Res.* **58** Suppl. 3 (2002), 49–55.

Javaid, M. K. and Cooper, C. Prenatal and childhood influences on osteoporosis. *Best Practice and Res. Clin. Endocrinol. Metab.* **16** (2002), 349–67.

Wajchenberg, B. L. Subcutaneous and visceral adipose tissue: their relation to the metabolic syndrome. *Endocr. Rev.* **21** (2000), 697–738.

## Other diseases

Courchesne, E., Carper, R. and Akshoomoff, N. Evidence of brain overgrowth in the first year of life in autism. *JAMA* **290** (2003), 337–44.

Creswell, J., Fraser, R. P., Bruce, C., *et al.* Relationship between polycystic ovaries, body mass index and insulin resistance. *Acta Obstet. Gynecol. Scand.* **82** (2003), 61–4.

Gale, C. R., O'Callaghan, F. J., Godfrey, K. M., Law, C. M., Martyn, C. N. Critical periods of brain growth and cognitive function in children. *Brain* **127** (2004), 321–9.

Gale, C. R., Walton, S., Martyn, C. N. Fetal and postnatal head growth and risk of cognitive decline in old age. *Brain* **126** (2003), 2273–8.

Hill, E. L. and Frith, U. Understanding autism: insights from mind and brain. *Phil. Trans. R. Soc. Lond. B* **358** (2003), 281–9.

Shibata, Y., Yamashita, S., Masyakin, V. B., Panasyuk, G. D. and Nagataki, S. 15 years after Chernobyl: new evidence of thyroid cancer. *Lancet* **358** (2001), 1965–6.

Vila, M. and Przedborski, S. Targeting programmed cell death in neurodegenerative diseases. *Nat. Rev. Neurosci.* **4** (2003), 365–75.

## Prenatal induction

*General reading*

Aplin, J. Maternal influences on placental development. *Seminars in Cell & Dev. Biol.* **11** (2000), 115–25.

*Barker, D. *The Best Start in Life.* (London: Arrow 2003.)

Barker, D. J., Gluckman, P. D., Godfrey, K. M. *et al.* Fetal nutrition and cardiovascular disease in adult life. *Lancet* **341** (1993), 938–41.

Barker, D. J. P., ed. Fetal Origins of Cardiovascular and Lung Disease. (New York, NY: Marcel Dekker, Inc., 2001.)

Bertram, C. E, Hanson, M. A. Animal models and the programming of the metabolic syndrome. In *Type 2 Diabetes: The Thrifty Phenotype*, ed. D. J. P. Barker. *Br. Med. Bull.* **60** (2001): 103–21.

Bertram, C. E. and Hanson, M. A. Prenatal programming of postnatal endocrine responses by glucocorticoids. *Repro.* **124** (2002): 459–67.

Bloomfield, F. H. and Harding, J. E. Experimental aspects of nutrition and fetal growth. *Fetal and Maternal Med. Rev.* **10** (1998), 91–107.

Cianfarani, S., Geremia, C., Scott, C. D., and Germani, D. Growth, IGF system and cortisol in children with intrauterine growth retardation: is catch-up growth affected by reprogramming of the hypothalamic–pituitary–adrenal axis? *Pediatr. Res.* **51** (2002), 94–9.

Gluckman, P. D. and Hanson, M. A. The developmental origins of the metabolic syndrome. *Trends in Endocrinology and Metabolism* (Hormones and the Heart Symposium) **15** (2004), 183–7.

Hales, C. N. and Barker, D. J. Type 2 (non-insulin-dependent) diabetes mellitus: the thrifty phenotype hypothesis. *Diabetologia* **35** (1992), 595–601.

Hales, C. N. and Barker, D. J. The thrifty phenotype hypothesis. *Br. Med. Bull.* **60**, 5 (2001), 20.

Hanson, M. A. and Gluckman, P. D. The effects of pre-natal nutrition on cardiovascular function in offspring: some insights from comparative biology. *Havemeyer Foundation Monograph Series*, **No. 10** (2003a): 51–4.

Hanson, M. A. and Gluckman, P. D. The human camel: the concept of predictive adaptive responses and the obesity epidemic. *Pract. Diabetes Int.* **20**, 8 (2003b): 267.

Harding, J. E. and Gluckman, P. D. Growth, metabolic and endocrine adaptations to fetal under-nutrition. In *Fetal Origins of Cardiovascular Disease and Lung Disease. Lung Biology in Health and Disease,* ed. D. J. P. Barker (New York, NY: Marcel Dekkar, 2001), pp. 181–97.

Hoet, J. J. and Hanson, M. A. Intrauterine nutrition: its importance during critical periods for cardiovascular and endocrine development. *J. Physiol.* **514** (1999), 617–27.

Ingelfinger, J. R. Is microanatomy destiny? *New Engl. J. Med.* **348** (2003), 99–100.

Law, C. M. Significance of birth weight for the future. *Arch. Dis. Child. Neonatal Edn.* **86** (2002), F7–8.

Moritz, K. M., Dodic, M. and Wintour, E. M. Kidney development and the fetal programming of adult disease. *Bioessays* **25**, 3 (2003), 212–20.

Robinson, R. The fetal origins of adult disease. *BMJ* **322** (2001), 375–6.

Silverman, B. L., Cho, N. H., Rizzo, T. A. and Metzger, B. E. Long-term effects of the intrauterine environment. *Diabetes Care* **21** (1998), B142–9.

Wells, J. C. K. The thrifty phenotype hypothesis: thrifty offspring or thrifty mother? *J. Theor. Biol.* **221** (2003), 143–61.

Wintour, E. M., Johnson, K., Koukoulas, I. *et al.* Programming the cardiovascular system, kidney and the brain: a review. *Placenta* **24** (2003), Suppl. A Trophoblast Res., S65–71.

## *Clinical and epidemiological studies*

Adair, L. S., Kuzawa, C. W., and Borja, J. Maternal energy stores and diet composition during pregnancy program adolescent blood pressure. *Circulation* **104** (2001), 1034–9.

Anderson, P. and Doyle, L. W. Neurobehavioral outcomes in school-age children born extremely low birth weight or very preterm in the 1990s. *JAMA* **289** (2003), 3264–72.

Barker, D. J. P. The foetal and infant origins of inequalities in health in Britain. *J. Public Health Med.* **13** (1991), 64–8.

* Barker, D. J. P. *Mothers, Babies and Health in Later Life.* (Edinburgh: Churchill Livingstone, 1998.)

Barker, D. J. P. Intrauterine nutrition may be important. *BMJ* **318** (1999), 1477–8.

Barker, D. J. P., Bull, A. R., Osmond, C. and Simmonds, S. J. Fetal and placental size and risk of hypertension in adult life. *BMJ* **301**(1990), 259–62.

Barker, D. J. P., Eriksson, J. G., Forsén, T., and Osmond, C. Fetal origins of adult disease: strength of effects and biological basis. *Int. J. Epidemiol.* **31**(2002), 1235–9.

Barker, D. J. P., Forsen, T., Eriksson J. G., and Osmond, C. Growth and living conditions in childhood and hypertension in adult life: a longitudinal study. *J. Hypertens.* **20** (2002), 1951–6.

Barker, D. J. P., Forsen, T., Uutela, A., Osmond, C., and Eriksson, J. G. Size at birth and resilience to effects of poor living conditions in adult life: longitudinal study. *BMJ* **323** (2001), 1273–6.

Barker, D. J. P., Godfrey, K. M., Osmond, C., and Bull, A. The relation of fetal length, ponderal index and head circumference to blood pressure and the risk of hypertension in adult life. *Paediatr. Perinatal Epidemiol.* **6** (1992), 35–44.

Barker, D. J. P. and Lackland, D. T. Prenatal influences on stroke mortality in England and Wales. *Stroke* **34** (2003), 1598–602.

Barker, D. J. P., Osmond, C., Simmonds, S. J., and Weild, G. A. The relation of small head circumference and thinness at birth to death from cardiovascular disease in adult life. *BMJ* **306** (1993), 422–6.

Barker, D. J. P., Winter, P. D., Osmond, C., Margetts, B. and Simmonds, S. J. Weight in infancy and death from ischaemic heart disease. *Lancet* **2** (8663) (1989), 577–80.

Barker, M., Robinson, S., Osmond, C. and Barker, D. J. P. Birth weight and body fat distribution in adolescent girls. *Arch. Dis. Child.* **77** (1997), 381–3.

Bavdekar, A., Yajnik, C. S., Fall, C. H. *et al.* Insulin resistance syndrome in 8-year-old Indian children: small at birth, big at 8 years, or both? *Diabetes* **48** (1999), 2422–9.

Bolt, R. J., van Weissenbruch, M. M., Popp-Snijders, C. *et al.* Fetal growth and the function of the adrenal cortex in preterm infants. *J. Clin. Endocrinol. Metab.* **87** (2002), 1194–9.

Brenner, B. M. and Chertow, G. M. Congenital oligonephropathy and the etiology of adult hypertension and progressive renal injury. *Am. J. Kidney Dis.* **23** (1994), 171–5.

Brenner, B. M., Garcia, D. L., and Anderson, S. Glomeruli and blood pressure: less of one, more of the other? *Am. J. Hypertens.* **1** (1988), 335–47.

Campbell, D. M., Hall, M. H., Barker, D. J. *et al.* Diet in pregnancy and the offspring's blood pressure 40 years later. *Br. J. Obstet. Gynaecol.* **103** (1996), 273–80.

Cho, N., Silverman, B. L., Rizzo, T. A. and Metzger, B. E. Correlations between the intrauterine metabolic environment and blood pressure in adolescent offspring of diabetic mothers. *J. Pediatr.* **136** (2000), 587–92.

Chotai, J., Forsgren, T., Nilsson, L.-G. and Adolfsson, R. Season of birth variations in the temperament and character inventory of personality in a general population. *Neuropsychobiol.* **44** (2001), 19–26.

Chotai, J. and Salander-Renberg, E. Season of birth variations in suicide methods in relation to any history of psychiatric contacts support an independent suicidality trait. *J. Affect. Disorder.* **69** (2002), 69–81.

Clark, P. M., Atton, C., Law, C. M. *et al.* Weight gain in pregnancy, triceps skinfold thickness, and blood pressure in offspring. *Obstet. Gynecol.* **91** (1998), 103–7.

Cresswell, J. L., Egger, P., Fall, C. H. D. *et al.* Is the age of menopause determined in-utero? *Early Hum. Dev.* **49** (1997), 143–8.

Doblhammer, G. and Vaupel, J. W. Lifespan depends on month of birth. *Proc. Natl. Acad. Sci.* **98** (2001a), 2934–9.

dos Santos Silva, I., de Stavola, B. L., Mann, V. *et al.* Prenatal factors, childhood growth trajectories and age at menarche. *Int. J. Epidemiol.* **31** (2002), 405–12.

Eriksson, J. G., Forsén, T., Tuomilehto, J., Osmond, C. and Barker, D. J. P. Early growth, adult income, and risk of stroke. *Stroke* **31** (2000), 869–74.

Eriksson, J., Forsén, T., Tuomilehto, J., Osmond, C., and Barker, D. Size at birth, childhood growth and obesity in adult life. *Int. J. Obesity* **25** (2001a), 735–40.

Eriksson, J. G., Forsén, T., Tuomilehto, J., Osmond, C. and Barker, D. J. Early growth and coronary heart disease in later life: longitudinal study. *BMJ* **322** (2001b), 949–53.

Eriksson, J. G., Forsén, T., Tuomilehto, J., Osmond, C. and Barker, D. J. Early adiposity rebound in childhood and risk of Type 2 diabetes in adult life. *Diabetologia* **46** (2003), 190–4.

Eriksson, J. G., Forsén, T., Tuomilehto, J. *et al.* Catch-up growth in childhood and death from coronary heart disease: longitudinal study. *BMJ* **318** (1999), 427–31.

Eriksson, J. G., Lindi, V., Uusitupa, M. *et al.* The effects of the Pro12Ala polymorphism of the peroxisome proliferator-activated receptor-gamma2 gene on insulin sensitivity and insulin metabolism interact with size at birth. *Diabetes* **51** (2002), 2321–4.

Eriksson, J. G., Osmond, C., Lindi, V. *et al.* Interactions between peroxisome proliferator-activated receptor gene polymorphism and birth length influence risk for type 2 diabetes. *Diabetes Care* **26** (2003), 2476–7.

Fall, C. H., Barker, D. J., Osmond, C. *et al.* Relation of infant feeding to adult serum cholesterol concentration and death from ischaemic heart disease. *BMJ* **304** (1992), 801–5.

Fall, C., Hindmarsh, P., Dennison, E. *et al.* Programming of growth hormone secretion and bone mineral density in elderly men – a hypothesis. *J. Clin. Endocrinol. Metab.* **83** (1998a), 135–9.

Fall, C. H., Pandit, A. N., Law, C. M. *et al.* Size at birth and plasma insulin-like growth factor-1 concentrations in childhood. *Arch. Dis. Childhood* **73** (1995), 287–93.

Fall, C. H., Stein, C. E., Kumaran, K. *et al.* Size at birth, maternal weight, and Type 2 diabetes in South India. *Diabetic Med.* **15** (1998), 220–7.

Fewtrell, M. S., Doherty, C., Cole, T. J. *et al.* Effects of size at birth, gestational age and early growth in preterm infants on glucose and insulin concentrations at 9–12 years. *Diabetologia* **43** (2000), 714–17.

Flanagan, D. E., Vaile, J. C., Petley, G. W. *et al.* The autonomic control of heart rate and insulin resistance in young adults. *J. Clin. Endocrinol. Metab.* **84** (1999), 1263–7.

Forrester, T. E., Wilks, R. J., Bennett, F. I. *et al.* Fetal growth and cardiovascular risk factors in Jamaican schoolchildren. *BMJ* **312** (1996), 156–60.

Forsdahl, A. Are poor living conditions in childhood and adolescence an important risk factor for arteriosclerotic heart disease? *Br. J. Preventive Social. Med.* **31** (1977), 91–5.

Forsdahl, A. Living conditions in childhood and subsequent development of risk factors for arteriosclerotic heart disease. The cardiovascular survey in Finnmark 1974–75. *J. Epidemiol. Community Health* **32** (1978), 34–7.

Forsén, T., Eriksson, J. G., Tuomilehto, J., Osmond, C. and Barker, D. J. P. Growth in utero and during childhood among women who develop coronary heart disease: longitudinal study. *BMJ* **319** (1999), 1403–7.

Forsén, T., Eriksson, J., Tuomilehto, J. *et al.* The fetal and childhood growth of persons who develop type 2 diabetes. *Ann. Intern. Med.* **133** (2000), 176–82.

Forsén, T., Eriksson, J. G., Tuomilehto, J. *et al.* Mother's weight in pregnancy and coronary heart disease in a cohort of Finnish men: follow up study. *BMJ* **315** (1997), 837–40.

Gale, C. R., Martyn, C. N., Kellingray, S., Eastell, R. and Cooper, C. Intrauterine programming of adult body composition. *J. Clin. Endocrinol. Metab.* **86** (2001), 267–72.

Gale, C. R., Walton, S. and Martyn, C. N. Foetal and postnatal head growth and risk of cognitive decline in old age. *Brain* **126** (2003), 2273–8.

Godfrey, K. M., Barker, D. J., Robinson, S. and Osmond, C. Maternal birthweight and diet in pregnancy in relation to the infant's thinness at birth. *Br. J. Obstet. Gynaecol.* **104** (1997), 663–7.

Godfrey, K., Robinson, S., Barker, D. J., Osmond, C. and Cox, V. Maternal nutrition in early and late pregnancy in relation to placental and fetal growth. *BMJ* **312** (1996), 410–14.

Hales, C. H., Barker, D. J., Clark, P. M. *et al.* Fetal and infant growth and impaired glucose tolerance at age 64. *BMJ* **303** (1991), 1019–22.

Hardy, R. and Kuh, D. Does early growth influence timing of the menopause? Evidence from a British birth cohort. *Hum. Reprod.* **17** (2002), 2474–9.

Hattersley, A. T., Beards, F., Ballantyne, E. *et al.* Mutations in the glucokinase gene of the fetus result in reduced birth weight. *Nat. Genet.* **19** (1998), 209–10.

Hilakivi-Clarke, L., Forsén, T., Eriksson, J. G. *et al.* Tallness and overweight during childhood have opposing effects on breast cancer risk. *Br. J. Cancer* **85** (2001), 1680–4.

Hofman, P. L., Cutfield, W. S., Robinson, E. M. *et al.* Insulin resistance in short children with intrauterine growth retardation. *J. Clin. Endocrinol. Metab.* **82** (1997), 402–6.

Hokken-Koèlege, A. C. S. Timing of puberty and fetal growth. *Best Practice and Res. Clin. Endocrinol. Metab.* **16** (2002), 65–71.

Hultman, C. M., Sparén, P. and Cnattingius, S. Perinatal risk factors for infantile autism. *Epidemiology* **13** (2002), 417–23.

Huxley, R., Neil, A. and Collins, R. Unravelling the fetal origins hypothesis: is there really an inverse association between birthweight and subsequent blood pressure? *Lancet* **360** (2002), 659–65.

Ibáñez, L., Ferrer, A., Marcos, M. V., Hierro, F. R. and de Zegher, F. Early puberty: rapid progression and reduced final height in girls with low birth weight. *Pediatrics* **106** (2000), 72–4.

Ibanez, L., Potau, N., Enriquez, G. and de Zegher, F. Reduced uterine and ovarian size in adolescent girls born small for gestational age. *Pediatr Res.* **47** (2000), 575–7.

Ibáñez, L., Potau, N., Enriquez, G., Marcos, M. V. and DeZegher, F. Hypergonadotrophinaemia with reduced uterine and ovarian size in women born small-for-gestational-age. *Hum. Reprod.* **18** (2003), 1565–9.

Ibanez, L., Ong, K. K., Mongan, N. *et al.* Androgen receptor gene CAG repeat polymorphism in the development of ovarian hyperandrogenism. *J. Clin. Endocrinol. Metab.* **88** (2003), 3333–8.

Ibanez, L., Valls, C., Potau, N., Marcos, M. V. and de Zegher, F. Polycystic ovary syndrome after precocious pubarche: ontogeny of the low-birthweight effect. *Clin. Endocinol.* **55** (2001), 667–72.

Ijzerman, R. G., Stehouwer, C. D., de Geus, E. J. *et al.* Low birth weight is associated with increased sympathetic activity: dependence on genetic factors. *Circulation* **108** (2003), 566–71.

Jaquet, D., Tregouet, D. A., Godefroy, T. *et al.* Combined effects of genetic and environmental factors on insulin resistance associated with reduced fetal growth. *Diabetes* **51** (2002), 3473–8.

Jefferis, B. J. M. H., Power, C. and Hertzman, C. Birth weight, childhood socioeconomic environment, and cognitive development in the 1958 British birth cohort study. *BMJ* **325** (2002), 305–11.

Kaati, G., Bygren, L. O. and Edvinsson, S. Cardiovascular and diabetes mortality determined by nutrition during parents' and grandparents' slow growth period. *Eur. J. Hum. Genet.* **10** (2002), 682–8.

Kaufman, J., Birmaher, B., Perel, J. *et al.* The corticotropin-releasing hormone challenge in depressed abused, depressed nonabused, and normal control children. *Biol. Psychiatry* **42** (1997), 669–79.

Keen, R. W., Egger, P., Fall, C. *et al.* Polymorphisms of the vitamin D receptor, infant growth, and adult bone mass. *Calcif. Tissue Int.* **60** (1997), 233–5.

Kiserud, T. Liver length in the small-for-gestational-age fetus and ductus venosus flow. *Am. J. Obstet. Gynecol.* **182** (2000), 252–3.

Koziel, S. and Jankowska, E. A. Effect of low versus normal birthweight on menarche in 14-year-old Polish girls. *J. Paediatr. Child Health* **38** (2002), 268–71.

Kuh, D., Bassey, J., Hardy, R. *et al.* Birth weight, childhood size, and muscle strength in adult life: evidence from a birth cohort study. *Am. J. Epidemiol.* **156** (2002), 627–33.

Law, C. M., de Swiet, M., Osmond, C. *et al.* Initiation of hypertension in utero and its amplification throughout life. *BMJ* **306** (1993), 24–7.

Law, C. M., Egger, P., Dada, O. *et al.* Body size at birth and blood pressure among children in developing countries. *Int. J. Epidemiol.* **30** (2001), 52–7.

Law, C. M., Shiell, A. W., Newsome, C. A. *et al.* Fetal, infant, and childhood growth and adult blood pressure: a longitudinal study from birth to 22 years of age. *Circulation* **105** (2002), 1088–92.

Limosin, F., Rouillon, F., Payan, C., Cohen, J. M. and Strub, N. Prenatal exposure to influenza as a risk factor for adult schizophrenia. *Acta Psychiatr. Scand.* **107** (2003), 331–5.

Lindsay, R. S., Bennett, P. H., Hanson, R. L. and Knowler, W. C. Secular trends in birth weight, BMI, and diabetes in the offspring of diabetic mothers. *Diabetes Care* **23** (2000), 1249–54.

Lucas, A. (1991). Programming by early nutrition in man. In *The Childhood Environment, and Adult Disease*, ed. G. R. Bock and J. Whelan (Chichester: John Wiley), pp. 38–55.

Lucas, A., Morley, R. and Cole, T. J. Randomised trial of early diet in preterm babies and later intelligence quotient. *BMJ* **317** (1998), 1481–7.

Lumey, L. H. (1992). Decreased birthweights in infants after maternal in utero exposure to the Dutch famine of 1944–1945. *Paediatr. Perinatal Epidemiol.* **6**, 240–53.

Lurbe, E., Torro, I., Rodriguez, C., Alvarez, V. and Redon, J. Birth weight influences blood pressure values and variability in children and adolescents. *Hypertension* **38** (2001), 389–93.

Mackenzie, H. S. and Brenner, B. M. Fewer nephrons at birth: a missing link in the etiology of essential hypertension? *Am. J. Kidney Dis.* **26** (1995), 91–8.

Martyn, C. N., Gale, C. R., Sayer, A. A. and Fall, C. Growth in utero and cognitive function in adult life: follow up study of people born between 1920 and 1943. *BMJ* **312** (1996), 1393–6.

Martyn, C. N. and Greenwald, S. E. A hypothesis about a mechanism for the programming of blood pressure and vascular disease in early life. *Clin. Exp. Pharm. Physiol.* **28** (2001), 948–51.

McAllister, A. S., Atkinson, A. B., Johnston, G. D. and McCance, D. R. Relationship of endothelial function to birth weight in humans. *Diabetes Care* **22** (1999), 2061–6.

McNeil, T. F., Cantor-Graae, E., Nordstrom, L. G. and Rosenlund, T. Head circumference in 'preschizophrenic' and control neonates. *Br. J. Psychiatry* **162** (1993), 517–23.

Mednick, S. A., Machon, R. A., Huttunen, M. O. and Bonett, D. Adult schizophrenia following prenatal exposure to an influenza epidemic. *Arch. Gen. Psychiatry* **45** (1988), 189–92.

Mi, J., Law, C., Zhang, K.-L. and Osmond, C. Effects of infant birthweight and maternal body mass index in pregnancy on components of the insulin resistance syndrome in China. *Ann. Intern. Med.* **132** (2000), 253–60.

Moore, S. E., Cole, T. J., Collinson, A. C. *et al.* Prenatal or early postnatal events predict infectious deaths in young adulthood in rural Africa. *Int. J. Epidemiol.* **28** (1999), 1088–95.

Moore, V. M., Miller, A. G., Boulton, T. J. *et al.* Placental weight, birth measurements, and blood pressure at age 8 years. *Arch. Dis. Childhood* **74** (1996), 538–41.

Nilsson, P. M., Ostergen, P. O., Nyberg, P., Soderstrom, M. and Allebeck, P. Low birth weight is associated with elevated systolic blood pressure in adolescence: a prospective study of a birth cohort of 149 378 Swedish boys. *J. Hypertens.* **15** (1997), 1627–31.

O'Keefe, M. J., O'Callaghan, M., Williams, G. M., Najman, J. M. and Bor, W. Learning, cognitive, and attentional problems in adolescents born small for gestational age. *Pediatrics* **112** (2003), 301–7.

Ong, K. K., Preece, M., Emmett, P. M., Ahmed, M. L. and Dunger, D. B. Size at birth and early chidhood growth in relation to maternal smoking, parity and infant breast-feeding: longitudinal birth cohort study and analysis. *Pediatr. Res.* **52** (2002), 863–7.

Osmond, C. and Barker, D. J. P. Fetal, infant, and childhood growth are predictors of coronary heart disease, diabetes, and hypertension in adult men and women. *Environ. Health Perspect.* **108** (2000), 545–53.

Osmond, C., Barker, D. J. P. and Slattery, J. M. Risk of death from cardiovascular disease and chronic bronchitis determined by place of birth in England and Wales. *J. Epidemiol. Community Health* **44** (1990), 139–41.

Palinski, W. and Napoli, C. Pathophysiological events during pregnancy influence the development of atherosclerosis in humans. *Trends Cardiovasc. Med.* **9** (1999), 205–14.

Pastrakuljic, A., Derewlany, L. O. and Koren, G. Maternal cocaine use and cigarette smoking in pregnancy in relation to amino acid transport and fetal growth. *Placenta* **20** (1999), 499–512.

Pettitt, D. J. and Knowler, W. C. Long-term effects of the intrauterine environment, birth weight, and breast-feeding in Pima Indians. *Diabetes Care* **21** (1998), B138–41.

Phillips, D. I., Barker, D. J., Hales, C. N., Hirst, S. and Osmond, C. Thinness at birth and insulin resistance in adult life. *Diabetologia* **37** (1994), 150–4.

Phillips, D. I. W., Fall, C. H. D., Cooper, C. *et al.* Size at birth and plasma leptin concentrations in adult life. *Int. J. Obesity* **23** (1999), 1025–9.

Phillips, D. I. W., Handelsman, D. J., Eriksson, J. G. *et al.* Prenatal growth and subsequent marital status: longitudinal study. *BMJ* **322** (2001), 771.

Piven, J., Berthier, M. L., Starkstein, S. E. *et al.* Magnetic resonance imaging evidence for a defect of cerebral cortical development in autism. *Am. J. Psychiatry* **147** (1990), 734–9.

Poulsen, P., Andersen, G., Fenger, M. *et al.* Impact on two common polymorphisms in the PPARgamma gene on glucose tolerance and plasma insulin profiles in monozygotic and dizygotic twins: thrifty genotype, thrifty phenotype, or both? *Diabetes* **52** (2003), 194–8.

Rao, S., Yajnik, C. S., Kanade, A. *et al.* Intake of micronutrient-rich foods in rural Indian mothers is associated with the size of their babies at birth: Pune maternal nutrition study. *J. Nutr.* **131** (2001), 1217–24.

Ravelli, A. C. J. van der Meulen, J. H P., Michels, R. P J. *et al.* Glucose tolerance in adults after prenatal exposure to famine. *Lancet* **351** (1998), 173–7.

Ravelli, A. C., van der Meulen, J. H., Osmond, C., Barker, D. J. and Bleker, O. P. Obesity at the age of 50 y in men and women exposed to famine prenatally. *Am. J. Clin. Nutr.* **70** (1999), 811–16.

Rich-Edwards, J. W., Stampfer, M. J., Manson, J. E. *et al.* Birth weight and risk of cardiovascular disease in a cohort of women followed up since 1976. *BMJ* **315** (1997), 396–400.

Roberts, A. B., Mitchell, J. M., McCowan, L. M. and Barker, S. Ultrasonographic measurement of liver length in the small-for-gestational-age fetus. *Am. J. Obstet. Gynecol.* **180** (1999), 634–8.

Rogers, I. The influence of birthweight and intrauterine environment on adiposity and fat distribution in later life. *Int. J. Obesity* **27** (2003), 755–77.

Sayer, A. A., Cooper, C. and Barker, D. J. P. Is lifespan determined in utero? *Fetal and Neonatol.* **77** (1997), F162–4.

Sayer, A. A. and Cooper, C. Early life effects on ageing. *Nutrition and Ageing* **6** (2002), 33–48.

Singhal, A., Fewtrel, M., Cole, T. J. and Lucas, A. Low nutrient intake and early growth for later insulin resistance in adolescents born preterm. *Lancet* **361** (2003), 1089–97.

Sorenson, H. T., Sabroe, S., Olsen, J. *et al.* Birth weight and cognitive function in young adult life: historical cohort study. *BMJ* **315** (1997), 401–3.

Sorenson, H. T., Thulstrum, A. M., Norgdard, B. *et al.* Fetal growth and blood pressure in a Danish population aged 31–51 years. *Scand. Cardiovasc. J.* **34** (2000), 390–5.

Stanner, S. A., Bulmer, K., Andres, C. *et al.* Does malnutrition in utero determine diabetes and coronary heart disease in adulthood? Results from the Leningrad siege study, a cross sectional study. *BMJ* **315** (1997), 1342–8.

Stein, C. E., Fall, C. H., Kumaran, K. *et al.* Fetal growth and coronary heart disease in South India. *Lancet* **348** (1996), 1269–73.

Stevens, L. M. and Landis, S. C. Developmental interactions between sweat glands and the sympathetic neurons which innervate them: effects of delayed innervation on neurotransmitter plasticity and gland maturation. *Dev. Biol.* **130** (1988), 703–20.

Weindrich, D., Jennen-Steinmetz, C., Laucht, M. and Schmidt, M. H. Late sequelae of low birthweight: mediators of poor school performance at 11 years. *Dev. Med. Child Neurol.* **45** (2003), 463–9.

Weitz, G., Deckert, P., Heindl, S. *et al.* Evidence for lower sympathetic nerve activity in young adults with low birth weight. *J. Hypertens.* **21** (2003), 943–50.

Williams, J. H. G., Greenhalgh, K. D. and Manning, J. T. Second to fourth finger ratio and possible precursors of developmental psychopathology in preschool children. *Early Hum. Dev.* **72** (2003), 57–65.

Wohlfahrt, J., Melbye, M., Christens, P., Andersen, A.-M. N. and Hjalgrim, H. Secular and seasonal variation of length and weight at birth. *Lancet.* **352** (1998), 1990.

Yajnik, C. S., Coyaji, K. J., Joglekar, C. V., Kellingray, S. and Fall, C. Paternal insulin resistance and fetal growth: problem for the 'fetal insulin' and the 'fetal origins' hypotheses. *Diabetologia* **44** (2003a), 1197–201.

Yajnik, C. S., Fall, C. H. D., Coyaji, K. J. *et al.* Neonatal anthropometry: the thin–fat Indian baby. The Pune maternal nutrition study. *Int. J. Obesity* **27** (2003b), 173–80.

Yajnik, C. S., Fall, C. H. D., Pandit, A. N. *et al.* Fetal growth and glucose and insulin metabolism in four-year-old Indian children. *Diabetic Med.* **12** (1995), 330–6.

Yajnik, C. S., Lubree, H. G., Rege, S. S. *et al.* Adiposity and hyperinsulinemia in Indians are present at birth. *J. Clin. Endocrinol. Metab.* **87** (2002), 5575–80.

## Experimental and mechanistic studies

Benediktsson, R., Lindsay, R. S., Noble, J., Seckl, J. R., Edwards, C. R. Glucocorticoid exposure in utero: new model for adult hypertension. *Lancet* **341** (1993), 339–41.

Bennis-Taleb, N., Remacle, C., Hoet, J. J. and Reusens, B. A low-protein isocaloric diet during gestation affects brain development and alters permanently cerebral cortex blood vessels in rat offspring. *J. Nutr.* **129** (1993), 1613–19.

Bertram, C. E. and Hanson, M. A. Animal models and programming of the metabolic syndrome. *Br. Med. Bull.* **60**, 103–21.

Bloomfield, F. H., Oliver, M. H., Giannoulias, D. *et al.* Brief undernutrition in late-gestation sheep programmes the hypothalamic–pituitary adrenal axis in adult offspring. *Endocrinology* **144** (2003b), 2933–40.

Bloomfield, F. H., Oliver, M. H., Hawkins, P. *et al.* A periconceptual nutritional origin for non-infectious preterm birth. *Science* **300** (2003c), 606.

Brawley, L., Itoh, S., Torrens, C. *et al.* Dietary protein restriction in pregnancy induces hypertension and vascular defects in rat male offspring. *Pediatr. Res.* **54**(1) (2003): 83–90.

Brawley, L., Poston, L. and Hanson, M. Mechanisms underlying the programming of small artery dysfunction: review of the model using low protein diet in pregnancy in the rat. *Arch. Physiol. Biochem.* **111** (2003), 25–35.

Breier, B. H., Vickers, M. H., Ikenasio, B. A., Chan, K. Y. and Wong, W. P. Fetal programming of appetite and obesity. *Mol. Cell. Endocrinol.* **185** (2001), 73–9.

Burns, S. P., Desai, M., Cohen, R. D. *et al.* Gluconeogenesis, glucose handling, and structural changes in livers of the adult offspring of rats partially deprived of protein during pregnancy and lactation. *J. Clin. Invest.* **100** (1997), 1768–74.

Challis, J. R., Sloboda, D., Matthews, S. G. *et al.* The fetal placental hypothalamic–pituitary–adrenal (HPA) axis, parturition and post natal health. *Mol. Cell Endocrinol.* **185** (2001), 135–44.

Chowen, J. A., Goya, L., Ramos, S. *et al.* Effects of early undernutrition on the brain insulin-like growth factor-1 system. *J. Neuroendocrinol.* **14** (2002), 163–9.

Christensen, L. W. and Gorski, R. A. Independent masculinization of neuroendocrine systems by intracerebral implants of testosterone or estradiol in the neonatal rat. *Brain Res.* **146** (1978), 325–40.

Cooney, C. A., Dave, A. A. and Wolff, G. L. Maternal methyl supplements in mice affect epigenetic variation and DNA methylation of offspring. *J. Nutr.* **132** (2002), 2393S–400.

Davis, L., Roullet, J. B., Thornburg, K. L. *et al.* Augmentation of coronary conductance in adult sheep made anaemic during fetal life. *J. Physiol.* **547** (2003), 53–9.

Desai, M., Byrne, C. D., Zhang, J. *et al.* Programming of hepatic insulin-sensitive enzymes in offspring of rat dams fed a protein-restricted diet. *Am. J. Physiol.* **272** (1997), G1083–90.

Dodic, M., May, C. N., Wintour, E. M. and Coghlan, J. P. An early prenatal exposure to excess glucocorticoid leads to hypertensive offspring in sheep. *Clin. Sci.* **94** (1998), 149–55.

Dodic, M., Peers, A., Coghlan, J. P. *et al.* Altered cardiovascular haemodynamics and baroreceptor-heart rate reflex in adult sheep after prenatal exposure to dexamethasone. *Clin. Sci.* **97** (1999), 103–9.

Gardner, D. K., Pool, T. B. and Lane, M. Embryo nutrition and energy metabolism and its relationship to embryo growth, differentiation, and viability. *Sem. Reprod. Med.* **18** (2000), 205–18.

Gatford, K. L., Wintour, E. M., De Blasio, M. J. *et al.* Differential timing for programming of glucose homoeostasis, sensitivity to insulin and blood pressure by in utero exposure to dexamethasone in sheep. *Clin. Sci.* **98** (2000), 553–60.

Gotz, F., Stahl, F., Rohde, W. and Dorner, G. The influence of adrenaline on plasma testosterone in adult and newborn male rats. *Exp. Clin. Endocrinol.* **81** (1983), 239–44.

Hawkins, P., Hanson, M. A. and Matthews, S. G. Maternal undernutrition in early gestation alters molecular regulation of the hypothalamic–pituitary–adrenal axis in the ovine fetus. *J. Neuroendocrinol.* **13** (2001), 855–61.

Hawkins, P., Steyn, C., McGarrigle, H. H. G. *et al.* Cardiovascular and hypothalamic–pituitary–adrenal axis development in late gestation fetal sheep and young lambs following modest maternal nutrient restriction in early gestation. *Reprod. Fertil. Dev.* **12** (2001), 443–56.

Hoet, J. J., Ozanne, S. and Reusens, B. Influences of pre- and postnatal nutritional exposures on vascular/endocrine systems in animals. *Environmental Health Perspectives* **108** (2000), 563–8.

Jackson, A. A., Dunn, R. L., Marchand, M. C. and Langley-Evans, S. C. Increased systolic blood pressure in rats induced by maternal low-protein diet is reversed by dietary supplementation with glycine. *Clin. Sci.* **103** (2002), 633–9.

Khan, I. Y., Taylor, P. D., Dekou, V. *et al.* Gender-linked hypertension in offspring of lard fed pregnant rats. *Hypertension* **41** (2003), 168–75.

Khan I. Y., Hanson, M., Poston, L. and Tylor, P. Predictive adaptation to maternal high fat diet prevents endothelial dysfunction but not hypertension in adult rat offspring. *Circulation* (in press).

Kind, K. L., Clifton, P. M., Katsman, A. I., Tsiounis, M. and Owens, J. A. Restricted fetal growth and the response to dietary cholesterol in the guinea pig. *Am. J. Physiol.* **277** (1999), R1675–82.

Kwong, W. Y., Wild, A. E., Roberts, P., Willis, A. C. and Fleming, T. P. Maternal undernutrition during the preimplantation period of rat development causes blastocyst abnormalities and programming of postnatal hypertension. *Development* **127** (2000), 4195–202.

Langley-Evans, S. C. Hypertension induced by foetal exposure to a maternal low-protein diet, in the rat, is prevented by pharmacological blockade of maternal glucocorticoid synthesis. *J. Hypertens* **15** (1997), 537–44.

Langley-Evans, S. C. Critical differences between two low protein diet protocols in the programming of hypertension in the rat. *International Journal of Food Sciences and Nutrition* **51** (2000), 11–17.

Lingas, R., Dean, F. and Matthews, S. G. Maternal nutrient restriction (48 h) modifies brain corticosteroid receptor expression and endocrine function in the fetal guinea pig. *Brain Res.* **846** (1999), 236–42.

Liu, D., Diorio, J., Day, J. C., Francis, D. D. and Meaney, M. J. Maternal care, hippocampal synaptogenesis and cognitive development in rats. *Nat. Neurosci.* **3** (2000), 799–806.

Liu, D., Diorio, J., Tannebaum, B. *et al.* Maternal care, hippocampal glucocorticoid receptors, and hypothalamic–pituitary–adrenal responses to stress. *Science* **277** (1997), 1659–62.

Lonergan, P., Rizos, D., Kanka, J. *et al.* Temporal sensitivity of bovine embryos to culture environment after fertilization and the implications for blastocyst quality. *Reproduction* **126**, 337–46.

Mallard, C., Loeliger, M., Copolov, D. and Rees, S. Reduced number of neurons in the hippocampus and the cerebellum in the postnatal guinea-pig following intrauterine growth-restriction. *Neuroscience* **100** (2000), 327–33.

Mallard, E. C., Rehn, A., Rees, S., Tolcos, M. and Copolov, D. Ventriculomegaly and reduced hippocampal volume following intrauterine growth-restriction: implications for the aetiology of schizophrenia. *Schizophr. Res.* **40** (1999), 11–21.

Marchand, M. C. and Langley-Evans, S. C. Intrauterine programming of nephron number: the fetal flaw revisited. *J. Nephrol.* **14** (2001), 327–31.

Mehta, G., Roach, H. I., Langley-Evans, S. *et al.* Intrauterine exposure to a maternal low protein diet reduces adult bone mass and alters growth plate morphology in rats. *Calcified Tissue Int.* **71** (2002), 493–8.

Merlet-Benichou, C., Gilbert, T., Muffat-Joly, M., Lelievre-Pegorier, M. and Leroy, B. Intrauterine growth retardation leads to a permanent nephron deficit in the rat. *Pediatr. Nephrol.* **8** (1994), 175–80.

Miller, S. L., Green, L. R., Peebles, D. M., Hanson, M. A. and Blanco, C. E. Effects of chronic hypoxia and protein malnutrition on growth in the developing chick. *Am. J. Obstet. Gynecol.* **186**, 2 (2002), 261–67.

Murotsuki, J., Challis, J. R., Han, V. K., Fraher, L. J. and Gagnon, R. Chronic fetal placental embolization and hypoxemia cause hypertension and myocardial hypertrophy in fetal sheep. *Am. J. Physiol.* **272** (1997), R201–7.

Nishina, H., Green, L. R., McGarrigle, H. H. *et al.* Effect of nutritional restriction in early pregnancy on isolated femoral artery function in mid gestation fetal sheep. *J. Physiol.* **553** (2003), 637–47.

Ozaki, T., Nishina, H., Hanson, M. A. and Poston, L. Dietary restriction in pregnant rats causes gender-related hypertension and vascular dysfunction in offspring. *J. Physiol.* **530** (2001), 141–52.

Petrik, J., Reusens, B., Arany, E. *et al.* A low protein diet alters the balance of islet cell replication and apoptosis in the fetal and neonatal rat and is associated with a reduced pancreatic expression of insulin-like growth factor-II. *Endocrinology* **140** (1999), 4861–73.

Plagemann, A., Harder, T., Rake, A. *et al.* Perinatal elevation of hypothalamic insulin, acquired malformation of hypothalamic galaninergic neurons, and syndrome x-like alterations in adulthood of neonatally overfed rats. *Brain Res.* **836** (1999), 146–55.

Plagemann, A., Heidrich, I., Gotz, F., Rohde, W. and Dorner, G. Obesity and enhanced diabetes and cardiovascular risk in adult rats due to early postnatal overfeeding. *Exp. Clin. Endocrinol.* **99** (1992), 154–8.

Sayer, A. A., Dunn, R. and Langley-Evans, S. Prenatal exposure to a maternal low protein diet shortens life span in rats. *Gerontology* **47** (2001), 9–14.

Seckl, J. R. Glucocorticoids, feto-placenta 11 beta-hydroxysteroid dehydrogenase type 2, and the early life origins of adult disease. *Steroids* **62** (1997), 89–94.

Shiels, P. G., Kind, A. J., Campbell, K. H. *et al.* Analysis of telomere lengths in cloned sheep. *Nature* **399** (1999), 316–7.

Simmons, R. A., Templeton, L. G. and Gertz, S. J. Intrauterine growth retardation leads to the development of type 2 diabetes in the rat. *Diabetes* **50** (2001), 2279–86.

Snoeck, A., Remacle, C., Reusens, B. and Hoet, J. J. Effect of a low protein diet during pregnancy on the fetal rat endocrine pancreas. *Biol. Neonate.* **57** (1990), 107–18.

Taylor, P. D., Khan, I. Y., Lakasing, L. *et al.* Uterine artery function in pregnant rats fed a diet supplemented with animal lard. *Exp. Physiol.* **88** (2003), 389–98.

Torrens, C., Brawley, L., Barker, A. C. *et al.* Maternal protein restriction in the rat impairs resistance but not conduit artery function in pregnant offspring. *J. Physiol.* **547** (2002), 77–84.

Vickers, M. H., Breier, B. H., Cutfield, W. S., Hofman, P. L. and Gluckman, P. D. Fetal origins of hyperphagia, obesity and hypertension and its postnatal amplification by hypercaloric nutrition. *Am. J. Physiol.* **279** (2000), E83–7.

Vickers, M., Breier, B., McCarthy, D. and Gluckman, P. Sedentary behavior during postnatal life is determined by the prenatal environment and exacerbated by postnatal hypercaloric nutrition. *Am. J. Physiol. Regul. Integr. Comp. Physiol.* **285** (2003), R271–3.

Vickers, M. H., Reddy, S., Ikenasio, B. A. and Breier, B. H. Dysregulation of the adipoinsular axis – a mechanism for the pathogenesis of hyperleptinemia and adipogenic diabetes induced by fetal programming. *J. Endocrinol.* **170** (2001), 323–32.

Weaver, I. C., Cervoni, N., D'Alessio, A. C. *et al.* Maternal behavior in infancy regulates methylation of the hippocampal glucocorticoid receptor promoter. 10th Annual Pharmacology Research Day, McGill University, Montreal, Quebec (2003a).

Weaver, I.C G., Cervoni, N., D'Alessio, A. C. *et al.* Transgenerational epigenomic imprinting by maternal behavior through DNA methylation. In press (2003b).

Welberg, L. A. M., Seckl, J. R. and Holmes, M. C. Inhibition of 11ß-hydroxysteroid dehydrogenase, the foeto–placental barrier to maternal glucocorticoids, permanently programs amygdala GR mRNA expression and anxiety-like behaviour in the offspring. *Eur. J. Neurosci.* **12** (2000), 1047–54.

Welberg, L. A. M., Seckl, J. R. and Holmes, M. C. Prenatal glucocorticoid programming of brain corticosteroid receptors and corticotrophin-releasing hormone: possible implications for behaviour. *Neuroscience* **104** (2001), 71–9.

Woodall, S. M., Johnston, B. M., Breier, B. H. and Gluckman, P. D. Chronic maternal undernutrition in the rat leads to delayed postnatal growth and elevated blood pressure of offspring. *Pediatr. Res.* **40** (1996), 438–43.

Zhang, J. and Byrne, C. D. Differential hepatic lobar gene expression in offspring exposed to altered maternal dietary protein intake. *Am. J. Physiol. Gastrointest. Liver Physiol.* **278** (2000), G128–36.

# Index

Note: page numbers in *italics* refer to figures and tables; 'n' suffix denotes footnote. 'Predictive adaptive responses' is abbreviated to PARs in subentries.